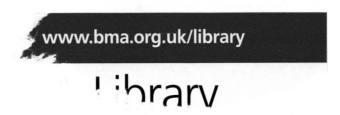
Ophthalmology in Primary Care

AMAR ALWITRY

BMedSci BM BS MRCS MRCS (Ed) MRCOphth FRCOphth

Ophthalmology in Primary Care

*Clinical Skills for GPs, Medical
Students & Allied Professionals*

ROYAL COLLEGE OF GENERAL PRACTITIONERS

LONDON · 2006

The Royal College of General Practitioners was
founded in 1952 with this object:

*'To encourage, foster and maintain the highest
possible standards in general practice and for that
purpose to take or join with others in taking steps
consistent with the charitable nature of that object
which may assist towards the same.'*

Among its responsibilities under its Royal Charter
the College is entitled to:

*'Diffuse information on all matters affecting general
practice and issue such publications as may assist
the object of the College.'*

British Library Cataloguing-in-Publication Data

A catalogue record for this book is available from the British Library

Published by the Royal College of General Practitioners, 2006
14 Princes Gate, Hyde Park, London sw7 1pu

Disclaimer
This publication is intended for the use of medical practitioners in
the UK and not for patients. The author, editors and publisher have
taken care to ensure that the information contained in this book
is correct to the best of their knowledge, at the time of publication.
Whilst efforts have been made to ensure the accuracy of the information presented, particularly that related to the prescription of
drugs, the author, editors and publisher cannot accept liability for
information that is subsequently shown to be wrong. Readers are
advised to check that the information, especially that related to drug
usage, complies with information contained in the *British National
Formulary*, or equivalent, or manufacturers' datasheets, and that it
complies with the latest legislation and standards of practice.

Designed & typeset at the Typographic Design Unit

Printed in the UK by Cromwell Press Ltd

Indexed by Carol Ball

ISBN: 0 85084 304 9

Dedicated to my father, the finest ophthalmologist I know, my mother, my lovely wife and my firstborn son Max.

With gratitude to my GP colleagues for their invaluable help, support and input into this book:

Dr Claudia Petillon
Dr Ola Alwitry
Dr Katie Spensley
Dr Gemma David
Dr Jane Partington
Dr Paul Spensley
Dr Heather Tasker
Dr James Threlfall
Dr Rebecca Hudson
Dr Joanna Durrant

With great thanks to my ophthalmology colleague and good friend for proofreading:

Tom Butler, *Consultant Ophthalmologist,* James Paget Hospital, Norfolk

I would also like to thank Lorraine Abercrombie, Richard Gregson, Richard Cragg and John Scrimgeour for their kind help in obtaining the images.

Contents

Contents | *continued*

Preface

Ophthalmology is particularly hard to teach and learn, as it is a fairly specialised subject. Many of you probably had no intention of lifting an ophthalmoscope ever again after you finished your eye attachment at medical school, but unfortunately this just isn't possible. Every GP becomes familiar with eye examinations and carries them out on a regular basis. You are often the first port of call for patients presenting with eye symptoms and are also expected to recognise ocular features of systemic disease; for example, examining diabetic fundi. As elements of secondary care are increasingly falling to GPs, this may become more important in the future.

Moreover, many of your patients will inevitably have some type of eye problem – glaucoma or cataract, for example – so it is important to understand these disorders and their implications.

I have written this book with several aims. I appreciate that many of you will not share my enthusiasm for ophthalmology and will not want to study it in detail. This book is not designed to teach ophthalmology but to help you manage your ophthalmic patients.

I have kept each section of the book short in order to keep your attention and not bog you down with unnecessary detail. Consequently, this book is fairly simplistic and definitely not exhaustive. There are volumes of texts about eyes, and this is but a small taster. Those of you who require a more in-depth understanding of ophthalmic pathology may benefit from referring to a more detailed text. I hope that this book demystifies ophthalmology and takes away some of the fear it evokes.

The minutiae and rarities are for ophthalmologists to deal with. I trust that this book will help you to recognise when to refer and will give you some guidance about the urgency of that referral.

I hope you enjoy the text, find it an easy read and, most importantly, a valuable reference.

The first part is designed to be a user-friendly reference book. The idea is that you will have it on your desk and refer to it whenever you receive a letter from an optometrist or ophthalmologist in order to understand exactly what is being said and, more importantly, what you need to do. Moreover, when faced with an ophthalmic patient, this book should give you a basic and intuitive management algorithm.

The second part is more in the nature of a formal text, designed to give you, in simple terms, an understanding of the basics of ophthalmology and of the pathological processes that may affect the eye. This section will be ideal for medical students preparing for their assessments and also helpful as an introductory text to doctors contemplating a career in ophthalmology, to ophthalmic nurses, optometrists, orthoptists and those in other allied specialities. Information in Part I is cross-referenced to Part II, allowing the reader to look up certain conditions in more depth if needed. Inevitably there is some repetition, as each part is designed to be used separately if desired.

This book has been written with the kind assistance of ten practising GPs in order to ensure that the text really is directed at primary care. It is easy for ophthalmologists to lose touch with the front line and misinterpret the needs and requirements of GPs in modern practice.

I hope this book is helpful to you all.

Amar Alwitry
BMedSci BM BS MRCS MRCS(Ed) MRCOphth FRCOphth

Practical applications

1 | Symptom-based approach

How to deal with patients presenting with these symptoms, and treatment algorithms.

Red eyes

Red eyes are a very common complaint and you probably see patients presenting with them at least once a week. *See also* Chapter 15.

Common causes

- Infection (conjunctivitis): bacterial, viral, chlamydial
- Subconjunctival haemorrhage
- Iritis
- Corneal foreign bodies and abrasions
- Episcleritis
- Allergy
- Trauma

Rarer but severe causes

- Acute angle-closure glaucoma
- Corneal ulcers
- Dendritic ulcers
- Endophthalmitis
- Scleritis
- Penetrating trauma
- Chemical burns
- Acute thyroid eye disease

Important points to elicit in the history

- Effect on vision
- Presence of stickiness
- Itching
- Laterality, i.e. affecting one or both eyes, and the presence (or absence) of pain
- Previous episodes (e.g. iritis, seasonal allergy)
- Contact lens use (increased risk of infection and allergy)

In the examination concentrate on

- Measuring the visual acuity (remember that serious conditions usually reduce vision)
- Assessing precisely where the redness is
- Staining the cornea
- Checking pupil reactions
- Assessing corneal clarity
- Looking at the appearance of the conjunctiva

What are you looking for?

HISTORY

Vision?

□ Patients often complain of reduced vision. Remember that blurring may be associated with excessive watering, so ask the patient to dry their eyes and blink before you test their vision. Patients who 'think' that their vision is reduced are unlikely actually to have reduced vision. If the vision is definitely blurred then the patient is usually acutely aware of it. (Beware of children – they very rarely complain unless the problem is bilateral!)

Stickiness?

□ Stickiness is usually an indicator of bacterial infection. The patient's eyelashes are often slightly matted together in the morning. Ask about purulent discharge throughout the day.

Itching?

□ Usually a symptom associated with ocular allergy. Think also: Is it seasonal? Do they have a history of atopy? Have they recently started using new eye drops or contact lenses?

Laterallity?

▢ Serious sight-threatening conditions are usually unilateral. Bilateral redness is often related to a form of conjunctivitis, whether bacterial, viral or allergic. Thyroid eye disease or injuries that affect both eyes simultaneously are exceptions.

Pain?

▢ Painful conditions are a concern. Sharp, well-localised pain usually indicates a corneal pathology. More diffuse pain occasionally referred to the eyebrow is related to intraocular pathology such as inflammation or raised intraocular pressure. A foreign-body sensation is a common symptom and usually relates to a corneal epithelial defect, such as an actual foreign body, an abrasion, or an infective corneal ulcer.

EXAMINATION

Visual acuity?

▢ Different conditions reduce vision to different degrees. Corneal pathology that involves the visual axis (central portion of the cornea that the patient 'looks' through) reduces vision markedly. Even a moderate-sized ulcer that is eccentric may not reduce vision to a great degree. Below is a rough indicator of how different pathologies reduce vision. Each assumes a pre-morbid normal 6/6 vision.

Where is the redness?

▢ It is important to fully assess the degree and localisation of the redness.

Concentrate on exactly where the redness is. Is it worse in the fornix or around the limbus? Use a magnifying glass to look at the blood vessels. Examination of the eye will clearly reveal the source of the problem. If a small segment of the limbus is injected (engorged) then there is probably a lesion within the cornea in that segment.

Viral conjunctivitis causes diffuse violet hue to the whole conjunctiva, with all the conjunctival blood vessels injected.

Bacterial conjunctivitis causes diffuse redness, which is usually worse in the inferior fornix, with the presence of pus.

Stain on cornea?

▢ If there is an epithelial defect on the cornea, it will stain with fluorescein. This will mean either the epithelium has rubbed off because of some form of injury or abrasion (including the multiple pinpoint abrasions related to dry eyes), or that there is some form of infective process of the cornea. Look at the cornea underneath the epithelial defect. If there is a localised white corneal opacity in a red eye, this is an infective keratitis. If the cornea is completely clear and the history fits with a traumatic aetiology, then there is less cause for concern.

Pupil?

▢ Check the pupil. If it is reacting normally, then this is not angle-closure glaucoma. In angle-closure glaucoma the pupil is fixed and mid-dilated. The presence of a relative afferent pupillary defect with reduced vision indicates optic nerve pathology (*see* Swinging flashlight test, Chapter 11).

Is the cornea clear?

▢ Use a magnifier to look at the cornea. Is it clear? Look at the details of the iris for an indication. If they are crystal clear, there is unlikely to be a significant pathology. A localised white opacity in a red eye indicates an ulcer or corneal abscess. If the cornea appears generally cloudy and 'lacklustre' there may be corneal oedema.

Conjunctival appearance?

▢ The conjunctiva should be flat and smooth with a few folds in the lower fornix. The best places to look are the inferior fornix or beneath the upper lid on the tarsal plate. If there is a localised raised red area over the sclera, it may be a nodular episcleritis.

Look for raised confluent 'bobbles' on the conjunctiva – these are papillae or follicles. You do not need to be able to differentiate follicles from papillae. They are present in viral, allergic or chlamydial infection, or in toxic conjunctivitis.

Bacterial conjunctivitis

Vision?

▢ Normal – watering or purulent matter may cause slight transient blurring.

Stickiness?

□ Yes – eyelashes will be 'matted together' in the mornings.

Laterality?

□ Usually begins as unilateral, but may become bilateral.

Pain?

□ No.

Visual acuity?

□ Normal.

Where is the redness?

□ Redness is more pronounced in the inferior fornix. The blood vessels around the limbus are not engorged.

Stain on cornea?

□ No stain on cornea unless a corneal ulcer has developed.

Pupil?

□ Normal.

Is the cornea clear?

□ Yes.

Conjunctival appearance?

□ Flat but erythematous.

Viral conjunctivitis

Vision?

□ Usually normal, although excessive watering may cause blurring. Adenoviral keratoconjunctivitis, which affects the cornea and the conjunctiva, may result in genuine slight reduction in vision.

Stickiness?

□ Not usually present. Eyelashes may be slightly 'matted' in the morning with mucous discharge.

Condition	Generalised effect on visual acuity	Exceptions
Bacterial/chlamydial conjunctivitis	Usually unaffected	
Viral conjunctivitis	Often unaffected (but an associated keratitis may occur)	If a dendritic ulcer affects the central corneal epithelium, the vision will be reduced
Subconjunctival haemorrhage	Unaffected	
Iritis	Slightly reduced: 6/9–6/12	
Corneal foreign body and abrasions	Unaffected, unless central cornea affected	
Episcleritis	Unaffected	
Acute angle-closure glaucoma	Reduced – approx. 6/36, dependent on degree of corneal oedema	
Corneal ulcers	Dependent on position of ulcer	If central or severe then vision will be markedly down, e.g. to hand motion
		If small and peripheral, vision may be normal
Dendritic ulcers	Slightly reduced, dependent upon location	
Endophthalmitis	In established cases then markedly reduced, e.g. to hand motion or even perception of light	
Scleritis	Vision usually slightly reduced	Posterior scleritis may cause some folds in the macula, reducing vision to around 6/18

Laterality?

□ Begins unilaterally but then often becomes bilateral.

Pain?

□ No, although the patient may experience some ache.

Visual acuity?

□ Usually normal, but in adenovirus the visual acuity may be reduced to about 6/12.

Where is the redness?

□ Redness more apparent in the inferior fornix. Limbal vessels are not engorged. Eye appears diffusely violaceous.

Stain on cornea?

□ Usually none. In adenoviral keratoconjunctivitis the cornea may have scattered areas of 'pinpoint' staining.

Pupil?

□ Normal.

Is the cornea clear?

□ Yes.

Conjunctival appearance?

□ Follicles ('bobbles') may be present.

Chlamydial conjunctivitis

Vision?

□ Normal.

Stickiness?

□ No, but there may be mild stickiness, increasing slowly with time. Usually chronic conjunctivitis with a history of several weeks' duration, resistant to usual treatment. The major features are redness, irritation and watering.

Laterality?

□ Often bilateral.

Pain?

□ No.

Visual acuity?

□ Usually normal.

Where is the redness?

□ Redness is more prominent in the inferior fornix.

Stain on cornea?

□ No.

Pupil?

□ Normal.

Is the cornea clear?

□ Yes.

Conjunctival appearance?

□ Numerous pronounced follicles ('bobbles').

Subconjunctival haemorrhage

Vision?

□ Normal.

Stickiness?

□ No.

Laterality?

□ Unilateral.

Pain?

□ No, but there may be slight ache coinciding with the onset of the haemorrhage.

Visual acuity?

□ Normal.

Where is the redness?

□ Redness is solid, due to blood rather than the engorged vessels seen in true conjunctival injection. Redness may be localised or diffuse.

Stain on cornea?

□ No.

Pupil?

□ Normal.

Is the cornea clear?

□ Yes.

Conjunctival appearance?

□ Flat and blood red. If the subconjunctival haemorrhage is marked, it may cause the conjunctiva to 'balloon' forward.

Iritis

Vision?

□ Usually normal if the condition is mild. If the inflammation is marked, vision may be slightly reduced.

Stickiness?

□ No.

Laterality?

□ Unilateral.

Pain?

□ Photophobia and ocular ache.

Visual acuity?

□ May be slightly reduced to about 6/9 or 6/12.

Where is the redness?

□ Most marked around the corneal limbus. Look closely at the vessels running up to the corneal periphery – they will be dilated.

Stain on cornea?

□ No.

Pupil?

□ Reacts normally but may be an abnormal shape because of inflammatory adhesions between the pupil margin and the lens behind it. This abnormality may be more obvious when the pupil is dilated.

Is the cornea clear?

□ Unless the pressure goes up in relation to the iritis, the cornea will stay clear. On close examination, you may notice some opacities on the lower inner surface of the cornea, related to collections of inflammatory debris, called keratic precipitates. The iris detail may be partially obscured by a hazy anterior chamber.

Conjunctival appearance?

□ Usually normal.

Corneal foreign bodies and abrasions

Vision?

□ If the visual axis is involved, vision will be reduced.

Stickiness?

□ No, but usually marked epiphora (watering eye).

Laterality?

□ Unilateral.

Pain?

□ Can be extremely painful, resulting in marked blepharospasm and difficulty in opening the eyes. Patients will feel they have something in their eye.

Visual acuity?

□ If the central corneal epithelium is lost in the abrasion, the vision will be reduced to approximately 6/12.

Where is the redness?

□ The limbal vasculature will be engorged.

Stain on cornea?

□ Yes, corresponding to area of epithelial cell loss.

Pupil?

□ Normal.

Is the cornea clear?

□ In the staining area (i.e. where the corneal epithelium has been rubbed off) the underlying corneal stroma will retain its clarity. If the area under and around the abrasion is whitish, this may indicate an infective keratitis.

Conjunctival appearance?

□ Normal, but erythematous.

Episcleritis

Vision?

□ Normal.

Stickiness?

□ No.

Laterality?

□ Unilateral.

Pain?

□ There may be a slight ache and the eye may be tender when pressure is applied over the injected area.

Visual acuity?

□ Normal.

Where is the redness?

□ Redness is usually very localised, involving a small area of the conjunctiva.

Stain on cornea?

□ No.

Pupil?

□ Normal.

Is the cornea clear?

□ Yes.

Conjunctival appearance?

□ The area of redness may be slightly elevated and nodular.

Acute angle-closure glaucoma

Vision?

□ Blurred.

Stickiness?

□ No.

Laterality?

□ Unilateral.

Pain?

□ Yes. Nausea is a predominant accompaniment to this pain, related to raised intraocular pressure. The pain is often localised to the eyebrow.

Visual acuity?

□ Reduced to approximately 6/36 or even worse, depending on the degree of ensuing corneal oedema.

Where is the redness?

□ More marked around the limbus.

Stain on cornea?

□ No, although there may be diffuse pinpoint staining over the cornea related to the corneal oedema and resulting in an unhealthy corneal epithelium.

Pupil?

□ Fixed and mid-dilated. If the pupil reacts normally, then the condition is not angle-closure glaucoma.

Is the cornea clear?

□ No, hazy with a 'ground-glass' appearance.

Conjunctival appearance?

□ Normal, but erythematous.

Corneal ulcers

Vision?

□ If the central cornea is involved, vision will be dramatically reduced.

Stickiness?

□ Not necessarily, but there may be marked purulent discharge.

Laterality?

□ Unilateral.

Pain?

□ Yes. Small, mild ulcers may present solely with a foreign-body sensation. Ulcers related to herpes virus, however, may be fairly painless because of damage to the corneal nerves.

Visual acuity?

□ If the ulcer is peripheral, then vision may be perfect. If the central cornea is involved, vision may be reduced only to the ability to count fingers or worse.

Where is the redness?

□ Small ulcers will be pinpointed by the presence of limbal injection in the quadrant adjacent to the position of the ulcer. If the ulcer is larger, the whole limbus will be red.

Stain on cornea?

□ Yes. The ulcer area will be stained, and the cornea around and under this area will be whitish.

Pupil?

□ Reacts normally.

Is the cornea clear?

□ No. The corneal tissue near to the ulcer will be whitish.

Conjunctival appearance?

□ Normal, but erythematous.

Dendritic ulcers

Vision?

□ Usually slightly reduced.

Stickiness?

□ No.

Laterality?

□ Always unilateral.

Pain?

□ Usually some slight pain. Often a foreign-body sensation.

Visual acuity?

□ Usually about 6/12.

Where is the redness?

□ Around the limbus (the junction of the sclera and cornea).

Stain on cornea?

□ Yes – in dendritic branching pattern. If long-standing or if the patient has inadvertently been given topical steroids, the branching patterns may coalesce and form a geographic ulcer.

Pupil?

□ Normal.

Is the cornea clear?

□ Under the staining linear ulcerations, the cornea tends to be clear, i.e. there is no whitening within the substance of the cornea itself.

Conjunctival appearance?

□ Normal, but erythematous.

Endophthalmitis

Vision?

□ Usually profoundly reduced.

Stickiness?

□ No.

Laterality?

□ Unilateral, usually in an eye with a history of surgery or trauma.

Pain?

□ Yes, although debilitated patients may not experience severe pain.

Visual acuity?

□ Usually reduced to 6/60 or worse.

Where is the redness?

□ Diffuse.

Stain on cornea?

□ No.

Pupil?

□ Reactive but usually sluggish.

Is the cornea clear?

□ Yes.

Conjunctival appearance?

□ Markedly red.

Scleritis

Vision?

□ May be normal.

Stickiness?

□ No.

Laterality?

□ Unilateral.

Pain?

□ Yes, the pain tends to be marked.

Visual acuity?

□ Normal or slightly reduced.

Where is the redness?

□ Localised redness of the sclera. It can be hard to differentiate this from episcleritis, but the engorged vessels tend to be more 'beefy' and appear deeper than in episcleritis.

Stain on cornea?

□ No.

Pupil?

□ Normal.

Is the cornea clear?

....

□ Yes.

Conjunctival appearance?

....

□ Normal, but the underlying sclera is inflamed and may have a white, avascular, necrotic patch.

Important points

If conjunctivitis does not improve after one week of treatment, it is important to reconsider the diagnosis. Assess the red eye again and look for features of any of the severe causes of redness described above.

If the patient's condition appears to have worsened after starting topical treatment, they may have developed an allergy to the antibiotic drops or ointment. The typical example is a patient who comes to see you with a mildly red eye. You prescribe an antibiotic and after one week the eye is much redder. If any worrying signs have developed, then treat or refer appropriately. If not, stop all treatment and wait to see if the condition improves.

Contact lens wearers are at risk of bacterial corneal infections. Examine the cornea thoroughly and stain it. If there is any sign of an ulcer refer *immediately*. Don't start treatment as it may cause a false negative when the cornea is scraped and cultured. Make sure the patient takes their contact lens out as soon as possible. Ask patients to take their contact lenses and case with them to the hospital as a culture may help isolate the infective organism.

See Chapter 2 for definitions of the terms 'immediate', 'urgent', 'soon', 'soon via letter' and 'routine' in relation to referrals.

Decreased vision (*see also* Chapter 16)

Sudden loss of vision (*unilateral*)

WHOLE FIELD OF VISION AND PERMANENT?

Is this giant cell arteritis (GCA)?

....

Indications

- Patient over 60 years of age.
- Headache/temporal pain.
- Temporal tenderness.
- Pain on chewing/talking – jaw claudication. If a patient volunteers this symptom, strongly consider a diagnosis of temporal arteritis.

What do I find?

- Vision is reduced markedly in one eye.
- Temporal artery tender, thickened and non-pulsatile.
- There will be a relative afferent pupillary defect (RAPD); see below. Shine the light into one pupil and then the other – you will see one does not react as well (*see* Swinging flashlight test, Chapter 11).
- The optic disc will be swollen.

What do I do?

- Check erythrocyte sedimentation rate/C-reactive protein (ESR/CRP) and full blood count (FBC). Refer *urgently*.

Is this a central retinal artery occlusion (CRAO)?

....

Indications

- Older patient.
- Very sudden onset.
- Cardiovascular or cerebrovascular risk factors.

What do I find?

- Vision is reduced, usually markedly in one eye.
- There will be an RAPD.
- On fundoscopy, the retinal arterioles will be extremely thin and attenuated. You may see the 'cherry-red spot' or even an embolus lying at the disc within the retinal artery.

What do I do?

- Refer *urgently*.

Is this a vitreous haemorrhage?

....

Indications

- Patient may describe clouds of reddish brown floaters.
- Patient may describe thick 'cobwebs' or fog across the vision.
- Patient may be diabetic.

What do I find?

- Ophthalmoscopy will be impossible with a dense vitreous haemorrhage. You may be tempted to assume that you simply cannot get a view because of your technique. Check by looking into the other eye: if you can see the fundus then there is nothing wrong with your technique and the problem (probably a vitreous haemorrhage) is with the other eye.
- The pupils will react normally.

What do I do?

- Patients who are known to have significant diabetic retinopathy will already be under follow up at the hospital. They should be re-referred *soon via letter*.
- Patients who have diabetes but are not known to have diabetic retinopathy should be referred *soon/urgently* for formal assessment.
- Patients who do not have diabetes may have sustained a retinal tear involving a blood vessel and thus caused a vitreous haemorrhage. Refer *urgently*.

Is this a retinal vein occlusion?

Indications

- Older patient.
- May have cardiovascular risk factors, e.g. hypertension.
- May be a smoker, diabetic or have glaucoma.
- If the cause is central vein occlusion, then the whole field of vision may be involved. If the problem is only a branch vein occlusion, then only the superior or lower part of the visual field will be affected.

What do I find?

- There may be an RAPD (*see* Chapter 11), particularly if this is a central retinal vein occlusion.
- There will be haemorrhages throughout the retina.
- You will be able to see the retina. In the case of a vitreous haemorrhage, the retina would not be visible.

What do I do?

- Patients need to be referred *soon via letter*.
- Check blood pressure.

Is this an anterior ischaemic optic neuropathy?

□ This simply means infarction of the posterior ciliary artery that supplies the optic nerve, presumed secondary to a microembolic event, but also a common manifestation of GCA (see above).

Indications

- Sudden onset.
- Patient may have an altitudinal defect (i.e. upper or lower half of vision gone).

Prognosis is poor although only part of the visual field may be involved.

What do I find?

- Disc may be swollen.
- RAPD present.

What do I do?

- Check ESR/CRP – in case this is GCA.
- Consider antiplatelet treatment.
- Refer *urgently* for exclusion of other causes.

CENTRAL FIELD DEFECT AND PERMANENT?

Is this optic neuritis?

Indications

- Patient usually young and female.
- Onset usually sudden, but may get progressively worse over a two-week period, and then improves over the next four to six weeks.
- Often described as a central black blob in vision.

What do I find?

- There will be a central field defect.
- There will be an RAPD.
- The optic disc is swollen in one-third of cases. (Look closely at the macula to ensure that there is no haemorrhage there causing the central field defect.)

What do I do?

- The patient should be referred *soon*. There is a significant risk that the patient is developing multiple sclerosis – check neurology.

Is this wet/haemorrhagic age-related macular degeneration (AMD)?

Indications

- Usually older patient.
- May have long history of gradual mild blurring of vision (pre-existing dry AMD).
- Often begins with distortion followed by rapid reduction of vision associated with a macular haemorrhage.
- Peripheral vision is normal.

What do I find?

- Visual acuity is reduced.
- There may be a significant haemorrhage at the macula.

What do I do?

- If the patient has a large macular haemorrhage, the prognosis is poor. If there is no haemorrhage or limited haemorrhage, the patient may be eligible for photodynamic therapy. These patients should be referred *immediately via letter* to the nearest photodynamic therapy (PDT) service for assessment. If the diagnosis is uncertain the patient should be assessed at eye casualty.

AFFECTING THE WHOLE FIELD OF VISION AND TEMPORARY?

Is this amaurosis fugax?

□ This is a transient ischaemic attack (TIA) of the retinal circulation.

Indications
- Patient is usually elderly with cardiovascular risk factors.
- Sudden onset.
- Grey/black curtain coming down or up across vision, obscuring vision, which usually disappears within 30 minutes. Vision is back to normal after an attack.

What do I find?
- Usually no ocular abnormality. May have carotid bruit.

What do I do?
- Assess risk factors for embolic stroke.

Rare but important – GCA can manifest as amaurosis fugax – worth checking ESR/CRP.

Is this ocular migraine?

Indications
- Patient usually younger.
- Patient usually complains of missing patches of vision, flashes, scintillating colours or lights, typically lasting 20 minutes.
- Headache not always present.
- Episodes may recur.

What do I find?
- Usually nothing.

What do I do?
- Reassure as long as the vision continues to return to normal.

Sudden loss of vision (bilateral)

TOTAL LOSS OF VISION

In order suddenly to lose all vision in both eyes the patient would have to sustain a cerebrovascular occlusive event compromising both occipital lobes (visual cortices), optic tracts or radiations simultaneously.

The patient may have previously lost vision in one eye but only noticed it when they lost the vision in their other eye. They become concerned, check their vision in both eyes and notice that vision is poor bilaterally.

Very rarely patients will have pathology affecting both eyes in rapid succession (may occur in untreated GCA).

Occasionally malingerers present claiming to have complete vision loss; watch how they walk and act. If the patient is completely blind they will not fixate on you and will struggle to negotiate obstacles.

PARTIAL LOSS OF VISION

An occipital CVA will infarct the visual cortex on one side, resulting in a homonymous hemianopia of the contralateral side to the lesion. Often the macula is spared, leaving the visual acuity intact.

If just a portion of the visual cortex is lost, the patient may only lose one corresponding quadrant of vision in each eye – a homonymous quadrantanopia.

Sudden blurring of vision (one eye)

The degree of visual loss associated with the above conditions may vary, depending on the degree of the pathology. For example, a patient with a mild case of central retinal vein occlusion may have vision of 6/12, while another patient's vision may be reduced to hand motions. All of the above may cause blurring rather than visual loss.

Is this wet AMD?

Indications
- Usually older patient.
- May have long history of gradual mild blurring of vision (pre-existing dry AMD).
- Patients often say that straight lines do not appear straight (metamorphopsia). Ask the patient to look at a window frame or any form of grid and to describe what they see.
- Peripheral vision is normal.

What do I find?
- Visual acuity is reduced.
- There may be haemorrhage at the macula. If you are skilled at fundoscopy you may see a greyish/green lesion below the retina.

What do I do?
- Such patients may be eligible for photodynamic laser therapy to minimise the degree of visual loss. These patients should be referred *immediately via letter* to the closest PDT service for assessment. [As above.]

Is this central serous retinopathy?

Indications
- Usually affects young or middle-aged men.
- Relatively rapid onset of distortion and reduced vision in one eye.
- Vision is not excessively reduced – usually in the region of 6/12.

What do I find?
- Usually hard to see anything abnormal with the ophthalmoscope.

What do I do?
- Refer *urgently/soon via letter* for confirmation of the diagnosis.

Gradual blurring of vision

May be related to cataract or AMD.

Patients who have had previous cataract surgery may have developed posterior capsular opacification, which warrants *routine* referral.

Sending the patient to their optician for assessment is prudent.

Flashes and floaters

Flashes and floaters are common symptoms, and in most cases represent no significant pathology, especially if they are long-standing. Possible causes include a posterior vitreous detachment (PVD), ocular migraine and vitreous haemorrhage.

Sometimes the PVD causes a retinal hole to form, with the subsequent risk of retinal detachment.

Is this a PVD?

□ Probably. The key question is whether this has caused a retinal tear.

PVD is a normal ageing phenomenon – it may occur without symptoms or cause flashes and floaters.

The flashes are usually short-lived but floaters may persist.

Classically, patients describe a single spider's web or floater complex that 'wobbles' in and out of vision.

Often flashes persist, particularly at night or on eye movement.

Is there a retinal tear or hole?

□ The only way to know is for an ophthalmologist to examine the retina with specialised lenses and visualise every part. Ideally, this should be done for every patient but resources are not available for such blanket screening.

Optometrists are skilled at fundoscopy and many use slit lamp biomicroscopy to assess the retina. They are thus a good initial port of call for such patients.

General guidelines

□ Long-standing flashes and floaters – no need to refer.

Flashes and floaters of under six weeks' duration – refer *soon via letter*.

Flashes and floaters with decreased vision – refer *urgently*.

Judge each case on its merits.

Certain risk factors should be taken into account, and these features will increase the suspicion of pathology:

- Myopia, particularly if highly myopic – look at the thickness of the lenses in the patient's glasses
- Younger age, i.e. under 55 years
- Pseudophakia/aphakia (previous cataract extraction – pseudophakia means replacement lens placed, aphakia means no lens placed).

All patients should be warned about the symptoms of retinal detachment and advised to contact the hospital eye service urgently if they experience the following:

- Sudden increase in floaters ('swarm of tadpoles')
- Solid or grey curtain encroaching across peripheral field of vision
- Central visual loss.

Double vision

Is it really double vision or blurry vision? In other words, does the patient see a haze or 'halo' around objects or do they truly see two images?

If they truly see two images, do they go away if they close one eye? If yes, then this is true double vision (diplopia). If they have monocular diplopia, they probably have a cataract in the affected eye.

Is it intermittent or constant?

....

□ If intermittent, consider decompensation or manifestation of a latent squint. Everyone has some degree of latent squint, and sometimes older patients lose the ability to control it, causing the squint to come on and off.

Also consider myasthenia gravis (*see* p. 192).

If it is constant, consider a cranial nerve palsy.

Note

....

□ A third nerve palsy (an eye pointing 'down and out' with a ptosis) and a dilated pupil is considered to be a cerebral aneurysm compressing the third nerve, until proven otherwise by imaging – refer *immediately*.

If the eyes are red as well, consider thyroid eye disease or trauma-related pathology.

Occasionally GCA patients may present with a cranial nerve palsy. Maintain an 'index of suspicion' as outlined above.

Are the two images seen side by side or one above the other?

Problems with vertical muscles or their nerve supply produce images one above the other. Images side by side are caused by problems with horizontal muscles or by palsies of the nerves supplying them.

2 | Diagnoses

When ophthalmologists write to GPs we aim to convey information about the patient and their condition. The other point of the letter is to ensure that the information in the notes is legible, as opposed to our handwriting, which must rank amongst the worst of all medical professionals. In an ideal world we would include only information that is directly relevant to you but we are often overzealous and end up writing what must appear gibberish, using terms that you may have never heard before.

Usually the letters are simply scanned and then filed away in the notes. You do not particularly care about the intricacies of management, but do care about major changes in the treatment regimen and when the next follow up is due.

A patient may sometimes consult you about an unrelated issue, but then ask about their eyes. They often find it difficult to ask questions in a busy hospital clinic and do not want to 'waste the consultant's valuable time'. Instead, they come to you during your busy list and expect you to spend the 10-minute slot explaining their eye condition as well as dealing with their hypertension, depression and weight problem.

This section is designed to demystify some of the key acronyms and terminology. The aim is not to teach you about all of the conditions in depth but to give you a simple explanation of the pertinent factors, and how they may affect your patient. This section will also guide you on how to take an active part in the systemic management of your patients with eye problems.

When you receive a diagnosis from an ophthalmologist or a question from a patient, you should then be able to look up the condition in this text and get a general understanding of what is happening. If you need more information or have an interest in the underlying principles of a disorder then Part II goes into more depth.

The list of diagnoses addressed is far from exhaustive but covers most conditions you are likely to face. If you are asked about a disorder not on this list then it is perfectly reasonable to say that you do not know

and recommend that the patient ask for more details when they next attend hospital.

I have also included a section on what to do if you diagnose certain ophthalmic conditions, particularly on the need and urgency of referral to the hospital eye service.

Please be aware that these are general guidelines to assist you in making clinical decisions about referral. Each patient should be thoroughly assessed and managed according to their particular clinical situation. As with every branch of medicine, there are no hard and fast rules.

I have used the following terminology with regard to the urgency of referral:

Immediate □ Patient should be sent to the hospital eye service without delay. If an eye casualty department is available, the patient should attend immediately. You should phone the eye service to arrange for fast assessment and management.

Urgent □ Patient should be seen by the hospital eye service as soon as possible. If the patient is diagnosed over night, then assessment the following morning is acceptable in most cases. A phone call to the on-call hospital team is appropriate.

Soon □ Patient should be seen by the eye service in the next day or so. If the diagnosis is made at the weekend, then a review on Monday morning is acceptable in most cases.

Urgent via letter □ A referral letter should be faxed to the hospital eye service, preferably to the primary care/eye casualty department, to ensure speedy triage and appropriate call for patient review. The eye casualty department will then usually send for the patient or a clinic appointment will be booked for the next available slot.

Soon via letter □ A referral letter should be posted to the hospital eye service, but should request a review 'soon'.

Routine □ A referral letter should be sent to the hospital eye service for triage. The patient will then be given an appointment for a review in the main eye clinic.

Conditions

Age-related macular degeneration (see *Chapter 17*)

DRY AGE-RELATED MACULAR DEGENERATION

What's going on?

□ Age-related wear and tear is affecting the macula and thus central vision. Central vision is affected very gradually over years, with progressive blurring and difficulty with small print. Near vision is generally affected more than distance vision, especially in the early stages.

If I examine the patient, what will I find?

□ You may see drusen (calcific deposits), pigment changes or atrophic patches in the macula (figure 17.2).

What if I've diagnosed it?

□ Dry AMD is extremely common and virtually a universal finding in the elderly population. It does not need referral in isolation if the vision is relatively well maintained and the patient is happy. If there is evidence of significant but gradual progression, then the patient should be referred *routinely*.

What will the hospital do?

□ The patient will be counselled and may be given what is known as an Amsler chart with which to check their vision regularly, in order to detect early onset of metamorphopsia (image distortion).

What do I need to do?

□ Dry AMD is a risk factor for wet AMD. If the patient develops image distortion in either eye, it is important to refer them to hospital *urgently/soon*, as they may have developed a subretinal neovascular membrane, which may be amenable to photodynamic laser therapy (PDT).

What to tell the patient

□ They will never go blind, but their central vision will be affected to a variable extent. Dry AMD progresses very slowly but the concern is conversion to wet AMD. If the wear and tear progresses, vision can be markedly reduced, even in the absence of wet changes.

Problems that may arise, and how to deal with them

□ Development of definite metamorphopsia (distortion) warrants an *urgent/soon* referral, ideally to your local PDT service for assessment.

WET AGE-RELATED MACULAR OEDEMA

□ Also: subretinal choroidal neovascular membrane; subretinal membrane; choroidal neovascularisation.

What's going on?

□ New vessels have grown from the choroid into the space beneath the retina. These vessels are abnormal and leak fluid or haemorrhage. If untreated, vision will deteriorate rapidly, and the patient may eventually be left with a macular scar, with resulting poor central vision.

If I examine the patient, what will I find?

□ You may see haemorrhages, exudates, elevation of the retina or the yellowy-green membrane itself (figures 17.3 and 17.4).

What if I've diagnosed it?

□ Patients should be referred *urgently/soon*, ideally to your local photodynamic therapy (PDT) service for assessment.

What will the hospital do?

□ The patient will usually have a fluorescein angiogram, whereby fluorescein dye is injected intravenously and photographs taken of the retinal and choroidal vasculature through the dilated pupil. This will detect the presence of the new blood vessels (choroidal neovascular membrane) and will determine the type of membrane. Membranes may be classic (well-defined) or occult (poorly defined), or both types may be present. Depending on the precise features of the membranes and certain patient characteristics, the patient may receive laser treatment in the form of PDT. If the abnormal vessels are situated away from the fovea, then ordinary argon thermal laser may be used.

What do I need to do?

□ The patient may benefit from being given a certificate of visual impairment (CVI). This may be requested from the hospital eye service. Recent onset of bilateral visual loss may pose a risk to the patient, especially if they are elderly and/or live alone. In these circumstances, it may be appropriate to involve social services at an early stage.

Controlling risk factors for the development of wet AMD in the other eye, such as smoking and hypertension, will be beneficial. Recent research has also looked at the role of vitamin supplements and antioxidants to help prevent wet AMD.

What to tell the patient

□ If they are amenable to treatment with argon laser, then their central vision may be spared, but they will have a scotoma (blank patch) in their vision in the area where the laser was applied. Recurrence rates are high.

If the patient has PDT, they may require approximately three treatments in the first year and two in the second. Treatment aims to prevent further deterioration, and so the patient should be made aware that it is not a cure and that they will inevitably have some loss of vision.

If no treatment is possible, then the news is bad and the vision will probably deteriorate to the 6/60/counting fingers/hand motion range. You can emphasise that peripheral (navigational) vision will not be lost; in other words, they won't go blind. There is a risk to the other eye.

Other eye involvement should be referred to the hospital *urgently/soon*.

Cataract (see *Chapter 18*)

What's going on?

□ The lens has become cloudy and the vision blurred. Alternatively, the vision is intact but the patient complains of 'haloes' and glare, particularly with night driving.

If I examine the patient, what will I find?

□ If you look at the patient through the ophthalmoscope and see the red reflex from a few feet away, you will notice black, spoke-like patches within the red glow itself (figures 18.2a and b).

What if I've diagnosed it?

□ Refer *routinely* if the patient is visually symptomatic.

What will the hospital do?

□ If the cataract is causing visual symptoms and the patient is motivated for surgery, they will be listed for cataract extraction.

What to tell the patient

□ The cataract can be removed with an operation that has a high chance of success if the eye is otherwise healthy. This is performed as a day case under local anaesthetic. Cataracts do not damage the eye, and only need to be removed if the patient is complaining of reduced vision and chooses to have surgery.

Problems that may arise, and how to deal with them

□ After cataract surgery, the patient will be given drops. It is important that they use these, and if they run out a single repeat prescription should be supplied. If the eye becomes red and painful with reduced vision, the patient may be developing infective endophthalmitis – refer *immediately*.

Traumatic cataract

What's going on?

□ Blunt or penetrating injury to the eye may result in cataractous lens changes. Blunt injury causes damage through the concussion wave spreading throughout the eye. A penetrating injury that causes the lens capsule to rupture will result in an early, dense cataract. Even minimal injury can cause a cataract. If cataract extraction is carried out, there will be an increased risk of complication due to damage to the suspensory ligaments (zonules).

If I examine the patient, what will I find?

□ If you look through the ophthalmoscope, the red reflex will be reduced or absent. The patient may also have a corneal scar or pupillary mydriasis (dilatation) or irregularity from the original trauma, which may have occurred many months before.

What if I've diagnosed it?

□ If the injury is recent and the eye is quiet, the patient should be referred *soon via letter/urgently via letter* for assessment to ensure there is no other associated ocular injury.

If the injury is long passed, the patient should be referred *routinely*.

What will the hospital do?

☐ The eye will be assessed for concurrent damage and surgical intervention will be planned if appropriate.

What to tell the patient

☐ The cataract can be treated with an operation, but this may be more complex as a result of the injury. If the eye sustained any other damage (e.g. to the retina) the potential for improvement in vision may be reduced.

Problems that may arise, and how to deal with them

☐ The postoperative course is much the same as for routine cataract surgery.

Posterior capsular opacification (see *p. 144*)

What's going on?

☐ When we remove a cataract, we leave the back capsule in place to support the new intraocular lens. In a proportion of patients, residual lens epithelial cells may grow across this posterior capsule, resulting in opacity and reduced vision. This process usually takes more than a year.

If I examine the patient, what will I find?

☐ If you look at the eye using the ophthalmoscope as a magnifying glass, you may see the cloudy posterior capsular opacification.

What if I've diagnosed it?

☐ If a patient has had a cataract extraction with lens implant and then develops reduced vision, they may have posterior capsular opacification. Remember though that there are other causes of visual deterioration after cataract surgery, including AMD and vascular occlusions.

Late gradual deterioration in vision thought to be due to posterior capsular opacification can be referred as *routine*. The optician is usually very helpful in making the diagnosis.

What will the hospital do?

☐ A YAG (yttrium aluminium garnet) laser may be used to make a hole in the thickened, opaque capsule with a piece of equipment like a slit lamp to allow clear vision (figure 18.6).

Problems that may arise, and how to deal with them

☐ Vision should improve virtually immediately after YAG laser treatment, and patients should go back to their optician for further refraction after the treatment. Rarely after the procedure, the intraocular pressure goes up dramatically or the eyes become inflamed.

Postoperative intraocular infection

☐ Also: infective endophthalmitis; postoperative endophthalmitis.

What's going on?

☐ Bacteria have infected the vitreous cavity in the eye in the early postoperative period. The aqueous and vitreous are ill-equipped to deal with bacterial invasion, so the infection can take hold rapidly and cause significant damage.

If I examine the patient, what will I find?

☐ The eye will be very red and the vision will be reduced. There may be a collection of pus at the bottom of the anterior chamber – a hypopyon.

What if I've diagnosed it?

☐ If a patient who has had recent intraocular procedure presents to you with a red eye and reduced vision they should be referred as *immediate* to the hospital.

What will the hospital do?

☐ It is sometimes impossible to differentiate between severe sterile inflammation and infection. Such cases are treated as infections as this is a potentially catastrophic complication that can result in loss of sight.

Typically, samples from the vitreous and the aqueous will be taken for culture. In addition, antibiotics for both gram-negative and gram-positive organisms (usually vancomycin and amikacin) will be injected into the vitreous cavity.

Vitrectomy will rarely be used in the acute phase in order to remove/debulk the infective load.

What to tell the patient

□ The visual prognosis for infective postoperative endophthalmitis is poor, but immediate treatment can be effective in restoring sight.

Problems that may arise, and how to deal with them

□ Rarely, the infection may occur in an eye that has never had an operation. This is called endogenous endophthalmitis, and is usually seen in an immuno-compromised, debilitated patient who has a severe sepsis with bacteraemia.

Conditions of the cornea (see Chapter 19)

BACTERIAL KERATITIS

What's going on?

□ The patient has an infection of the cornea. If untreated, a bacterial keratitis can result in significant visual loss related to perforation of the cornea.

If I examine the patient, what will I find?

□ The eye will be red. The cornea will have some degree of white opacity. Fluorescein will show an epithelial defect (ulcer). There may be a hypopyon (collection of pus at the bottom of the anterior chamber) (see figure 15.4). If the ulcer is small and peripheral, the eye will help you pinpoint its position by localised redness adjacent to the pathological area.

What if I've diagnosed it?

□ Refer *immediately/urgently*. If the patient is wearing contact lenses, tell them to take them out immediately, and bring their lenses, lens case and cleaning solution to the hospital with them. Unless the ophthalmology review is delayed, it is better not to start antibiotic treatment as this may affect the results of any microbiology scrape at the hospital.

What will the hospital do?

□ We will take a sample for microscopy and culture in the hope of identifying the infective organism. Before waiting for definitive culture results, however, we will commence intensive antibiotic treatment. The patient is usually started on one of two regimens: topical gentamicin and cefuroxime together or a quinolone, such as ciprofloxacin or ofloxacin, alone. Drops are usually administered hourly, including overnight, and then tapered off according to response. As a general rule, if the infection is severe, the patient is admitted to ensure compliance with drops and to facilitate continual 24-hour treatment.

What do I need to do?

□ Advise the patient about the need to prevent further episodes. *De novo* infection in an uncompromised patient is rare, and probably indicates an underlying, predisposing condition. The most important risk factor is wearing contact lenses. A patient who has had an infective complication caused by contact lenses needs to consider whether they are adhering to good lens-wearing practice and whether to carrying on wearing them. The lenses, cases and cleaning solutions should all be discarded. Often patients escape lightly from an ocular infection. Any ulcer leaves a scar when it heals; but if it is on the peripheral cornea the patient will not experience any damage to their sight. It should be emphasised that if they have another infection, they may develop an ulcer over that part of the cornea that they look through, which would result in a significant loss of vision.

What to tell the patient

□ The infection will eventually clear up, but will leave a scar, which could result in some damage to their sight. They should not wear contact lenses until the infection has been completely clear for at least a month (some ophthalmologists recommend stopping contact lens wear altogether after a proven infection) and they should ensure that they pay great attention to hygiene with their lenses. Recommend that they go back to their contact lens practitioner, who can reassess their lenses and hygiene practice. Emphasise that the disorder can result in blindness.

HERPES SIMPLEX KERATITIS

□ Also: dendritic ulcer; geographic ulcer.

What's going on?

□ This is herpes virus infection of the corneal epithelium. Patients will usually have had some exposure to the herpes virus in the past. The infection may have been subclinical or in the form of a blepharoconjunctivitis. The virus lies dormant in the trigeminal ganglia and then reactivates and spreads to involve the eye.

If I examine the patient, what will I find?

□ If you put fluorescein on the eye you will see the classical branching linear ulcer staining (figures 19.1a and b).

What if I've diagnosed it?

□ Topical aciclovir five times daily should result in rapid resolution. If there is a classical dendritic lesion on the cornea, referral should be *soon*. If there is doubt about the diagnosis and a bacterial ulcer is suspected, the patient should be referred *urgently*.

What will the hospital do?

□ Treat with topical aciclovir.

What do I need to do?

□ Avoid any topical steroids, and refer as above.

What to tell the patient

□ They have a herpes virus infection that should resolve quickly with few long-lasting consequences. If the patient has multiple episodes, some corneal scarring and therefore visual loss may result. If they have a recurrent red eye in the future, therefore, they should seek prompt medical attention.

Problems that may arise, and how to deal with them

□ The virus can never be eliminated, and thus a future recurrence is a definite possibility.

ACANTHAMOEBA KERATITIS

What's going on?

□ Acanthamoebae are free-living protozoa found in water. Contaminated contact lens fluid or washing contact lenses in tap water can lead to significant corneal infection. The infection does not resolve with the usual antibiotic treatment regimens and the delay in recognition and effective treatment can be sight threatening.

If I examine the patient, what will I find?

□ Your findings will be similar to those seen with other corneal infections.

What if I've diagnosed it?

□ Such patients have usually already been referred to the hospital as this is a specialist diagnosis typically made in the hospital setting. The diagnosis is made by the clinical features and by isolating the organism from the eye and/or contact lenses or case.

What will the hospital do?

□ If acanthamoeba keratitis is suspected, the superficial corneal epithelium is sent for specialised culture and staining. Treatment is with specialised topical therapy, as acanthamoebae are resistant to all other fortified antibiotics.

What do I need to do?

□ Emphasise that contact lens hygiene is vital.

What to tell the patient

□ Those with an established diagnosis will need to be on topical treatment for many months, and will need regular follow up at the eye clinic.

Problems that may arise, and how to deal with them

□ Acanthamoeba infection can relapse, in which case *urgent* re-referral is required. Other complications include scleritis, and drop toxicity.

PTERYGIUM

What's going on?

□ The conjunctiva begins to grow and encroach upon the cornea. The condition is thought to be related to excessive exposure to ultraviolet (UV) light and is thus more commonly seen in those who have worked out of doors. It tends to affect the cornea at the three o'clock and nine o'clock positions, but is more common on the nasal side. The conjunctiva grows over the cornea in a triangular fashion.

If I examine the patient, what will I find?

□ A triangular wedge of conjunctiva pointing into the cornea from the nasal or temporal side (figure 19.2).

What if I've diagnosed it?

□ A pterygium is a fairly common condition. If it is minor, peripheral and has the classical triangular appearance extending on to the cornea, it does not require referral.

If the patient is troubled by their appearance then referral should be *routine*.

If the patient is untroubled by the cosmesis but feels some irritation, try topical lubricant drops, because sometimes the cornea adjacent to the pterygium dries up slightly. If this does not work, then refer *routinely*.

If the pterygium extends almost to the centre of the cornea the patient should be referred *soon via letter*.

What will the hospital do?

□ If indicated, the patient will be given surgery.

What to tell the patient

□ They have a benign growth of the conjunctiva that can be static or slowly progressive. It does no harm, but can affect vision if it gets too close to the visual axis.

Problems that may arise, and how to deal with them

□ Pterygia may recur after surgical excision. They usually do so within the first six months, and can be more aggressive than the original lesion. They should be re-referred *soon via letter*.

BAND KERATOPATHY

What's going on?

□ Chronic eye disease (such as persistent intraocular inflammation) affects the metabolic milieu of the cornea. There is deposition of calcium into the superficial corneal stroma, occurring in the interpalpebral band, running horizontally between the upper and lower lids across the centre of the cornea. Gradually, vision is reduced by the white corneal opacity.

If I examine the patient, what will I find?

□ There will be a band of white across the middle of the cornea extending horizontally but with a clear 1 mm strip at the limbus, both nasally and temporally.

What if I've diagnosed it?

□ There must be an underlying pathology so the patient needs investigating. Referral should be *soon via letter*. The exception is children, who should be referred *urgently*.

What will the hospital do?

□ An underlying aetiology will be determined and appropriate management initiated. If the band keratopathy affects vision, the calcium may be leached out with topically applied chelating agents in theatre.

What do I need to do?

□ Rarely, this condition occurs secondary to systemic hypercalcaemia, so it may be worth checking serum calcium level.

What to tell the patient

□ The calcium deposition can be removed but will recur if the underlying pathology is not addressed.

CORNEAL ARCUS

What's going on?

□ This is lipid deposition in the peripheral cornea. It is a normal finding in the elderly.

If I examine the patient, what will I find?

□ A white circumferential band around the whole cornea, separated by a small clear area from the limbus.

What if I've diagnosed it?

□ In someone over 50 years of age, it is a normal finding and does not warrant referral.

What will the hospital do?

□ Nothing.

What do I need to do?

□ If seen in someone under 50 years of age, the patient should have a lipid screen to detect hypercholesterolaemia.

What to tell the patient

□ This is a normal finding, unless the patient is under 50 and needs screening for hypercholesterolaemia.

KERATOCONUS

What's going on?

□ This is a progressive condition whereby the cornea loses its spherical shape and gradually develops a central protrusion (ectasia), forming a cone. The gradual distortion of the front surface of the cornea results in significant astigmatism as the focusing function of the cornea is disrupted. Initially, this astigmatism can be corrected by spectacles, but as it worsens the patient will need a hard contact lens to achieve adequate vision. If the cone becomes too advanced, corneal grafting surgery may be required. This is more likely in patients presenting in their teens. It is a bilateral condition but can be markedly asymmetrical in severity.

If I examine the patient, what will I find?

□ If you look from the side you may see the cornea protruding abnormally and forming a slight point or cone (figure 19.3).

What if I've diagnosed it?

□ The patient should be referred *routinely*. If you are unsure, optometrists are skilled in making this diagnosis.

What will the hospital do?

□ Initially, contact lenses will be prescribed but corneal grafting surgery may be required. It is also important to treat any allergic eye disease, so that patients do not rub their eyes because this makes the condition worse.

What to tell the patient

□ This condition causes blurred vision because of an abnormal distortion of the front of the eye. Most patients manage with contact lenses, although the prescription may need to be changed over time, so regular check-ups at the hospital or the opticians will be needed. If the condition gets worse an operation may be necessary. This is most likely in patients who are affected in their teens or early 20s.

It is important not to rub the eyes because this will make the condition worse. This diagnosis is an absolute contraindication to laser refractive surgery.

Problems that may arise, and how to deal with them

□ Rarely, the progressive changes in the cornea weaken the endothelial cell layer. The descemets membrane underlying the endothelial cells can rupture, and aqueous can enter the cornea, resulting in sudden visual blurring and pain. The central cornea will be cloudy. This is called acute hydrops. It will resolve but leave a scar. Patients will normally already be under hospital follow up. However, they should be re-referred *soon via letter*.

PSEUDOPHAKIC BULLOUS KERATOPATHY

What's going on?

□ The cornea stays clear by maintaining a relative level of dehydration through the action of its endothelial cells. Throughout life there is gradual attrition on these cells. When the cell density drops below a certain critical level (usually less than $500/mm^2$), the cornea fills with water derived from the aqueous, and corneal oedema develops, with consequent drop in vision due to excessive light scatter. Intraocular procedures such as cataract surgery inevitably kill some endothelial cells and, if their density drops too low, corneal oedema ensues. This is called pseudophakic (false lens) bullous (small microcysts of fluid called bullae develop in the cornea) keratopathy (corneal pathology).

If I examine the patient, what will I find?

□ The cornea will have a ground-glass appearance and look slightly cloudy. If you put fluorescein on the eye you may see small pinpoint areas of staining, corresponding to the areas where the bullae have burst (figure 19.4).

What if I've diagnosed it?

□ Refer *routinely*.

What will the hospital do?

□ Topic hyperosmotic ointments or drops may be used to try to dehydrate the cornea and restore some clarity of vision. These are short-term measures and are unlikely to maintain a prolonged remission.

Sometimes the cysts/bullae burst on the corneal surface and cause pain. If this happens, lubricants or a bandage contact lens may be used for comfort.

A corneal graft procedure is often required.

What to tell the patient

□ The problem is unlikely to resolve without surgery, but corneal grafting tends to have a good visual prognosis. If the patient declines an operation, then keeping the eye comfortable is of key concern.

Problems that may arise, and how to deal with them

□ These patients often suffer recurrent pain from ruptured corneal bullae. They are at increased risk of corneal infection as a result of this and also through the use of bandage contact lenses. It is therefore important to be alert to this possibility, and refer *urgently* any patient with suspected infection.

CORNEAL DYSTROPHIES

What's going on?

□ These are inherited bilateral conditions that may affect any of the layers of the cornea.

Epithelial dystrophies (the commonest is epithelial basement membrane dystrophy, also called Cogan's microcystic dystrophy or map-dot-fingerprint dystrophy) affect the corneal epithelium and can cause recurrent erosion syndrome (see below).

Stromal dystrophies result in deposits of opaque abnormal material within the corneal substance. Lattice dystrophy results in linear deposits, while the deposits seen in granular dystrophy are more 'clump'-like.

Endothelial dystrophies involve the endothelial cells and result in malfunction of the pump required to keep the cornea clear. The commonest is Fuchs' endothelial dystrophy, which results in corneal oedema and may require corneal grafting.

If I examine the patient, what will I find?

□ If the patient is pain free and if the eyes are white and there appear to be white or grey opacities within both corneas, then this may be a dystrophy.

What if I've diagnosed it?

□ Referral should be *routine*.

What will the hospital do?

□ If the vision is unaffected, nothing will be done. If vision is adversely affected, the patient will be offered a corneal graft.

What to tell the patient

□ They have an inborn error in their corneal metabolism, causing abnormal depositions that are affecting their vision. Such disorders are often hereditary.

Problems that may arise, and how to deal with them

□ Apart from reduced vision, many corneal dystrophies also cause recurrent erosion of the corneal epithelium, which becomes unstable over the area of the abnormal deposits. This can cause recurrent pain. Topical lubricants may help, especially at night.

RECURRENT EROSION SYNDROME

What's going on?

□ This condition can occur if the patient has some form of corneal epithelial dystrophy, or following a superficial corneal abrasion. The epithelial cells fail to form their usual attachments to their basement membrane, and are thus prone to dislodging. The continual movement of the lids over the cornea may rub off some of these cells, particularly if the eye is dry. When the cells come away, the patient experiences sudden pain and a foreign-body sensation. Classically this occurs in the morning, as nocturnal dehydration of the ocular surface causes the upper lid to adhere to the cornea. When patients open their eyes, they feel sudden pain as the lid causes a spontaneous abrasion.

Often the patient does not have a dystrophy but may have had some corneal trauma in the past. Corneal abrasions caused by nail or paper injuries are common culprits. The initial abrasion heals, but the epithelial cells that move in to cover the area of the abrasion never quite stick down properly.

If the recurrent erosion is minor, the patient may only have a transient red eye with watering that settles within an hour. If severe, they may have a large corneal abrasion, which requires a course of chloramphenicol ointment to prevent secondary infection and facilitate healing.

If I examine the patient, what will I find?

□ If the patient has recently had an attack, you will see staining on the cornea corresponding to the abrasion.

If the patient has had no recent attack you will not see anything.

What if I've diagnosed it?

□ If the history is classical, commence lubricant drops for acute episodes and lubricant ointment at night. If the diagnosis is in doubt or if the patient is symptomatic despite the lubrication ointment, refer *routinely*.

What will the hospital do?

□ Acute corneal abrasions are treated with antibiotic ointments. Prophylactic lubricant ointment every night will be advised to stop the nocturnal drying and prevent the recurrent morning erosions. Other options are available if the attacks are persistent and frequent.

What to tell the patient

□ This is a chronic problem, but topical lubricants usually help. These may have to be used indefinitely. Where the cause is trauma rather than a dystrophy, tell the patient that half of all cases resolve within 12 months.

Problems that may arise, and how to deal with them

□ Acute episodes may be treated with lubricant drops or antibiotic ointments.

CORNEAL MELT

What's going on?

□ This condition is related to systemic vasculitides. Deposits of immune complexes at the end of the limbal blood vessels result in collagenolysis. The collagen of the cornea literally melts away, thinning progressively, usually just within the corneal limbus. This can lead to perforation, which is potentially sight threatening.

If I examine the patient, what will I find?

□ You will notice a trough of thinning in the peripheral cornea that will stain or pool with fluorescein dye (figure 19.8).

What if I've diagnosed it?

□ Refer *urgently*.

What will the hospital do?

□ Systemic immunosuppression is usually started or increased. The mainstay of topical treatment is frequent, liberal application of preservative-free lubricant drops. Topical steroids are used with caution as they can make the melt worse. Sometimes oral collagenase inhibitors, such as oxytetracycline or doxycycline, are given.

What do I need to do?

□ The corneal problem is related to systemic disease. These patients are usually suffering from active rheumatoid arthritis. Their systemic immunosuppression needs addressing in order to limit their on-going systemic pathology and facilitate healing of the cornea.

It is important to keep the cornea moist, so the patient must not run out of drops. These patients are often elderly: general dehydration will make the condition worse and increase the renal toxicity of some immunosuppressives. It is therefore important to educate patients and carers about the importance of maintaining hydration through moderate fluid intake.

Any immunosuppression commenced by the hospital eye service may result in complications.

What to tell the patient

□ Their cornea is at risk if their systemic autoimmune disease is not controlled. The lubricant drops must be administered very frequently, and general hydration must be maintained.

Problems that may arise, and how to deal with them

□ If the vision suddenly deteriorates or the eye suddenly waters copiously, the patient may have had a corneal perforation warranting *urgent* referral.

DRY EYES

What's going on?

□ Tears are vital to lubricate and maintain the health of the ocular surface. Patients with deficient tear production may have problems keeping their cornea wet and healthy. The superficial corneal epithelium becomes unhealthy and some cells fall away, leaving areas of pinpoint staining. These small mini-abrasions lead to a gritty or burning sensation. Paradoxically, the eyes may water, as the cornea dries up so much that the lacrimal gland releases a big bolus of 'reflex' tears, causing intermittent watering.

If I examine the patient, what will I find?

□ Usually nothing. If you stain the cornea with fluorescein you may see pinpoint areas of staining corresponding to the drying of the cornea and point loss of corneal epithelial cells. These drying changes typically occur in the inferior third of the cornea (figure 22.4).

What if I've diagnosed it?

□ Topical lubricants are the mainstay of treatment. There are many types of artificial tears available, some liquid and some gel-like. The gels last longer and thus tend to give longer-lasting symptomatic relief, but, because of their viscous nature, may temporarily blur vision when first instilled. Ointment may be used overnight to protect the ocular surface and make the eye more comfortable on waking.

Any concurrent blepharitis (see below) with worsening symptoms should be treated with lid hygiene and warm bathing.

What will the hospital do?

□ The hospital will probably assess tear function with a Schirmer's test. This involves placing a strip of blotting paper over the lid margin to measure tear production.

Artificial tears will be prescribed. If these do not bring symptomatic relief, then the tear drainage puncti may be occluded with temporary or permanent plugs. These plugs block tear drainage and allow the small amount of tears produced to linger longer on the eye.

What do I need to do?

□ Dry eyes may be a feature of Sjogren's syndrome (dry eye and dry mouth), or a manifestation of a systemic autoimmune disorder.

What to tell the patient

□ Unfortunately dry eye tends to be a lifelong problem.

Symptoms tend to be worse with reading or looking at a computer screen as the patient's blink rate slows. Prophylactic drops before such activities may help, as will conscious, regular blinking.

Problems that may arise, and how to deal with them

□ If the dry eye is very severe a corneal ulcer may develop.

These patients are also at increased risk of infection and tolerate contact lenses poorly. Dry eye is a contraindication to laser refractive surgery, which may make it worse.

Conjunctiva

HERPES ZOSTER OPHTHALMICUS

What's going on?

□ This is herpes zoster infection of the ophthalmic division of the trigeminal nerve. The vesicles occur on the forehead and around the eye. If the tip of the nose is involved, this indicates that the nasociliary nerve has been infected, and thus the risk of eye involvement is increased (called Hutchinson's sign).

Rarely, patients develop corneal problems and an anterior uveitis with concurrent inflammatory glaucoma.

If I examine the patient, what will I find?

□ The conjunctiva may be injected and the cornea may be stained, perhaps even as a precursor to a dendritic-type ulcer.

What if I've diagnosed it?

□ Prescribe systemic aciclovir in the early stages to minimise the risk of complications such as encephalitis.

What will the hospital do?

□ The eye will be assessed, and topical antivirals may be given as prophylaxis.

What to tell the patient

□ The virus cannot be eliminated, but lies dormant and can reactivate at any time.

The condition may affect the eye in a number of ways, and patients should seek medical attention if they notice problems with their vision or their eye.

Problems that may arise, and how to deal with them

□ Watch for the signs of secondary bacterial infection, which can cause a superimposed cellulitis.

Be aware that some patients may suffer trigeminal neuralgia in the distribution of the affected nerve for many months afterwards. This can respond to amitriptyline or carbamazepine if severe and/or prolonged.

ALLERGIC CONJUNCTIVITIS

What's going on?

□ The conjunctival mucosa has numerous patches of lymphoid tissue. In addition, tears have a large amount of immunoglobulin E (IgE). These defence mechanisms are designed to detect and destroy foreign material. Inappropriate reaction to airborne allergens results in mast cell degranulation and allergic conjunctival reaction.

If I examine the patient, what will I find?

□ The eyes will be red and watering. Itchiness is usually a predominant feature, and the condition tends to be bilateral. If you ask the patient to look up and pull the lower lid down, you will see that the reddened conjunctiva is not smooth but raised and 'bobbly'. These are follicles or papillae, and represent an allergic response. It is important to look at the cornea, as severe reactions can result in a corneal ulcer.

What if I've diagnosed it?

□ Topical antihistamines or mast cell stabilising drops are the mainstay of treatment. Once the allergy has taken hold, it is often hard to suppress it and hence pre-emptive prevention (see below) should be carried out if possible. Cold compresses may benefit the patient symptomatically. If the condition is very severe or if there is a corneal ulcer, the patient should be referred *soon* or *urgently*, respectively.

What will the hospital do?

□ Occasionally, the hospital may calm the allergy with a short course of steroids. If the allergy has caused an ulcer on the cornea, topical or even systemic immunosuppressants such as cyclosporin may be used. The diagnosis in this situation is usually a vernal allergic conjunctivitis, which tends to occur in younger patients. Vernal is effectively a worse variant of seasonal allergic conjunctivitis.

What do I need to do?

□ If the patient has significant morbidity, then it is prudent to advise about prevention. Prophylactic topical antihistamines a month or so before the patient usually begins to suffer may cut the risk, or even prevent recurrence.

INFECTIVE CONJUNCTIVITIS

What's going on?

□ This is bacterial or viral conjunctival infection.

If I examine the patient, what will I find?

□ If bacterial, the fornices will be redder than the corneal limbus and pus may be present.

In viral conjunctivitis, the eye tends to have a violaceous/diffuse violet tinge. Eyes are also watery, and pre-auricular lymph nodes are often palpable. Classically, the patient has a history of a recent upper respiratory tract infection. Viral conjunctivitis often begins in one eye but spreads to the other within days. If you ask the patient to look up or, alternatively, evert the upper lid you will see that the conjunctiva is not flat but 'bobbly'. These 'bobbles' are follicles and are commonly seen in viral or allergic conjunctivitides.

If it is clearly a bacterial conjunctivitis, treat with a topical antibiotic such as chloramphenicol.

If it is viral, then advise cold compresses for comfort.

Clinically evident conjunctivitis with no worrying features such as visual loss or failure to respond to treatment (*see* Chapters 1 and 15) does not require referral.

What if I've diagnosed it?

□ If bacterial, treat with topical antibiotics.

Do not treat viral conjunctivitis with antibiotics. Cold compresses will help symptoms.

What will the hospital do?

□ Bacterial conjunctivitis is treated with topical antibiotics, usually after a swab is taken for culture.

There is no effective treatment for viral conjunctivitis. Occasionally we prescribe a gentle steroid for symptomatic relief. This does not alter the duration of disease and is usually reserved for cases where there is some corneal viral involvement.

What do I need to do?

□ If the patient wears contact lenses, ask them to leave their lenses out until the infection has been completely cleared for a few weeks.

In recurrent conjunctivitis, look for a cause. Are the lids in a normal position? Is the eye excessively dry? Is there a collection of mucus or pus in the nasolacrimal sac (dacrocystitis)? Press it and see if any pus comes through the puncti.

What to tell the patient

□ If bacterial, tell them the topical antibiotics should result in speedy resolution.

If viral, tell them that there is no cure and their condition will simply have to run its course. Typically, it takes two weeks to improve, and patients may have systemic symptoms. Infectivity is high, so warn them to avoid transferring it to their other eye or passing it on to cohabitants (e.g. use separate face towels). Cold compresses may give symptomatic relief, as may topical lubricant drops (although these eyes are usually wet anyway).

Problems that may arise, and how to deal with them

□ Sometimes a patient is given a topical antibiotic for a mildly red eye and then presents back to you a few days later with a much redder eye and significant itching and lid swelling. Either the condition is more than simple bacterial conjunctivitis or they have developed an allergy and made it worse. It is sometimes prudent to stop the antibiotic (it is not working anyway) and await improvement. Naturally, if there is any evidence of visual loss, proptosis (eye protruding forward), excessive lid chemosis (swelling of the conjunctiva) or ocular motility disturbance, the possibility of orbital cellulitis should be considered. *See* section on red eyes, Chapters 1 and 15.

SUBCONJUNCTIVAL HAEMORRHAGE

What's going on?

□ A blood vessel has ruptured under the conjunctiva. The degree of haemorrhage can be quite marked, causing the conjunctiva to balloon up over the lids with no visible white sclera.

If I examine the patient, what will I find?

□ There will be confluent redness with no white sclera visible. It will be easy to distinguish this from inflammation, where the vessels are increased in calibre and the white sclera is still visible between them (figure 15.5).

Check that the eye is not obviously proptosed, that the pupil is reacting normally and that vision is normal. If the eye has moved forward or ocular movement is restricted, the patient may have had a retrobulbar haemorrhage, which needs *urgent* referral. If this is a retrobulbar haemorrhage, the entire conjunctiva will be red and probably ballooning forward.

What if I've diagnosed it?

□ If it is related to minor trauma, such as being poked in the eye with a finger, and the vision is normal with a comfortable eye, there is no need to refer. If there is a concern that the globe is injured then *urgent* referral is warranted.

What will the hospital do?

□ Nothing, if there is no injury to the globe.

What do I need to do?

□ Reassure the patient that the condition will resolve gradually over several weeks, first going yellow and then gradually fading. The haemorrhage may spread slowly to the lower lid to form a black eye.

Most spontaneous subconjunctival haemorrhages have no underlying cause. If there is a cause, the most common is hypertension, so it is important to check the blood pressure.

It is also prudent to look for other predisposing factors, e.g. a bleeding diathesis (if recurrent), chronic cough or constipation.

If the patient is anticoagulated, check that their international normalised ration (INR) is not excessively high.

What to tell the patient

□ Although the appearance is dramatic, it is of no real significance.

Diabetic eye disease

□ *See* Appendix 6.

BACKGROUND DIABETIC RETINOPATHY

□ Also: non-proliferative diabetic retinopathy.

What's going on?

□ Background diabetic changes, including dot and blot haemorrhages, exudates and 'cotton-wool' spots.

If I examine the patient, what will I find?

□ Dot and blot haemorrhages, exudates and cotton-wool spots (figures 20.1, 20.2 and 20.3).

What if I've diagnosed it?

□ If there is no maculopathy, no referral is required. The patient should be entered into an optometry-led screening programme if available.

What will the hospital do?

□ Patients with simple background diabetic retinopathy are not routinely followed up in the hospital. If they have advanced changes or maculopathy they are followed up so that they may be given argon laser treatment as soon as they reach treatment threshold (see below).

What do I need to do?

□ Optimal diabetic control reduces the risk of progression to sight-threatening diabetic eye disease.

Controlling blood pressure is also known to be as important as glycaemic control in reducing the risk of progression of diabetic eye disease.

Hyperlipidaemia should also be controlled.

What to tell the patient

□ They have some diabetic changes at the back of their eyes that are not affecting vision at present. If their diabetes is not strictly controlled, however, they may go on to have sight-threatening complications.

Problems that may arise, and how to deal with them

□ Diabetic patients have an increased incidence of cataract.

SEVERE NON-PROLIFERATIVE DIABETIC RETINOPATHY

□ Also: preproliferative diabetic retinopathy.

What's going on?

□ Several studies have found features of diabetic retinopathy that indicate a high risk of progression to proliferative diabetic retinopathy. These are severe haemorrhages in all four quadrants of the retina, venous beading in two quadrants or intraretinal microvascular anastomoses (IRMA). IRMA are seen as flat complexes of dilated capillary anastomoses lying within the retina.

If I examine the patient, what will I find?

□ There will be marked and florid changes of background diabetic retinopathy but no neovascularisation.

What if I've diagnosed it?

□ If the patient has not been seen before by the hospital eye service they should be referred *urgently via letter/soon via letter.*

What will the hospital do?

□ Patients will be followed up closely to detect the onset of proliferative diabetic retinopathy. If patient compliance or re-attendance is in doubt, early laser treatment may be given to prevent progression.

What do I need to do?

□ These patients are at high risk of significant visual loss. Optimal diabetic and blood pressure control should minimise the risk of progression.

What to tell the patient

□ They have severe diabetic eye disease, which is one step away from compromising their vision. They need to carry out the best possible diabetic control.

Problems that may arise, and how to deal with them

□ Sometimes the rapid stringent control of blood glucose from an uncontrolled state can actually worsen diabetic retinopathy. Watch out for this.

If the patient has sudden visual loss, they may have developed a vitreous haemorrhage due to undetected progression to proliferative diabetic retinopathy.

PROLIFERATIVE DIABETIC RETINOPATHY

What's going on?

□ The retinal ischaemia caused by the diabetic micro-vasculopathy results in release of vasoproliferative factors, which cause new blood vessels to form. These new vessels do not have the normal blood-retinal barrier function. They therefore leak and are highly prone to haemorrhage with consequent severe visual loss.

If I examine the patient, what will I find?

□ There may be fine new blood vessels at the optic disc or elsewhere within the retina. If the new vessels have already ruptured, there will be a vitreous haemorrhage and the view of the fundus will be obscured. If patients have had previous laser treatment, there will be scattered chorioretinal scars (white areas of retinal atrophy with pigmentary proliferation) throughout the retina (figure 20.4).

What if I've diagnosed it?

□ Referral should be *urgent via letter*.

What will the hospital do?

□ The ischaemic retina that is producing the factors driving the neovascularisation process must be obliterated. Argon laser burns are applied to the peripheral retina destroying retinal tissue. This is known as pan-retinal photocoagulation (PRP). Once the biochemical drive is removed, the new blood vessels will regress.

What do I need to do?

□ Diabetic and blood pressure control is vital to minimise further progression of diabetic retinopathy.

What to tell the patient

□ They are at significant risk of visual loss and will require laser treatment and close follow up at the hospital. Strict diabetic control is vital.

Problems that may arise, and how to deal with them

□ Despite PRP laser treatment, the patient may develop further neovascularisation requiring even more laser treatment, obliterating the remaining peripheral retina (called fill-in PRP).

This sometimes affects peripheral vision enough to prevent the patient being able to drive.

MACULOPATHY

What's going on?

□ Diabetic changes are affecting the macula.

Leakage from abnormal retinal vessels will lead to thickening and malfunction of the retina, secondary to oedema. If the oedema affects the fovea, the vision is usually slightly reduced (this is called clinically significant macular oedema – see below). Persistence of this oedema with exudation at the fovea will lead to permanent damage and visual loss. Treatment, therefore, is required (see below).

If I examine the patient, what will I find?

□ Exudates and haemorrhages within the macula.

What if I've diagnosed it?

□ Patients should be referred *soon via letter* if there are signs of maculopathy close to the centre of the macula. If the vision is unaffected and diabetic changes within the macula are minimal, the referral may be *routine*.

What will the hospital do?

□ The patient will be followed up closely to detect the presence of clinically significant macular oedema (see below).

What do I need to do?

□ Diabetic and blood pressure control must be optimised.

What to tell the patient

□ They have diabetic changes in the macula that, if they progress, could affect vision. The patient will need long-term hospital follow up to detect changes that will warrant laser treatment.

CLINICALLY SIGNIFICANT MACULAR OEDEMA (CSMO)

What's going on?

□ The patient has diabetic maculopathy that has reached a threshold for laser treatment. There is oedema and/or exudates very close to the fovea, and, if these changes persist or worsen, the vision will be permanently compromised. Large studies have indicated that this situation requires laser retinal photocoagulation to prevent visual loss. Once vision has been lost, laser treatment is seldom able to restore it – the emphasis is on prevention.

If I examine the patient, what will I find?

□ Changes such as haemorrhages and/or exudates at, or very close to, the fovea.

What if I've diagnosed it?

□ Refer *urgently via letter.*

What will the hospital do?

□ Apply argon laser photocoagulation to the area of leaky retina. This procedure is called a macular grid because a regular grid of laser is applied to the macula. Only mild burns are required to alter the blood-retinal barrier, but they do reduce vision in the area where they are applied. If the laser is inadvertently applied to the fovea, the central vision will be damaged. Sometimes the exudates surround a focal leaking microaneurysm (dot haemorrhage) in a circular (circinate) pattern (figure 20.2). Laser may be applied focally to the centre of the circinate to dry it up.

What do I need to do?

□ Optimisation of diabetic and blood pressure control is required.

What to tell the patient

□ They have a severe problem with their retina related to their diabetes and need laser treatment to preserve their sight. If the condition is left unchecked their vision will get worse.

Problems that may arise, and how to deal with them

□ Sometimes the macular oedema is related to capillary occlusion, resulting in an ischaemic maculopathy. This is not amenable to treatment.

Glaucoma (see *Chapter 21*)

CHRONIC OPEN-ANGLE GLAUCOMA

What's going on?

□ Raised intraocular pressure (IOP) results in compression of the optic nerve head/optic disc with consequent loss of retinal nerve fibres. With progressive neural cell death, the patient loses patches of their visual field. Because the loss is gradual the patient does not notice the deterioration, and the brain fills in the lost patch. This is an example of a negative scotoma similar to that of the blind spot. The optic disc becomes more and more cup-shaped as it loses neural fibres, eventually appearing extremely pale due to unmasking of the underlying sclera.

The patient is usually asymptomatic, and the condition is classically picked up as an incidental finding at a routine optometrist check.

The drainage angle of the anterior chamber is wide open, so it is thought that there is some blockage and resistance to aqueous outflow at a microscopic level within the trabecular meshwork.

If I examine the patient, what will I find?

□ The optic disc will be cupped (figure 9.3). If the glaucoma is advanced, testing the visual field will reveal markedly constricted vision.

What if I've diagnosed it?

□ It may be appropriate for the patient to be examined by an optometrist involved in glaucoma shared care in the first instance, if this is available. Otherwise refer *routine via letter* direct to the hospital.

What will the hospital do?

□ The patient will have formal visual field assessment with automated perimetry. The intraocular pressure will be measured using the gold standard of Goldmann applanation tonometry and the optic disc assessed with three-dimensional, slit lamp fundoscopy to confirm the diagnosis of glaucoma.

We know that reducing the IOP by at least 30% cuts or even eliminates the risk of damage progression. A target pressure is usually set that is one-third less than the pressure initially measured (their presenting IOP). Treatment will be started to bring the IOP down to this arbitrary target. Subsequent follow up will be aimed at ensuring that the target is indeed reached and that there is no further progression of the glaucoma. If progression persists, the target pressure is lowered further.

What do I need to do?

□ Such patients require lifelong follow up by the hospital eye service or specially trained community optometrists in a glaucoma shared care initiative.

Compliance with drops is essential in order to maintain a reasonable level of IOP reduction.

If the drops do not control the IOP, the patient may need an operation (trabeculectomy) or laser treatment (laser trabeculoplasty).

What to tell the patient

□ They have a chronic problem that will never be cured but can be controlled, usually by drops. They need lifelong follow up in order to monitor the pressure in their eyes. Even if the drops have worked for years, checks are still necessary because the pressure may build up gradually over a long period with consequent damage to the vision. If the drops do not control the pressure, then surgery may be necessary. With appropriate management and follow up, the prognosis is excellent. Few people diagnosed in recent years are likely to go blind because of their disease.

Problems that may arise, and how to deal with them

□ Drop allergy may occur at any stage of therapy, even if the patient has been using the drops for years (*see* Glaucoma drop problems, Chapter 21).

Topical beta blockers may exacerbate systemic conditions such as asthma, chronic obstructive pulmonary disease and heart failure.

Systemic acetazolamide can affect many systems of the body in many ways, potentially leading to hypokalaemia and dehydration.

ACUTE ANGLE-CLOSURE GLAUCOMA

□ Also: closed angle glaucoma; phacomorphic glaucoma.

What's going on?

□ The front of the patient's eye is shallow and cramped. The anterior chamber is not as deep as in other individuals, which means that the cornea is flatter and the angle between the peripheral iris and the peripheral inner surface of the cornea is reduced. Within this angle lies the trabecular meshwork that drains aqueous from the eye. If the pupil dilates, the iris ruffles up into the angle and blocks drainage of aqueous, with a resultant rapid and sudden rise in IOP.

If I examine the patient, what will I find?

□ The patient will have a red eye, pain, nausea and decreased vision, with a fixed mid-dilated pupil (figure 15.3). If you palpate the affected eye it will feel extremely firm like a cricket ball, particularly when compared to the other eye. The patient is usually longsighted.

What if I've diagnosed it?

□ Refer *immediately*.

What will the hospital do?

□ The acute attack will be reversed by aggressive topical and systemic antiglaucoma medication. Once the pressure has been reduced medically to below approximately 30 mmHg, the blood flow to the iris and the iris sphincter will be restored, and the pupil will begin to respond to topical miotic drops (e.g. pilocarpine). When the pupil begins to constrict, it pulls the peripheral iris out of the angle and allows the aqueous to drain. Naturally, if the pupil dilates again the problem will recur. To avoid this, the patient will have a YAG laser peripheral iridotomy (*see* Surgery, Chapter 28). Essentially a hole is 'blown' in the iris by several bursts of laser energy. Once the hole is patent it allows aqueous to flow through it, thereby equalising the pressure in front of and behind the peripheral iris, opening the angle and preventing acute closure.

Sometimes despite the above measures, the pressure is still uncontrolled and the patient will require long-term glaucoma drops and/or a glaucoma operation.

What to tell the patient

□ They have had an acute form of glaucoma, which has been treated with laser. The other eye is usually treated to prevent glaucoma in that eye.

Problems that may arise, and how to deal with them

□ These patients may be discharged from hospital follow up at some stage. They still need to see their optician for an annual pressure check as they may develop the other (chronic) form of glaucoma eventually.

Angle-closure glaucoma may be iatrogenic caused by pharmacologically dilating a predisposed angle (*see* Glaucoma drop problems, Chapter 21).

OCULAR HYPERTENSION

What's going on?

□ The pressure in the eye is high but there is no evidence of pressure-associated damage. The optic disc is normal with no evidence of cupping and there is no visual field defect.

If I examine the patient, what will I find?

□ Nothing, by definition.

What if my patient has been diagnosed with this?

□ Optometrists sometimes diagnose this at routine check-ups. In this case, refer *routinely*.

What will the hospital do?

□ The decision to lower the IOP with medication is not straightforward. Each patient should be assessed individually and several factors taken into account. Treatment should aim to reduce the risk of developing glaucoma.

If the IOP is very high (e.g. > 30 mmHg) it is reasonable to treat.

If the IOP is only moderately raised, the decision to treat should be based on the patient's age, the patient's views and feelings about lifelong therapy, and the thickness of the cornea. Corneal thickness (as measured by a technique called pachymetry) affects the accuracy of IOP measurements. If the cornea is thin then we know that we may be underestimating the true pressure inside the eye, so treatment is more likely to be beneficial. If the cornea is thick, the IOP measurements may be overestimates. The pressure may, indeed, be closer to normal but we are measuring it too high. Such patients may not require IOP-lowering therapy but may still warrant follow up to detect the development of any glaucoma damage.

What to tell the patient

□ They do not have glaucoma (i.e. they have no visual field loss) but have high pressure inside the eye, which is known to be related to glaucoma. The pressure may be 'normal for them' but above the recognised normal ranges. Any treatment will be prophylactic to prevent progression to glaucoma. Once the damage is done, there is no recovery of the visual field so prevention is important.

Problems that may arise, and how to deal with them

□ *See* Glaucoma drop problems, Chapter 21.

NORMAL-TENSION GLAUCOMA (NTG)

□ Also: normal-pressure glaucoma.

What's going on?

□ Despite normal IOP measurements, the patient is developing signs of glaucomatous pathology. There may be optic disc cupping and/or visual field defects. Therefore this IOP is still too high for the patient's optic disc and needs reducing.

If I examine the patient, what will I find?

□ Fundoscopy will reveal a cupped optic disc.

What if I've diagnosed it?

□ This diagnosis is sometimes made by optometrists at routine check-ups. In this case, refer *routinely via letter*.

What will the hospital do?

□ It is first important to establish the diagnosis and exclude other causes of optic neuropathy.

These cases are difficult as the patient's pressure is already 'normal'. Topical glaucoma medication will be required initially, but if there is still evidence of progression of visual field loss they may require a glaucoma operation.

What do I need to do?

□ NTG is sometimes related to systemic conditions such as migraine and Raynaud's syndrome. Vascular reactivity is thought to have a part to play.

Nocturnal hypotension has also been implicated in transient hypoperfusion of the optic disc and subsequent stepwise glaucomatous deterioration in visual fields. If the patient is on antihypertensive therapy it may be worth undertaking 24-hour blood pressure

(BP) measurement. If there are any nocturnal dips, then reducing the evening BP therapy may help prevent further glaucoma damage.

What to tell the patient

□ They have glaucoma despite normal pressures in their eyes. They will progressively lose vision unless the pressures are lowered and there is adequate follow up.

Problems that may arise, and how to deal with them

□ *See* Glaucoma drop problems, Chapter 21.

INFLAMMATORY GLAUCOMA

What's going on?

□ Inflammation within the eye causes blockage of the drainage angle with fibrous membranes. The intraocular pressure increases and the patient develops glaucoma.

If I examine the patient, what will I find?

□ You may see evidence of the previous inflammation or surgery within the eye.

What will the hospital do?

□ The source of the inflammation will be determined and, it is to be hoped, managed optimally. The inflammation will be suppressed with topical and/or systemic therapy. Once the inflammation is cured, the raised pressure may resolve, but sometimes the inflammatory debris causes permanent blockage of the trabecular drainage network. Such patients can be very difficult to manage. They require initial therapy with topical glaucoma drops, but a significant proportion require surgery.

What do I need to do?

□ Sometimes patients are treated with oral steroids to control the inflammation. Control of any dyspepsia and osteoporosis prophylaxis may be prudent.

What to tell the patient

□ They have raised IOP because of inflammation in the eye. It is very important to keep the inflammation under control, and they should seek medical attention if they have any symptoms in either eye. It is important to keep taking the medication to control the inflammation and the pressure, and so minimise the risk of long-term damage to their sight.

Problems that may arise, and how to deal with them

□ Recurrences of the inflammation should be dealt with promptly to prevent further blockage to the drainage mechanisms of the eye.

PIGMENTARY AND PSEUDO-EXFOLIATIVE GLAUCOMA

What's going on?

□ The trabecular meshwork in the drainage angle of the anterior chamber has become blocked with pigment or pseudo-exfoliative material. This pigment liberation is thought to come from rubbing of the dark rear surface of the iris on to the lens zonules, a phenomenon that occurs in pigment dispersion syndrome. In pseudo-exfoliative glaucoma, the abnormal matter is composed of an amyloid type material also liberated pathologically from the iris. The blockage to aqueous outflow results in glaucoma.

If I examine the patient, what will I find?

□ If you look closely with a magnifying glass you may notice some pigment or white flaky substance in the anterior chamber.

What will the hospital do?

□ Pressure management is with topical drops initially, but laser/surgery may be contemplated if the pressure is not controlled.

What to tell the patient

□ They have clogging of the drainage channels of their eyes, related to the release of abnormal material into the front of their eye. There is nothing that can be done to stop the release of this material, but the pressure may be controlled with drops.

RUBEOTIC/NEOVASCULAR GLAUCOMA

□ Also: rubeosis iridis.

What's going on?

□ An ischaemic process has affected the retina, causing the hypoxic retinal tissue to pathologically release growth factors in a fruitless attempt to stimulate vascular proliferation in order to increase blood supply and thus oxygen. These growth factors spread throughout the anterior and posterior segments of the eye and stimulate fibrovascular proliferation. New blood vessels (rubeosis) and their associated fibrous scaffold grow on the iris and within the drainage angle blocking drainage causing glaucoma (rubeotic glaucoma).

If I examine the patient, what will I find?

□ The eye may be red due to the high pressure. Palpating the eye will reveal a very firm globe. The patient may have a significant relative afferent pupillary defect (RAPD) due to the widespread retinal damage.

What will the hospital do?

□ The commonest causes of this pathology include central retinal vein occlusions and advanced diabetic retinopathy.

If the rubeosis is not advanced or long-standing, aggressive pan-retinal laser therapy may be enough to kill off the ischaemic retina. This will remove the stimulus for neovascularisation and, it is hoped, cause the new vessels to regress and eventually disappear in the anterior segment.

If the damage is too advanced, the patient will require glaucoma drops to treat the pressure. Glaucoma operations tend to have poor success in these cases.

Often such eyes are blind due to the underlying pathology. Here the pressure level is not as important as patient comfort. In a blind eye, a pressure of 50 mmHg (i.e. very high) may be treated conservatively, as long as the patient is pain free. Conversely, if the pressure is 40 mmHg but the patient is in pain, they should have therapy to bring this pressure down.

If the pressure is out of control and the eye is uncomfortable, patients may be given laser therapy to the ciliary body (cyclodiode laser) to reduce aqueous production and bring the pressure down. Sometimes an eye is surgically removed due to chronic intractable pain.

What to tell the patient

□ Explain that in their blind eye comfort is more important than the exact pressure. If the eye becomes painful, however, they will need treatment.

Problems that may arise, and how to deal with them

□ These eyes may become inflamed repeatedly. Often treatment with short courses of steroid therapy and atropine resolves inflammation and improves comfort. Long-term, once-a-day steroid and atropine drops are sometimes required for comfort. The risks of prolonged steroid use (cataract and glaucoma) are obviously not relevant in this situation, but these eyes are more vulnerable to infection.

Lids and lacrimal apparatus (see Chapter 22)

ECTROPION

What's going on?

□ The lower eyelid is not opposed to the globe but is rolled out. This means that the eye may dry up because the tears pool in the lower fornix rather than being spread over the ocular surface. The patient's eye may water because the normal pumping of tears towards the medial puncti for drainage into the nasolacrimal system does not occur. Cosmesis may also be a concern to patients.

If I examine the patient, what will I find?

□ The patient's lower lid will be rolled out (figure 22.1). The lid margin will not be opposed to the globe. There may be a scar on the skin beneath the eye that is pulling the lid out or the cause may be related to laxity of the lid skin. If you pull the lower lid out from the globe you will see that it is lax and does not bounce back. This lower-lid laxity is an involutional ageing change and is the commonest cause of ectropion.

What if I've diagnosed it?

□ If the cornea is healthy, referral should be *routine*.

What will the hospital do?

□ The abnormal position of the lid will be corrected with surgery.

What do I need to do?

□ Lubricant drops may be required to protect the cornea and keep it moist. A watering eye may still require lubricating ointments or drops to maintain the health of the cornea. It is always worth putting fluorescein dye on to the eye to assess the health of the corneal surface. Fluorescein will stain any areas of epithelial loss on the cornea. Shining a blue light on the eye after staining will cause these areas to show up as bright green.

What to tell the patient

□ They will need an operation to correct the lid position.

ENTROPION

What's going on?

□ The lower lid is turning in, causing the lashes to abrade the cornea.

If I examine the patient, what will I find?

□ The lower lid is turned in and the lashes may be in contact with the ocular surface (figure 22.2).

What if I've diagnosed it?

□ Initiate the temporary measures (see below) and refer *routinely*.

What will the hospital do?

□ An operation will be carried out to return the lid to its anatomical condition.

What do I need to do?

□ While waiting for surgery, simple measures will prevent the lashes irritating and damaging the cornea. Taping of the lower lid, from just below the lashes to the cheek, will pull the lid out temporarily. The eyelashes may even be plucked to give temporary relief. Lubricant eye drops and ointment will coat the cornea and minimise damage from any abrading lashes.

It is worth applying fluorescein to the eye to detect any corneal damage.

Problems that may arise, and how to deal with them

□ Bacterial keratitis may ensue because of the on-going corneal attrition. If there is an ulcer on the cornea, the patient should be referred *urgently*.

TRICHIASIS

What's going on?

□ Some eyelashes are pointing backwards and rubbing up and down the ocular surface with each blink. The lid position, however, is normal.

If I examine the patient, what will I find?

□ Lashes will be pointing backwards and making contact with the ocular surface. They are often clearly visible with a magnifying glass.

What if I've diagnosed it?

□ Sometimes lashes are simply too long and curl back towards the eye. Simply plucking these lashes may allow them to regrow in the correct direction. If they recur frequently or if there is associated abnormality of the lid position, the patient should be referred *routinely*.

What will the hospital do?

□ First the lashes will be plucked. Then electrolysis (an electric current passed down the hair follicle after local anaesthesia), cryotherapy (freeze/thaw cycles applied to the lid margin) or laser (argon laser applied down the hair follicle) are all tried to prevent the lashes regrowing.

If the lashes are all pointing backwards but the lid is in the correct position, an operation may be needed to split the lid into front and back halves, and redirect the front (with the lashes) more anteriorly (called a lid-splitting and lamellar rotation procedure).

What do I need to do?

□ Keep the cornea healthy with lubricant drops and watch out for ulcers.

What to tell the patient

□ If the patient has had numerous recurrences, simple epilation is unlikely to prevent long-term problems. If they are happy with simple removal every few months then that is a reasonable course of action, but if they want definitive treatment they will require a small operation.

Problems that may arise, and how to deal with them

□ If lashes are simply plucked they will regrow, but can be plucked again with ordinary tweezers and a magnifying glass.

CHALAZION

What's going on?

□ One of the meibomian gland orifices (in the eyelids) has become blocked. The fatty secretions build up within it and create a cyst. This is usually painless and does not cause many symptoms. If the cyst ruptures or leaks into the surrounding lid tissue, it causes an inflammatory reaction with localised redness and pain.

Infective cellulitis may also develop where the redness spreads beyond the margins of the lump.

If I examine the patient, what will I find?

□ A firm lump, usually the size of a pea or grape, within the upper or lower lid (figure 22.5).

What if I've diagnosed it?

□ Warm bathing is the key to management. Heating the fatty secretion should cause it to flow more freely and discharge spontaneously. If the patient has a quiet cyst that has failed to disappear completely and is symptomatic, they may warrant *routine* referral. If possible, patients should be referred directly to a minor operations or lid surgery list.

If despite warm bathing, the cyst gets bigger and becomes extremely painful and red, the patient may require incision and drainage. There is no hard and fast rule about how large a cyst must be before it warrants surgical intervention. Conservative measures should be used initially, with or without systemic antibiotics, and if, despite this, the patient's conditions worsen, they should be referred *soon*.

There is no need for topical antibiotics.

What will the hospital do?

□ If incision and curettage is required, local anaesthetic will be given around the cyst, the lid everted, a stab incision made into the body of the cyst and its contents removed.

What to tell the patient

□ The condition can recur so the patient should warm bathe the eyes regularly (usually daily), to prevent further episodes.

CAUTION. Beware of a chalazion that has been operated on and comes back in *exactly* the same place. It may be a sebaceous gland carcinoma.

PTOSIS

What's going on?

□ The eyelid is droopy. Most commonly, this is involutional related to ageing of the levator aponeurosis (the tendon connecting the levator muscle to the tarsal plate). It can also be myogenic (as seen in myotonic dystrophy or myasthenia gravis), neurogenic (as seen in Horner's syndrome or third nerve palsy), or mechanical (related to a mass lesion pulling down on the upper lid).

The normal upper lid lies 2 mm below the upper border (limbus) of the cornea. If the lid is lower than this, there is a ptosis.

Sometimes excessive skin on the upper lid creates a fold drooping over the upper lid and giving the impression of a ptosis; however, this condition is dermatochalasis.

If I examine the patient, what will I find?

□ The lid will be droopy. It may also be symmetrical or markedly asymmetrical (figure 22.6).

If the patient is asked to sustain an upward gaze for a time, the upper lid will be seen gradually to droop further if there is fatigability (*see* Section 4).

If there appears to be excessive skin on the upper lid, hold this skin up and see whether the ptosis disappears, in other words if the underlying position of the lid is normal. This is dermatochalasis.

What if I've diagnosed it?

□ Check the eye movements and pupil sizes/reactions to ensure that the ptosis is not part of a third nerve palsy or a Horner's syndrome.

If there is fatigability or any other symptoms to raise a suspicion of myasthenia gravis, it is worth checking serum acetylcholine receptor antibodies.

If the ptosis appears purely involutional, and the patient is motivated for surgery, then they should be referred to the hospital as *routine*.

What will the hospital do?

□ If appropriate, the patient will be listed for surgery.

What to tell the patient

□ Their droopy lid can be corrected but there are risks. The operation is usually done under local anaesthetic so that the height of the lid can be adequately assessed per-operatively.

Problems that may arise, and how to deal with them

□ Following ptosis surgery, the eyes occasionally have more difficulty closing, particularly at night. This exposure can lead to red eyes in the morning. If mild, this can be treated with lubricant ointment at night; otherwise re-refer *soon*.

WATERING EYE (EPIPHORA)

What's going on?

□ The eye is watering, possibly because of oversecretion of tears or poor drainage from the ocular surface.

Curiously, a watering eye may be a manifestation of a dry eye. The cornea rapidly dries up owing to excessive evaporation. This is worse in a windy or hot environment. The neural reflex response sends an impulse to the lacrimal gland, releasing a bolus of tears and thus causing sudden watering.

Other forms of ocular irritation, such as foreign bodies, allergy or inflammatory eye disease, may also cause excessive 'physiological' watering. Trichiatic (inward-turning) lashes or an entropion (turning in) of the lower lid (see p. 37) may result in corneal irritation and reflex watering.

Tears drain into the nasolacrimal system, which begins at the puncti located medially on the upper and lower lid. They then run horizontally into the nasolacrimal sac and down the nasolacrimal duct into the nose. Obstruction at any of these levels will result in watering in most patients. A patient may have a totally blocked nasolacrimal system and still produce no tears, however, because their baseline tear secretion is low.

Part of the physiological drainage system is the approximation of the lids during closure to pump the tears nasally. If the lower lid is ectropic (turned out) the tears will pool there and overflow.

If I examine the patient, what will I find?

□ There may be an underlying cause (see above) for the watering, which should be clear on careful examination.

What if I've diagnosed it?

□ It is important to exclude any obvious irritation causing the watering. Examine the lid margins for blepharitis and put some fluorescein on the eye to assess the health of the cornea.

Check the position of the lids and check for any trichiasis.

If the watering is intermittent, try treating with lubricant drops initially.

If the patient is markedly troubled by their symptoms and motivated for surgery to try to restore patency to their nasolacrimal system, refer *routinely*.

What will the hospital do?

□ The puncti will be dilated and the nasolacrimal system irrigated directly with fluid. If the patient feels fluid at the back of the throat, the nasolacrimal system is patent. If there is no fluid to the throat, the system is blocked and the patient may be offered surgery, either endonasally or externally via a skin incision on the side of the nose.

What to tell the patient

□ They have a blocked tear drainage system, which may require an operation. Many people tolerate their symptoms as an inconvenience rather than a major problem, so the decision to operate is not clear-cut.

Problems that may arise, and how to deal with them

□ Sometimes the patients are more bothered by the effect of the watering on the skin of their lower lid and cheek. Application of petroleum jelly to the skin may protect it and prevent irritation and redness.

The patient may have a mucocele, which predisposes them to a bacterial infection (see below).

MUCOCELE AND DACROCYSTITIS

□ Also: dacrocystocele.

What's going on?

□ Tears drain into the puncti on the medial aspects of upper and lower lid margins, and then move medially through the canaliculi to the lacrimal sac and drain down into the nose via the nasolacrimal duct. If the duct is blocked, the tears and mucus from the ocular surface may collect, causing the sac to dilate, resulting in a mucocele. Stagnation within the lacrimal sac predisposes to infection (dacrocystitis).

If I examine the patient, what will I find?

□ There will be a cystic swelling inferomedial to the medial canthus. If there is dacrocystitis, the overlying skin may be erythematous and cellulitic (figure 22.7). Firm pressure on the swelling may cause mucus to pass back through the canaliculus on to the eye.

What if I've diagnosed it?

□ If there is frank infection, then systemic antibiotics may be required. If the sac is markedly dilated and infected, the patient may require incision and drainage, although this is rare. In such a case, the patient should be referred *soon*. Occasionally pressure on the sac may cause pus to be regurgitated back through the canaliculi on to the eye. If the sac can be kept empty then topical antibiotics (usually chloramphenicol) may be able to enter the sac and clear the infection.

Patients with a mucocele may elect simply to keep it empty by regular massage or pressure upon it. This will minimise the risk of bacterial infection. If the patient experiences a concurrent watery eye and is motivated for surgical intervention, they should be referred *routinely*.

What will the hospital do?

□ Incision and drainage if required will be carried out under local anaesthesia.

Problems that may arise, and how to deal with them

□ If the patient has a mucocele or has developed dacrocystitis, then the nasolacrimal duct is blocked, and even after resolution of the acute condition, the patient will probably be left with a watery eye. If they are significantly troubled by it and are motivated for surgery, they should be referred to the oculoplastic ophthalmology team *routinely*.

BLEPHARITIS

□ Also: seborrhoeic blepharitis; anterior blepharitis; posterior blepharitis; meibomian gland dysfunction.

What's going on?

□ There is a problem with the lid margin, usually caused by a collection of dandruff-like skin flakes around the bases of the lashes. This is often associated with some inflammation and low-grade infective colonisation with bacterial organisms (usually staphylococci). This inflammation results in irritation of the ocular surface with consequent dryness, burning and foreign-body sensation. Bacteria may release exotoxins, which can cause an immune-mediated peripheral corneal ulcer.

There is another form of blepharitis, often called posterior blepharitis, where the meibomian glands are dysfunctional. Approximately 20 lipid-secreting glands line the upper and lower lids. These secrete fat on to the ocular surface to coat the tear film and prevent evaporation. These fatty secretions can stagnate and block the meibomian gland orifices. They are seen as a line of small domes of yellowish material overlying each meibomian gland pore. This form of blepharitis (meibomian gland dysfunction) is often associated with cutaneous rosacea.

If I examine the patient, what will I find?

□ The lid margins will be red, with some flaky material around the bases of the lashes. The orifices of the meibomian glands may have an overlying cap of fat.

What if I've diagnosed it?

□ The mainstay of therapy is lubricant drops to minimise ocular irritation and lid hygiene. The lid margins should be cleaned daily. First the lids should be warmed with a hot flannel to loosen any flakes and liquefy the meibomian gland secretions. An eggcup of water should be boiled and allowed to cool, and a drop of specialised non-irritant baby shampoo (to avoid stinging) should be added. The upper and lower lid margins at the lash bases should be cleaned with a cotton bud moistened with the water.

What will the hospital do?

□ The patient should be given a leaflet on lid hygiene. If patients show any evidence of rosacea or have significant meibomian gland dysfunction, they may benefit from a course of oral oxytetracycline or doxycycline. These drugs work by their anticollagenase activity rather than their antibiotic properties, and thus a minimum of a six-week course is usually required.

What do I need to do?

□ Patients will usually have been advised about the importance of regular lid hygiene, and the need for compliance should be emphasised.

What to tell the patient

□ This is likely to be a chronic condition. Topical lubricant drops will alleviate symptoms to some degree, but the underlying pathology will only be resolved by long-term adherence to regular lid hygiene.

Problems that may arise, and how to deal with them

□ Blepharitis can cause an ulcer on the cornea through the release of exotoxins. This will present as a red eye with a fluorescein staining area on the peripheral cornea, typically at the five o'clock or seven o'clock positions.

INFLAMMATORY IRITIS

□ Also: anterior uveitis.

What's going on?

□ The patient has inflammation of the iris. It is usually of an autoimmune aetiology, but in most patients no cause is identified. If it is bilateral or recurrent, a search must be made for a systemic autoimmune/ inflammatory cause such as HLA-B27-related disease. The inflammation within the anterior chamber results in redness, mildly blurred vision and photophobia. If the condition is unchecked, the patient may develop a cataract or glaucoma.

If I examine the patient, what will I find?

□ A red eye with ciliary injection (redness more around the limbus than in the inferior fornix) (figure 15.1). The pupil may be an abnormal shape due to adhesions between the iris and lens.

What if I've diagnosed it?

□ If patients have had many recurrences of iritis, they usually recognise the condition early (see below). Patients should ideally be referred *soon* for assessment. In the interim, it is reasonable to give a cycloplegic agent for comfort (NOTE: ensure the pupil is reactive and the eye is not firm, i.e. this is not angle-closure glaucoma). Topical steroids may, in limited cases, be given if you and the patient are confident of the diagnosis. Ideally, the patient should still be assessed by the hospital eye service to confirm the diagnosis.

What will the hospital do?

□ Examine the anterior chamber with a slit lamp. When we see cells floating around we can make the diagnosis. We will assess the fundus to ensure that the inflammation we see at the front of the eye is not related to an inflammatory/infective process at the back of the eye. The mainstay of treatment is intensive, topical, steroid drops and dilatation of the pupil to ensure the iris does not stick to the lens. If the inflammation is severe, we may give a subconjunctival injection of steroids or even commence oral steroids. Such patients are usually reassessed after approximately two weeks to ensure the inflammation has been suppressed and to check the intraocular pressure. Long-term steroids should be avoided if possible, but sometimes when the steroids are reduced the inflammation recurs.

What do I need to do?

□ If the patient has had multiple episodes or has bilateral disease, they should be evaluated for an underlying systemic disorder. An autoimmune screen (HLA-B27) and chest and sacroiliac X-rays are prudent. If the patient is known to have a generalised disease, their disease control should be evaluated, as a flare-up of iritis may indicate loss of systemic control. HLA-B27-positive patients have a risk of aortic insufficiency and aortitis.

What to tell the patient

□ They have an autoimmune process in the eye whereby their body reacts against their own iris tissue. In most cases the cause is unknown and peculiar to the individual, but it is sometimes related to an underlying systemic cause. It will get better with steroids but may recur. Long-term topical steroids can cause glaucoma or cataracts and so should be avoided if possible.

Problems that may arise, and how to deal with them

□ Recurrence is a concern. Patients tend to recognise the symptoms quite early and can usually diagnose recurrence. Do not treat with steroids based solely upon symptoms, as the red eye may have a different cause whose symptoms will be exacerbated by steroids. If patients are started on topical steroids before the diagnosis is certain, they should be referred on for definitive diagnosis by an ophthalmologist within a few days. If the symptoms do not rapidly improve with steroids or if they worsen, the treatment should be stopped and an *urgent* ophthalmology review arranged. Before any topical steroids are given, the cornea should be stained with fluorescein to ensure there is no ulcer.

Children with juvenile idiopathic arthritis (JIA) are also at risk of this condition. Children present differently: the eye is white and pain free, despite significant intraocular inflammation. For this reason, children with JIA should be screened regularly by an ophthalmologist.

EPISCLERITIS

What's going on?

□ The connective tissue layer between the sclera and the conjunctiva is inflamed. The condition may be idiopathic or, rarely, related to a connective tissue or autoimmune disorder. It may be localised and nodular (raised nodules lifting the overlying conjunctiva) or flat. Rarely, the episcleritis is diffuse, affecting all the visible episclera. Patients may feel some slight discomfort.

If I examine the patient, what will I find?

□ Localised redness of the conjunctiva, which may appear slightly elevated. The adjacent cornea will be clear with no fluorescein staining.

What if I've diagnosed it?

□ There is usually no need for referral if the diagnosis is clear.

If you are concerned that the patient has a scleritis (see below) refer *soon/urgently*.

What will the hospital do?

□ Often no treatment is necessary. Occasionally, a short course of topical steroids will be given.

What do I need to do?

□ Reassure the patient that the condition will resolve without treatment. Any discomfort may be treated with lubricant drops or oral non-steroidal anti-inflammatory drugs (NSAIDs).

What to tell the patient

□ Reassure them that this is a benign condition and recurrent episodes do not cause any long-term damage.

Problems that may arise, and how to deal with them

□ If the hospital has given the patient steroid drops, ensure that it is a short course and not a prolonged treatment. Patients may find that after they taper off and finally stop the drops, the condition recurs. If this happens, it is inadvisable to give further steroids as complications may arise from long-term use.

Unfortunately, this is a recurrent condition.

SCLERITIS

What's going on?

□ The sclera is firmly packed collagen. It is thus susceptible to involvement with system collagen vascular disorders. Scleritis is inflammation of the sclera and has significant associated ocular morbidity. An associated systemic disease is identified in 50% of patients with scleritis.

Pain is an important feature in differentiating scleritis from episcleritis. In episcleritis there is some discomfort but not the boring, aching pain and tenderness associated with scleritis.

If I examine the patient, what will I find?

□ This condition may be necrotising or non-necrotising.

In the necrotising variety, there is scleral inflammation with 'beefy'-red dilated scleral blood vessels surrounding a white avascular area of sclera. Necrotising scleritis is the more severe type and is associated indirectly with significant subsequent mortality from on-going systemic vasculitis.

In the non-necrotising type, there will be marked localised 'beefy' dilated vasculature.

What if I've diagnosed it?

□ Patients should be referred *soon/urgently.*

What will the hospital do?

□ We will assess the patient's systemic inflammatory status. If there is no underlying diagnosis, blood will be taken for an autoimmune screen and a chest X-ray will be carried out.

Some patients respond to systemic NSAIDs, while others require systemic immunosuppression.

What do I need to do?

□ The presence of scleritis can be a reflection of active systemic disease. If the patient is already known to have a collagen vascular disorder such as rheumatoid arthritis, their disease activity should be reassessed and re-referral to a rheumatologist considered. The patient may require systemic immunosuppression.

What to tell the patient

□ They have severe inflammation of the wall of the eye (sclera) that needs to be calmed with tablets (sometimes strong immunosuppression drugs). The condition of the eye indicates that their systemic disease (if they have one) is active, so that also needs attention.

Problems that may arise, and how to deal with them

□ Severe active scleritis is correlated with increased mortality in the subsequent years from systemic disease activity. The patient's systemic disease control should be carefully monitored and optimised.

Conditions of the orbit

PROPTOSIS

What's going on?

□ One or both eyes is protruding. Usually this is related to increased retro-orbital pressure secondary to inflammation (e.g. thyroid eye disease), infection (e.g. orbital cellulitis), vascular engorgement or blood (e.g. retro-orbital haemorrhage).

If I examine the patient, what will I find?

□ The eye(s) will be bulging forward. The upper and lower lids may be retracted. Usually the lower lid lies at the lower edge of the cornea and the upper lid lies 2 mm below the upper limbus. If sclera is showing above or below the cornea, then there is some degree of lid retraction (figure 23.2).

Looking from the top or up from beneath the chin is often the easiest way to do a rough assessment of proptosis. Lift the upper lids with both hands and look at the protrusion of the eye and cornea, comparing the two sides.

Checking pupil reactions and vision may reveal evidence of optic nerve compromise.

What if I've diagnosed it?

□ These patients require referral to the hospital eye service. The urgency of the referral depends on other clinical features.

If the proptosis is long-standing (take a careful history, ask friends and relatives how long they have noticed the problem, look at old photos) and the vision is uncompromised, then the patient should be referred *soon via letter.*

If the proptosis is acute and the vision is compromised, the patient should be referred *immediately/ urgently.*

What will the hospital do?

□ A computed tomography (CT) scan will be done and appropriate management arranged, according to the underlying pathology. If the optic nerve is compromised, the orbit needs decompressing, either medically or surgically, as a matter of urgency.

What do I need to do?

□ Check thyroid function and other markers of autoimmune disease.

What to tell the patient

□ They have a problem with the structures behind the eye. If the optic nerve becomes too squeezed or stretched, the result can be permanent visual loss. The pressure must be taken off the nerve as soon as possible.

Problems that may arise, and how to deal with them

□ Depending upon the particular pathology, the condition may recur. Often patients are discharged from hospital on oral corticosteroids. If the course of drugs is long term, it is worth considering gastric protection and osteoporosis prophylaxis, particularly in older patients.

Because the eyes are protruding too much, the lids cannot fulfil their normal protective, lubrication function, and the cornea may dry. Early symptoms of dryness may be alleviated by lubricant drops, but if the eye becomes red or painful, it may indicate that the cornea has been compromised (exposure keratopathy).

ORBITAL CELLULITIS

What's going on?

□ This term is often used incorrectly. The orbit consists of the loose connective tissue that surrounds and cushions the globe. It is separated from the tissue lying just behind the upper and lower lids by a fibrous sheet called the orbital septum. Infection within the orbit is called true orbital cellulitis and is sight threatening because of significant proptosis and optic nerve compromise.

If the infection involves only the skin of the lid anterior to the orbital septum, the condition is called preseptal cellulitis.

Preseptal cellulitis is of much less concern than true orbital cellulitis. Differentiating between the two is relatively straightforward, but it is always prudent to err on the side of caution when dealing with this condition.

Both orbital and preseptal cellulitis manifest as erythematous, swollen and cellulitic lids. The lids may be so swollen as to preclude a view of the eye itself. After opening the lids (you may have to prise them apart), if you find that the patient's eye is white, the pupils are reacting normally, ocular movements are full and the vision is unaffected, then the patient has preseptal cellulitis (figure 23.4). If any of the above is impaired or the eye is frankly red, the patient is assumed to have orbital cellulitis (figure 23.3).

Many patients affected by preseptal and orbital cellulitis are children.

Patients with true orbital cellulitis tend to be systemically unwell with pyrexia.

If I examine the patient, what will I find?

□ See above.

What if I've diagnosed it?

□ If the patient has mild preseptal cellulitis, a short trial of oral antibiotics may resolve it.

Always remember that preseptal cellulitis may rapidly progress to orbital cellulitis. If at any stage the eye itself becomes red, the patient should be assumed to have orbital cellulitis and referred *urgently*.

If the lids are so swollen as to preclude an adequate examination of the eye, then the patient should be assumed to have sight-threatening orbital cellulitis and referred *urgently*.

Children can progress rapidly to true sight-threatening orbital cellulitis, so it is wise to use a lower index for referral to a paediatrician, so that a short course of intravenous antibiotics can be considered. In general, children under five years with preseptal cellulitis should be admitted for intravenous antibiotics.

What will the hospital do?

□ Practice varies. The ideal approach is multidisciplinary, with the patient being assessed by paediatricians and the ear, nose and throat and ophthalmology teams. Preseptal cellulitis may be managed by intravenous antibiotics and daily review to pick up early development of orbital cellulitis. In orbital cellulitis, CT imaging should be carried out urgently and further management decided upon this basis. If there is pus in the orbit (usually from sinus extension), then early surgical drainage is required.

What do I need to do?

□ The sinuses are often the source of any bacterial inoculum that enters the orbit. Once the event has resolved it is worth assessing the patient for indolent chronic sinusitis.

What to tell the patient

□ In preseptal cellulitis, the infection is localised to the lid, so the prognosis is good, although there is a significant risk of developing sight-threatening orbital cellulitis. Tell the patient that if their vision deteriorates or the eye itself becomes red, they should re-attend your surgery or hospital eye casualty department immediately.

Problems that may arise, and how to deal with them

□ Chronic sinus disease should be addressed, as it may predispose to further orbital or preseptal infective episodes.

THYROID EYE DISEASE

□ Also: thyroid ophthalmopathy; dysthyroid eye disease; Graves' disease.

What's going on?

□ In autoimmune thyroid disease (Graves' disease), pathological antibodies attack the thyroid tissue, causing an initial overstimulation of thyroid hormone production. These antibodies also cross-react with antigen found on cells within the orbit. This leads to an autoimmune inflammatory reaction involving all the orbital structures.

The accumulation of inflammatory cells and by-products results in significant increase in orbital volume and proptosis. Proptosis due to thyroid eye disease is called exophthalmos.

There are two phases: the initial active phase and the long-standing, quiescent phase. In the active phase, the eye is red and inflamed, with the potential for significant optic nerve-threatening proptosis. Once this phase has settled, the patient is left with the consequences of the severe inflammation and scarring.

Often the globe fails to return to its original position but remains proptosed (see above). The extraocular muscles, which are usually involved in the inflammatory process, become fibrosed and do not function, resulting in a squint with double vision. The upper and lower lids are often retracted as they are forced further apart by the forward displacement of the globe. Scarring and sympathetic hyperstimulation may worsen this lid retraction. The quiescent phase is dominated by oculomotility disturbance, proptosis, lid retraction, corneal drying and poor cosmesis. Often cosmesis is a major concern, particularly as this disease can affect young females.

Thyroid eye disease may occur before, during or even long after the onset of frank thyroid disease.

If I examine the patient, what will I find?

□ If this is the active phase, the eye(s) will be proptosed and red, and the conjunctiva may be ballooned up, creating a jelly-like appearance called chemosis. Also, eye movement may be disturbed and the pupils may react abnormally (RAPD). Visual acuity and colour vision may be reduced in one or both eyes. The lids will be retracted, with scleral show superiorly and inferiorly. The eyes are often described as having a staring appearance (figure 23.2).

What if I've diagnosed it?

□ If you suspect the patient has thyroid eye disease, it is worth doing thyroid function tests and referring to the hospital eye service. The urgency will depend on the severity of symptoms. If the patient's eyes are obviously proptosed then a referral *soon via casualty* is warranted. If the patient's vision is compromised, then *urgent/immediate* referral is warranted for rapid assessment of optic nerve integrity.

What will the hospital do?

□ Once the diagnosis is made, the patient's thyroid function will be assessed and referral made to an endocrinologist, if appropriate.

If the optic nerve is compromised, the patient will require decompression, either medically or surgically. Medical decompression relies on immune-mediation to reduce the inflammatory reaction within the orbit. This is usually done with high-dose, pulsed corticosteroids. Surgical decompression involves breaking up to four of the orbital walls, allowing the orbital contents to prolapse into the sinuses and thus reducing retro-orbital pressure and proptosis.

Even if the optic nerve is not compromised, early intervention with high-dose corticosteroids may reduce the risk of sight-threatening complications and may indeed reduce the residual problems in the quiescent phase.

What do I need to do?

□ Certainly the patient's thyroid status needs to be assessed and thyroid function optimised. Stop the patient smoking (easier said than done!).

What to tell the patient

□ They have a problem affecting their eyes that is often linked to an autoimmune thyroid disorder. Tell them about the active and quiescent phases, and that future problems may occur. Advise smokers strongly to give up, as smokers have a much worse prognosis for final outcome.

Problems that may arise, and how to deal with them

□ Corneal exposure remains a concern, so if the patient has significant proptosis or is symptomatic with a red or irritable eye, they should be given topical artificial teardrops. Watch out for progressive proptosis and visual compromise. Loss or disturbance of colour vision is an early feature of optic nerve compromise and may be assessed with Ishihara test plates.

Patients who have significant cosmetic problems related to their eye disease may warrant surgical rehabilitative intervention.

Ocular oncology (see *Chaper 24*)

SEBACEOUS CELL CARCINOMA

What's going on?

□ This is a nasty but rare form of cancer. It has a bad prognosis because of its late diagnosis. It often manifests as a lump within the lid with surrounding apparent erythema. It is frequently mistaken for a chalazion, and thus any chalazion that recurs in exactly the same place after apparently successful incision and curettage should be viewed with suspicion. The surrounding erythema may actually be pagetoid spread (spread along the skin, similar to that seen in breast cancer) of sebaceous gland carcinoma.

If I examine the patient, what will I find?

□ There may be a lump, and the surrounding skin may be scaly and erythematous.

What if I've diagnosed it?

□ The patient should be referred *urgently by letter* for assessment.

What will the hospital do?

□ A biopsy will be done and a wide excision planned, depending on the extent of the disease. Sometimes an exenteration (removal of all orbital contents) is required.

INTRAOCULAR MALIGNANT MELANOMA/ CHOROIDAL NAEVI

What's going on?

□ Choroidal naevi are not uncommon and may, rarely, develop into malignancy in the form of a choroidal melanoma. Such lesions may metastasise.

If I examine the patient, what will I find?

□ You should be able to see the pigmented lesion in the fundus (figure 24.3).

What if I've diagnosed it?

□ If you have seen a pigmented lesion in the back of the eye, it is worth sending the patient to their optician for assessment. A key feature of the lesion is its elevation from the retina. With a direct ophthalmoscope, it can be difficult to see whether a lesion is markedly elevated or flat. The optometrist will use binocular ophthalmoscopy to assess whether a lesion is raised and suspicious. If a lesion is completely flat and quite small, it may simply be observed with regular yearly assessment by the optometrist. If a lesion is elevated, it is reasonable to refer to hospital for assessment *soon*.

The likelihood of malignancy is increased with the degree of elevation, the size of the lesion, the presence of orange pigment (called lipofuscin) on the surface and the presence of a surrounding retinal detachment.

What will the hospital do?

□ The patient will be clinically assessed and an ultrasound scan (called a B-scan) undertaken to determine elevation and internal reflectivity.

If the lesion is highly suspicious, the patient will be referred to a regional ocular oncology unit.

If the lesion is less suspicious, the patient will be reviewed by the ophthalmology service on a regular (usually yearly) basis.

If the lesion is clinically benign, it should ideally be photographed and the patient discharged. Recommend regular yearly ophthalmoscopy by the optometrist to detect any changes.

What to tell the patient

□ They have a mole at the back of their eye. If it were on their arm they could monitor it for change themselves, but naturally in this case their optometrist will need to check it regularly for them.

METASTASES

What's going on?

□ The choroid is the most vascular tissue in the body and thus is a frequent site of metastases. Often metastases remain clinically silent or the visual loss caused by the mass is overshadowed by the patient's morbidity. If the mass underlies the macula, the vision will be reduced. Sometimes the metastasis causes a retinal detachment, resulting in rapid visual loss. Very rarely, the ocular metastasis may be the presenting feature of an occult systemic malignancy.

If I examine the patient, what will I find?

□ Multiple, elevated, yellowish choroidal lesions are usually scattered throughout the retina.

What if I've diagnosed it?

□ A thorough search must be made for an underlying primary carcinoma.

What will the hospital do?

□ The decision to treat will depend upon the patient's condition. If this is good, the aim should be to maintain vision as long as possible. Radiotherapy may be used to good effect to shrink the lesion and prevent visual loss.

What to tell the patient

□ The visual prognosis tends to be poor as the metastasis will cause progressive vision loss as it grows.

Neuro-ophthalmology (see Chapter 25)

PAPILLOEDEMA

What's going on?

□ Raised intracranial pressure results in compromised axonal flow along both optic nerves. Both discs become swollen. Vision is often normal but the blind spot is increased. Patients may complain of transient visual disturbance often associated with movement, such as on standing up, for example. Prolonged raised intracranial pressure with papilloedema will result in permanent constriction of the visual field.

If I examine the patient, what will I find?

□ The disc margins will be blurred and indistinct. The striations of the engorged retinal nerve fibres will be noticeable, radiating from the optic disc (figure 25.1).

What if I've diagnosed it?

□ Refer to physicians/neurologists *urgently*.

What will the hospital do?

□ Neuro-imaging will be used to determine whether there is a mass lesion in the brain, and a lumbar puncture may be done.

What to tell the patient

□ The nerve at the back of the eye appears swollen. This can be a sign of raised pressure in the head, which needs investigating. There are multiple causes.

Problems that may arise, and how to deal with them

□ Differentiating true optic disc swelling from 'pseudo-swelling' can be difficult – see below.

PSEUDOPAPILLOEDEMA

What's going on?

□ The disc looks swollen but in fact is normal. The phenomenon can be related to buried optic nerve head drusen or to the appearance of the disc in a markedly long-sighted (hypermetropic) eye.

If I examine the patient, what will I find?

□ The disc will look swollen.

What if I've diagnosed it?

□ The patient should be referred to exclude true papilloedema.

What will the hospital do?

□ Sometimes an ultrasound scan will be carried out to look for a highly reflective disc consistent with disc drusen. A fluorescein angiogram can be the only way to tell whether the disc is truly swollen, however. A swollen disc will leak fluorescein.

What do I need to do?

□ Check for any associated neurological features that may contribute to the diagnosis – these will be absent in pseudopapilloedema.

What to tell the patient

□ If pseudopapilloedema is confirmed, the patient can be reassured that the eye is normal. However, if they are having a check-up for the first time with a new optician, they should explain the situation to avoid being wrongly referred to hospital.

OPTIC NEURITIS

What's going on?

□ This is inflammation of the optic nerve. It can be related to a demyelinative process, but can also be idiopathic or related to an inflammatory disease.

If I examine the patient, what will I find?

□ There will be an RAPD. The optic disc will be swollen in one-third of cases. The patient usually has a central scotoma; that is, their central vision is obscured or even lost, but their peripheral vision is usually intact. If you show the patient a red object, it will appear a normal colour when they look at it with their good eye but washed out or darker with their affected eye.

What if I've diagnosed it?

□ The patient should be referred to the hospital for assessment and confirmation of the diagnosis *soon/ urgently via letter*.

What will the hospital do?

□ Visual acuity, visual fields and pupil reactions will be documented.

Neuro-imaging is not usually indicated unless there are suspicious features.

The patient may or may not have other neurological deficits.

What do I need to do?

□ Examine the patient for any other neurological problems. If they do have other such problems, the likelihood of multiple sclerosis (MS) is increased and referral to a neurologist is indicated.

Often the hospital doctor will tell the patient the diagnosis but not explain the exact significance. These patients often (quite reasonably) look up the disease and are understandably concerned at the possibility of MS. They may require counselling (*see* What to tell the patient, below).

What to tell the patient

□ The vision usually gets progressively worse over a period of two weeks and may even go down to hand motion. The hospital should have told the patient to expect this, but the news could still be distressing. After two weeks, the vision tends gradually to improve, with most people recovering their pre-morbid Snellen chart reading vision within six months. They are however often left with some degree of difficulty with their colour vision or depth perception.

MS is indeed a concern, with a significant proportion of patients with optic neuritis (probably up to two-thirds) going on to develop demyelinating disease.

Problems that may arise, and how to deal with them

□ If the patient has another episode of optic neuritis or develops other neurological symptoms, refer to a neurologist for assessment with a provisional diagnosis of MS.

HOMONYMOUS HEMIANOPIA

What's going on?

□ The patient has a significant visual field defect and has lost either the left or right half of their visual field. Often the macula is spared, so the central vision should be completely normal. There must be an occipital or visual tract/radiation problem. A cerebrovascular accident (CVA) in the vertebrobasillar territory will cause a significant homonymous (matching) hemianopia.

If I examine the patient, what will I find?

□ The patient will have a significant visual field defect affecting the same side in both eyes, i.e. right field loss in both eyes (figure 10.3). They may demonstrate visual inattention to one side. Patients often deny they have a problem.

What if I've diagnosed it?

□ These patients have had a stroke and should be managed appropriately with referral to a physician if necessary. Referral to the eye service is not necessary once CVA assessment and modification of risk factors have been done.

What will the hospital do?

□ If this is an acute event, the patient could be referred to a physician for CVA assessment. If the defect is long-standing then little can be done except to advise the patient about the diagnosis and of the need to stop driving, and inform the Driver and Vehicle Licensing Agency (DVLA). Aspirin may be started as a prophylactic measure. The source of any embolus should be identified.

What do I need to do?

□ The patient has had a significant CVA and so management should aim to minimise the risk of further vascular events. Formal anticoagulation may be considered if there are significant risk factors.

What to tell the patient

□ They have had a stroke, and the likelihood of recovery decreases with the passage of time.

They are also at risk of a further CVA.

They should not drive and should inform the DVLA as soon as possible of their visual disability.

Problems that may arise, and how to deal with them

□ Patients may be very concerned about giving up driving.

BITEMPORAL HEMIANOPIA

What's going on?

□ The patient has lost the temporal visual field in both eyes. This is related to compression at the optic chiasm, leading to dysfunction of the fibres that decussate/cross there. The patient probably has a space-occupying lesion resulting in a compressive effect.

If I examine the patient, what will I find?

□ The patient will have a form of tunnel vision. They will have lost their right visual field in the right eye and their left visual field in the left eye (figure 10.7). Their vision may improve if a compressive lesion is excised.

What if I've diagnosed it?

□ The patient should be referred to the hospital eye services or physicians for neuro-imaging to exclude optic chiasm compression *urgently via letter*. It is worth checking prolactin levels urgently.

What will the hospital do?

□ The patient will have neuro-imaging. If a space-occupying lesion is present, they will then be referred to a neurosurgeon for evaluation and further management.

What do I need to do?

□ Assessment of pituitary function is sensible, with referral to an endocrinologist if indicated.

What to tell the patient

□ The patient should be advised not to drive as their visual field is unlikely to be adequate.

RELATIVE AFFERENT PUPILLARY DEFECT (RAPD)

What's going on?

□ The patient has a pupil abnormality, indicative of severe diffuse retinal disease or optic nerve disease. Patients do not get RAPDs with lesions behind the optic chiasm. The key is the underlying cause for the optic nerve or retinal malfunction. Optic nerve lesions may be inflammatory, compressive, infective or traumatic.

If I examine the patient, what will I find?

□ *See* Chapter 11, Pupil reactions.

What if I've diagnosed it?

□ Depending on the suspected cause, the patient should be referred to the hospital eye service.

If you suspect giant cell arteritis and the vision is reduced, the patient should be referred *immediately*. Taking blood for inflammatory indices – (ESR/CRP) – will be valuable, but send the blood samples with the patient, so they can be processed in the hospital and the results made immediately available.

If you suspect an optic neuritis, the patient should be referred *soon*.

What will the hospital do?

□ Try to find the cause of the retinal or optic nerve lesion. If a diffuse retinal disease is responsible, this is usually clinically evident from fundoscopy. Electro-diagnostic tests, which assess the function of the retina and optic nerve, may help find the exact location of the pathology. If a compressive lesion is suspected, then neuro-imaging is required.

What do I need to do?

□ The underlying cause may require an assessment from a systemic point of view.

HOLMES-ADIE PUPIL

What's going on?

□ This is an internal ocular muscle problem. The para-sympathetic supply to the pupilloconstrictor muscle has been interrupted by a presumed viral pathology. The patient's vision may be blurred due to their dilated pupil and poor accommodation.

If I examine the patient, what will I find?

□ Initially, the pupil is dilated but gradually becomes smaller over time. It is usually poorly reactive to light.

What if I've diagnosed it?

□ Refer *routinely* for confirmation of diagnosis.

What will the hospital do?

□ No need for treatment.

HORNER'S SYNDROME

What's going on?

□ There is an interruption in the sympathetic nerve supply to the eye. A lesion may occur anywhere along the route of the sympathetic nerves, i.e. the hypotha-lamus, the cervical spine, the thorax including the upper portion of the lung (Pancoast tumour, *see* Chap-ter 11) and the neck.

If I examine the patient, what will I find?

□ A small pupil (miosis) on the affected side with a small ptosis, anhidrosis (lack of sweating on the side of the face) and apparent enophthalmos because of a lowered upper lid and an elevated lower lid.

What if I've diagnosed it?

□ Refer *soon/urgently via letter*.

What will the hospital do?

□ Search for the cause. Now that imaging is easily accessible, scans of the entire sympathetic tract are recommended.

What do I need to do?

□ A thorough search should be made for a cause. The neck should be palpated and the nasopharynx thor-oughly examined.

What to tell the patient

□ This will depend on the underlying aetiology.

Problems that may arise, and how to deal with them

□ Very rarely, acute onset of unilateral Horner's syndrome may indicate an ipsilateral carotid artery dissection.

ARGYLL ROBERTSON PUPIL

What's going on?

□ The patient has a pupil abnormality classically related to neurosyphilis. The cerebral centres respon-sible for stimulating pupil constriction in response to a bright light and to looking at a near object (accom-modation) are separate. Lesions that block the light reflex may spare the accommodation reflex. Such lesions result in an Argyll Robertson pupil.

If I examine the patient, what will I find?

□ The pupils will not react to light, but when the patient is asked to read the pupils will miose (con-strict). This is called light-near dissociation.

What if I've diagnosed it?

□ Refer *soon via letter*.

What will the hospital do?

□ Screen for luetic disease. Neuro-imaging may be indicated to exclude a space-occupying lesion.

FOURTH NERVE PALSY

What's going on?

□ Most cases of fourth nerve palsy are caused by decompensation of a congenital fourth nerve deficit. These can present quite suddenly, often with no obvious cause, in mid-life and onwards. The fourth nerve can also be compromised by a diabetic or hypertensive mononeuropathy, or a compressive, traumatic, neoplastic or inflammatory process.

If I examine the patient, what will I find?

□ The patient may have a slight vertical squint when looking straight ahead. They may tilt their head slightly to try to line up their eyes. When they look down and towards their nose with the affected eye, the vertical double vision worsens (figure 12.3).

What if I've diagnosed it?

□ If the patient has other neurological problems, they should be referred to a physician for assessment and management.

If it is an isolated palsy, the referral should be to the hospital eye service *urgently via letter/soon via letter*.

What will the hospital do?

□ Undertake an orthoptic assessment to document and quantify the degree of oculomotility disturbance. If the lesion is isolated and there are no other suspicious features, the management may be expectant, with simple observation awaiting either stabilisation (if congenital) or spontaneous resolution. If there is evidence of multiple nerve palsy or other neurological features, then neuro-imaging will be done.

The patient may be given an occluding patch for their spectacles to prevent the troublesome double vision. Alternatively, a prism may be fitted to redirect the incoming light to match the position of their deviating eye. This stops the double vision while still allowing sight out of both eyes.

If the defect is long-standing and there is no sign of resolution, extraocular muscle surgery may be done.

What do I need to do?

□ The patient should have a neurological examination to elicit any other neurological abnormality. Progressive or changing neuropathies are a concern as they are not a feature of 'benign' mononeuropathies.

What to tell the patient

□ Most of these cases are related to a decompensated congenital weakness of the fourth nerve. Once settled, the double vision can be corrected with prisms, although occasionally surgery may be necessary.

If the patient is hypertensive or diabetic and the lesion is isolated, the patient can be told that the prognosis is good for complete recovery within about six months. If the lesion is the result of a compressive or traumatic problem, the prognosis is less certain.

Some people have congenital palsies and adapt to them by subconsciously altering the position of their head. A congenital or long-standing palsy should be left alone.

Problems that may arise, and how to deal with them

□ If the palsy worsens or other neurological problems manifest, the patient should be re-referred to the hospital eye service for possible neuro-imaging.

SIXTH NERVE PALSY

What's going on?

□ The sixth nerve is compromised by a diabetic or hypertensive mononeuropathy, or a compressive, traumatic, neoplastic or inflammatory process.

If I examine the patient, what will I find?

□ The patient may have a slight horizontal convergent squint (esotropia) when looking straight ahead. They may turn their head slightly away from the side of the lesion to try to line up their eyes. When they look towards the side of the lesion with the affected eye, the horizontal double vision worsens (figure 12.4).

What if I've diagnosed it?

□ If the patient has other neurological problems, refer to a physician for assessment and management.

If it is an isolated palsy, the referral should be to the hospital eye service *urgently via letter/soon via letter*.

What will the hospital do?

□ Undertake an orthoptic assessment to document and quantify the degree of oculomotility disturbance. If the lesion is isolated and there are no other suspicious features, the management may be expectant, with simple observation awaiting spontaneous resolution. If there is evidence of multiple nerve palsies or other neurological features, then neuro-imaging is indicated.

The patient may be given an occluding patch for their spectacles to stop the troublesome double vision. Alternatively, a prism may be fitted to redirect the incoming light to match the position of their deviating eye and prevent the double vision, while still allowing sight out of both eyes.

If the defect is long-standing and there is no sign of resolution, the lateral rectus muscle might be tightened by surgery (lateral rectus resection).

What do I need to do?

□ The patient should have a neurological examination to find any other neurological abnormality. Progressive or changing neuropathies are a concern, as they are not a feature of 'benign' mononeuropathies.

What to tell the patient

□ If the patient is hypertensive or diabetic and the lesion is isolated, the patient can be told that the prognosis is good for complete recovery within about six months. If the lesion is the result of a compressive or traumatic problem, the prognosis is less certain.

Problems that may arise, and how to deal with them

□ If the palsy worsens or other neurological problems develop, the patient should be re-referred to the hospital eye service for possible neuro-imaging.

THIRD NERVE PALSY

What's going on?

□ The third nerve is compromised by a diabetic or hypertensive mononeuropathy, or a compressive, traumatic, neoplastic or inflammatory process.

The neurones carrying the parasympathetic supply responsible for pupil constriction are carried around the outside of the third nerve. If these pupil fibres are compromised along with the rest of the third nerve fibres, resulting in a dilated pupil and third nerve palsy ('pupil-involving third'), then it must be assumed that a compressive lesion is the cause. A potentially life-threatening cerebral vascular aneurysm must be assumed until proven otherwise. Such patients need urgent imaging.

If the pupil is normal, the most likely cause is a microvascular event, which has compromised the vasa nervorum of the nerve, knocking off the oculomotor neurones. This spares the outer pupillomotor fibres that receive their blood supply from the pial plexus and thus the pupil is normally reactive.

If I examine the patient, what will I find?

□ The patient will have a ptosis (figures 12.5a–c). If you lift the lid the eye will be down and out. All ocular movement will be restricted except for sixth nerve mediated abduction (fourth nerve function will be difficult to assess without proper tests). The pupil may be reactive or dilated (pupil sparing or pupil involving, respectively).

What if I've diagnosed it?

□ If the pupil is involved the patient should be referred as *immediate*, particularly if pain is present.

If the pupil is spared, i.e. the pupil is still reacting normally despite all the other features of the third nerve palsy being present, the patient should be referred *urgently*. Although in these cases an aneurysm is less likely, it cannot be discounted, especially in patients under 50. The presence of pain is worrying. Neuro-imaging should be considered for all patients with a third nerve palsy.

What will the hospital do?

□ An orthoptic assessment will be undertaken to confirm the diagnosis and assess whether the third nerve palsy is indeed in isolation, or if the fourth and sixth cranial nerves are also involved. If the other oculomotor cranial nerves are involved, neuro-imaging to assess the orbital apex and cavernous sinus should be arranged urgently.

Usually prisms cannot correct the excessive degree of ocular position disturbance, so a patch is placed over the eye or an occlusive attached to the spectacle lens to prevent diplopia.

If the patient is pain free and the pupil is spared, management can be expectant, in the hope of recovery. Inflammatory indices may be measured in the older age group to exclude symptomatically silent giant cell arteritis (GCA).

If the pupil is involved, neuro-imaging is done as a matter of urgency, and management is based on the findings.

What do I need to do?

□ The patient should have a neurological examination to elicit any other neurological abnormality. Progressive or changing neuropathies are a concern as this is not a feature of 'benign' mononeuropathies. If a patient with a previously pupil-sparing third nerve palsy develops a dilated pupil, they should be referred *immediately*.

What to tell the patient

□ In the absence of a compressive or inflammatory lesion, the prognosis is quite good, with most people recovering within six months. If it is related to a compressive lesion, then the prognosis is more uncertain and depends on the amount of damage caused.

OPTIC ATROPHY

What's going on?

□ The optic nerve has been damaged to some degree, because of pathology such as a compressive or inflammatory condition. The optic disc appears extremely pale due to loss of nerve fibres and the consequent show-through of the underlying white sclera. The degree of visual loss depends upon the underlying problem.

If I examine the patient, what will I find?

□ The disc will be pale (white).

What if I've diagnosed it?

□ If you have noticed a pale disc and the pupil reactions are normal with no RAPD, it is worth referring the patient to their optician for a definitive check. If the vision is reduced and the history of visual loss short and progressive, then there may be a space-occupying lesion compressing the nerve. Such patients should be referred *soon via letter*.

Compare the right and left discs: if they are symmetrical in colour they are unlikely to be pathological.

What will the hospital do?

□ The patient's visual field will be assessed. If there is the suspicion of an infiltrative or compressive lesion, neuro-imaging will be done. The patient's vitamin B12 and folate levels may be checked.

What to tell the patient

□ Their optic nerve is damaged and there is little likelihood of recovery. The aim is now to stop it from getting worse.

ANTERIOR ISCHAEMIC OPTIC NEUROPATHY

What's going on?

□ The blood supply to the optic nerve has been compromised, resulting in loss of vision. The cause is either a microinfarct (non-arteritic anterior ischaemic optic neuropathy (NAION), or an inflammatory process, usually secondary to GCA (arteritic anterior ischaemic neuropathy). The patient may lose their whole field of vision or develop a pattern of visual loss, such as an altitudinal defect when only the upper or lower portion of the visual field is lost.

If I examine the patient, what will I find?

□ The vision will be reduced. They may have an upper or lower altitudinal visual field defect. The disc will be swollen. There will be a relative afferent pupillary defect (RAPD).

What if I've diagnosed it?

□ GCA needs excluding. Refer *urgently*.

What will the hospital do?

□ If there is a suspicion of GCA, the patient will undergo a temporal artery biopsy to exclude or confirm the diagnosis. Inflammatory indices will be assessed. If it is a non-arteritic process, there is no possible intervention and a conservative approach is taken in the hope of spontaneous recovery.

What do I need to do?

□ If the process is arteritic, the patient will be on long-term steroids. Consider osteoporosis prophylaxis and gastric protection.

If the process is non-arteritic, then assessment of cardiovascular and cerebrovascular risk factors is prudent. Consider antiplatelet treatment as a prophylactic measure if not contraindicated.

What to tell the patient

□ The prognosis is much better for the non-arteritic process. Visual recovery is extremely unlikely in the arteritic process.

Problems that may arise, and how to deal with them

□ Despite steroid treatment, the vision may deteriorate further due to the on-going inflammatory process. If vision deteriorates or the patient has a recurrence of GCA symptoms, their inflammatory indices should be measured urgently and the steroid dose increased.

Vascular diseases (see Chapter 26)

AMAUROSIS FUGAX

What's going on?

□ This is transient ischaemic attack (TIA) of the retinal circulation. An embolus has lodged in the central retinal circulation and caused ischaemia of the retina. The embolus either dislodges or is lysed, and blood flow is restored. Classically, patients describe the sudden, painless onset of complete visual loss in one eye. Often they describe a black or grey curtain falling or rising over their vision.

If I examine the patient, what will I find?

□ By definition after the resolution of the episode there should be no residual visual defect. There may be a carotid bruit on auscultation (although some clinicians believe this is a completely worthless sign) or the patient may have atrial fibrillation.

What if I've diagnosed it?

□ If the diagnosis is clear-cut and the vision is completely restored with no evidence of any visual field defect, then referral to the eye service is not required.

If the diagnosis is in doubt the patient should be referred soon via letter.

If there are multiple episodes, the possibility of GCA should be considered and an ESR/CRP obtained, even in the absence of GCA symptoms. If GCA symptoms are present, urgent assessment of inflammatory indices and urgent referral if the results are positive is required (see Is this giant cell arteritis (GCA)? Chapter 1).

Any predisposing factors should be addressed as described above.

If you have access to a TIA fast-track clinic, then refer according to local criteria.

What will the hospital do?

□ Carotid Dopplers and/or a cardiac echo will be organised. If carotid Dopplers indicate a significant stenosis, referral may be made directly to a vascular surgeon. Inflammatory indices should be checked in case the patient has occult asymptomatic GCA.

What do I need to do?

□ These patients are at risk of further embolic phenomena, which could result in a permanent occlusion (central retinal artery occlusion) or even a CVA. Cardiovascular risk factors should be addressed and carotid Dopplers or cardiac echo should be arranged to ensure there is no carotid or cardiac source of embolus. Antiplatelet medication should be considered as a prophylactic measure.

What to tell the patient

□ They have had a mini-stroke and are at risk of further ocular or cerebral embolic events.

HYPERTENSIVE RETINOPATHY

What's going on?

□ The normal response to raised blood pressure is vasoconstriction of the retinal vasculature. This vasoconstriction tends to manifest fully only in younger patients, however, as their vessels still have some elasticity. Older patients have pre-existing arteriolosclerosis, and therefore do not have this autoregulatory response. Sustained hypertension leads to rupture of blood vessels and breakdown of the blood-retinal barrier. Retinal haemorrhages, exudates and oedema occur, all of which results in blurred vision. In severe cases, the optic disc becomes swollen.

If I examine the patient, what will I find?

□ Marked thinning of the retinal arteries, 'cotton-wool' spots, exudates and arteriovenous nipping. If this is severe the disc will be swollen (malignant/accelerated hypertension).

What if I've diagnosed it?

□ Manage blood pressure appropriately.

What will the hospital do?

□ Once the diagnosis is made, the patient will be referred to a physician for management of their hypertension.

What do I need to do?

□ Check renal function and monitor the blood pressure carefully. A swollen disc indicates severe hypertension and the risk of significant end organ compromise. Treat as appropriate.

What to tell the patient

□ Any visual loss may be reversible to some degree once their blood pressure is controlled and the retinal changes subside.

CENTRAL RETINAL VEIN OCCLUSION

What's going on?

□ The central retinal vein has become occluded, resulting in back pressure and rupture of the veins throughout the retina. Arterial blood cannot enter the eye, the retina becomes ischaemic and part of it dies. The degree of ischaemia usually correlates well with the degree of visual loss. If the halt to blood flow is temporary, the vision may be fairly well preserved. With time the venous outflow returns, but the retinal ischaemia may persist. If the ischaemia is severe, the macula will be oedematous and neovascularisation may occur in the iris in response to release of vasoproliferative mediators. The new vessels on the iris may clog the drainage angle of the eye and cause rubeotic glaucoma. This can happen very quickly, typically within the first three months after the vein occlusion.

If I examine the patient, what will I find?

□ There will be extensive haemorrhages throughout the retina. The disc may be swollen and there may be an RAPD. Vision will be reduced (figure 26.2).

What if I've diagnosed it?

□ Refer *soon*.

What will the hospital do?

□ The patient will be monitored for glaucoma and for resolution of the retinal haemorrhages and oedema. If new vessels develop, the patient will have aggressive argon laser pan-retinal photocoagulation to remove the dead retina cells and stop the ischaemic process.

What do I need to do?

□ Check blood pressure. Consider aspirin as a prophylactic measure.

What to tell the patient

□ They have sustained severe damage to the eye. The visual prognosis is variable and the best indicator of final vision is the vision immediately after the event. Intuitively, if they have very poor vision immediately after the vein occlusion they will probably not do well.

Problems that may arise, and how to deal with them

□ If the eye becomes red and painful, the patient may have developed rubeotic glaucoma. Feel the eye – if it is rock-solid, the patient probably has markedly raised pressure and should be seen by the ophthalmologist *soon*.

BRANCH RETINAL VEIN OCCLUSION

What's going on?

□ One of the branch veins within the eye has become occluded. This usually happens at a point where a retinal arteriole and retinal vein cross each other, as they share a sheath and pressure from the adjacent artery blocks venous flow. Back pressure causes rupture of the veins in that part of the retina. Usually a whole quadrant of the retina is involved and the vision in that field is reduced. If the blockage is close to the macula, the central vision will be impaired and visual acuity will drop. If the blockage involves the nasal retina, it may be completely clinically silent and the patient will not know that anything has occurred. Sometimes a single vein in the macula is affected, resulting in visual loss in that area and also problems in the surrounding area with exudates and oedema.

If I examine the patient, what will I find?

□ There will be retinal haemorrhages localised to one quadrant of the retina. There may also be some exudates around the damaged area (figure 26.3).

What if I've diagnosed it?

□ Refer *soon via letter.*

What will the hospital do?

□ A fluorescein angiogram is sometimes done to assess the degree of ischaemia and damage. If the vision remains poor (worse than 6/12) at three months after the initial visual loss, the patient may be offered argon laser treatment to try to dry the leakage affecting the macula and thereby improve the vision.

What do I need to do?

□ Check for evidence of hypertension and treat as appropriate. Ensure the patient does not have some hypercoagulable condition.

Problems that may arise, and how to deal with them

□ These patients may develop rubeotic glaucoma, although this is less likely than in those with central retinal vein occlusion.

CENTRAL RETINAL ARTERY OCCLUSION (CRAO)

What's going on?

□ The central retinal artery has been blocked by an embolus or some compressive/inflammatory process. The retina dies within approximately 90 minutes, with concomitant severe visual loss.

If I examine the patient, what will I find?

□ The patient will have severe visual loss and an RAPD. On fundoscopy, a pale white fundus with marked arteriolar attenuation and a cherry-red spot will be visible (figure 26.4). An embolus may also be seen within the retinal vessels (figure 26.5).

What if I've diagnosed it?

□ If the history is short (i.e. less than 24 hours), the patient should be referred *immediately* to the hospital eye services and assessed as soon as possible (*immediately*). If the history is more than 24 hours, the patient should be referred but assessment is less urgent (*soon*). If the duration of visual loss is more than a few days soon referral by letter is acceptable (*soon via letter*).

This can be a manifestation of GCA – if any features suggest this, the patient needs *urgent* referral.

What will the hospital do?

□ In acute cases, management will depend on the duration of the visual loss. If this is more than 24 hours, little is likely to be done as the prognosis is poor. If the history is less than 24 hours, attempts may be made to dislodge any embolus by dramatic reduction of the pressure inside the eye. This will be done medically or by needle aspiration of aqueous from the anterior chamber. In chronic cases the patient can develop rubeosis iridis (p. 35), but this is rare.

GCA must be excluded unless there is an embolus obviously visible within the retinal vasculature. Patients over 50 years of age will have inflammatory indices measured.

What do I need to do?

□ Look for any source of embolus.
 Is the patient in atrial fibrillation (AF?)
 Is there a cardiac or carotid murmur?
 Antiplatelet therapy is a sensible precaution against further embolic phenomena if there are no contra-indications.
 If there is a definite cardiac arrhythmia or valvular defect, then formal anticoagulation with warfarin may be indicated.
 General cardiovascular risk factors should be addressed.

What do I tell the patient?

□ If there has been no recovery within 24–48 hours, the news is bad. The visual prognosis is poor and the likelihood of improvement is slim.

Problems that may arise, and how to deal with them

□ Other eye involvement is a great worry. As the patient has only one eye now, any problem with this good eye must be dealt with quickly.

There is also the possibility of new vessel formation and rubeotic glaucoma as a result of the ischaemia, although this is less common than with venous occlusive disease.

BRANCH RETINAL ARTERY OCCLUSION

What's going on?

□ The aetiology is similar to CRAO (above) but in this situation the embolus was small enough to impact further into the retina, away from the disc. It may affect half the retina or only one quadrant of the retina. That part of the retina will die and there will be corresponding visual loss in that sector of the visual field. If the embolus impacts proximally enough to affect the macula then some central vision will be lost. Rarely, only the cilioretinal artery (an artery running straight from the optic disc to the macula) is affected, knocking off a small section of the macula. If the fovea is involved, visual acuity will be markedly reduced.

If I examine the patient, what will I find?

□ You may be able to see the glistening cholesterol or greyish fibrinoplatelet embolus in one of the branches of the retinal artery. The area of retina radiating distal to this blockage will be whitish and oedematous in the early stages (figure 26.6).

What if I've diagnosed it?

□ As for CRAO (see above).

What will the hospital do?

□ Attempts may be made to move the embolus further downstream by reducing the intraocular pressure, as in CRAO management.

What do I need to do?

□ As for CRAO.

What to tell the patient

□ The chances of recovering vision depend upon exactly where the embolus has impacted and how much damage it has done to the retina. They are at risk of further problems with emboli and thus their cardiovascular risk factors need to be addressed.

Problems that may arise, and how to deal with them

□ The patient is at risk of formal stroke and so should be managed appropriately.

RETINAL MACROANEURYSM

What's going on?

□ There is an aneurysm of the retinal arteries usually related to systemic hypertension. The aneurysm walls stretch and leak to different degrees. Sometimes the leakage is minimal, but often the amount of retinal oedema and exudation related to the aneurysm results in reduced vision.

Spontaneous haemorrhage is a concern and can result in significant visual loss.

If I examine the patient, what will I find?

□ If you follow the blood vessels leading away from the optic disc you will see the dilated portion of artery, usually before the third branch of the vessel. Around this area, you may see the yellowish lipid deposit in the surrounding retina.

What if I've diagnosed it?

□ If vision is reduced, the patient should be referred *urgently via letter*. If the vision is unaffected, the patient should be referred *soon via letter*.

What will the hospital do?

□ These cases are difficult. If the leakage is marked and vision is poor, argon laser may be applied in order to reduce the leakage and try to close off the aneurysm. There is always a risk that the laser treatment itself may cause a haemorrhage.

What do I need to do?

□ Hypertension is the major predisposing factor for this disorder. Blood pressure should be measured and controlled.

What to tell the patient

□ They have an area of weakness caused by their high blood pressure resulting in a 'blow-out' of one of the retinal arteries. This may leak or rupture, causing reduced vision. Treatment itself may make things worse.

Problems that may arise, and how to deal with them

□ Sudden profound visual loss may indicate a spontaneous haemorrhage.

CAROTID-CAVERNOUS FISTULA

What's going on?

□ There is an abnormal communication between the carotid artery and the cavernous sinus. High-pressure, high-flow blood enters the sinus and causes marked dilatation. The venous vasculature of the orbit cannot drain effectively and the orbit becomes engorged. The eye becomes red and proptosed. The oculomotor nerves run through or close to the cavernous sinus, and thus a third, fourth or sixth nerve palsy is common. Vision may be compromised, and patients usually have pain.

This condition is often related to trauma but can occur sporadically in the elderly. The high-flow type is worse as there is a direct communication between the artery and the venous circulation. In the low-flow type, the connection is via the dural plexus, and the features and subsequent risks are less marked.

If I examine the patient, what will I find?

□ One or both eyes will be red and proptosed. If you look closely with a magnifying glass or ophthalmoscope, you will see that all of the conjunctival vessels are markedly dilated.

What if I've diagnosed it?

□ Such patients should be referred *immediately/urgently* to hospital.

What will the hospital do?

□ Neuro-imaging is carried out and the patient will often be referred to a neurosurgeon. An interventional radiologist may be able to occlude the aneurysm with an intravascular balloon or coil. This procedure carries significant risks of CVA.

Problems that may arise, and how to deal with them

□ Beware drying of the cornea due to proptosis.

Miscellaneous conditions

MYOPIA

What's going on?

□ Short sight in itself is not pathological. Light is focused too far in front of the retina, either because of the excessive focusing power of the front of the eye or because the eye is too long. The latter condition is pathological because the sclera is abnormally stretchy and degenerative. These eyes are highly prone to retinal detachments and may develop numerous areas of chorioretinal atrophy.

If I examine the patient, what will I find?

□ You may see patches of atrophy in the retina or a large area of circumferential atrophy surrounding the optic disc (peripapillary atrophy) (figure 27.1).

What if I've diagnosed it?

□ Myopia in itself is not a problem. The patient's spectacle prescription will give you an idea of how bad their myopia is. More than around –5 is quite myopic. Alternatively, look at their spectacles – if the lenses are thick, the patient is quite short-sighted. Remember that if the spectacles magnify, they are for long-sighted people.

What will the hospital do?

□ If the patient is referred to hospital, they will probably have either a retinal tear or a myopic maculopathy.

What to tell the patient

□ The major risk is retinal detachment and patients should be warned about the symptoms. Some patients develop a maculopathy where their central vision is progressively and irreversibly reduced.

Problems that may arise, and how to deal with them

□ If the patient develops flashes and floaters they should attend their optician or the hospital eye service as a matter of urgency as these are symptoms of a potential retinal detachment.

Patients may ask you about laser refractive surgery. This is an evolving field, and not suitable for everyone. Generally, the outcome is less predictable for higher refractive errors, and there are risks. These can be discussed at a laser refractive centre, and there is much information on the internet.

RETINITIS PIGMENTOSA

What's going on?

□ This is a dystrophy of the retina. The rods responsible for peripheral and night vision gradually deteriorate. Night vision is impaired and the patient's visual fields gradually constrict. This is a hereditary condition, inherited either recessively or dominantly. It may also be sporadic.

The retinal pigment epithelium reacts to the dysfunctional rods by releasing pigment clumps that give the retina its 'bone spiculed' appearance (resembling the spicules seen on light microscopy of the bone). The blood vessels become attenuated and the disc is pale.

If I examine the patient, what will I find?

□ Reduced field of vision. Bone-spicule pigmentation in the peripheral retina, sparing the macula, as well as a pale disc and attenuation of the blood vessels.

Progression is variable, but if the patient has a severe condition the vision can deteriorate rapidly.

What if I've diagnosed it?

□ Refer *routinely*.

What will the hospital do?

□ Diagnosis may be made by testing the electrical impulses generated by the retina. The patient is counselled and usually informed of the likely prognosis.

What to tell the patient

□ This condition is unfortunately progressive, but the degree of vision lost and the speed at which it happens varies between patients. Generally, the younger the age at which the patient notices symptoms, the more severe the vision loss will be. There are support groups for people with retinitis pigmentosa throughout the country.

Problems that may arise, and how to deal with them

□ These patients are also at risk of developing cataract

and open-angle glaucoma, for which they may need referral if they are not still under follow up.

VITREOUS HAEMORRHAGE

What's going on?

□ Blood has been released into the vitreous cavity resulting in a reduction in vision. This reduction may be minimal, in the form of black, stringy floaters, or complete, where vision is suddenly reduced to hand motion or perception of light.

If I examine the patient, what will I find?

□ The anterior segment will be normal and there will be no RAPD. When you dilate the pupil, you will not be able to see the fundus at all. Try fundoscopy in the other eye. If you can see the retina in the normal eye then your technique is sound and there is something blocking your view, i.e. a vitreous haemorrhage.

What if I've diagnosed it?

□ These patients should be referred with an urgency dependent upon the most likely underlying aetiology.

If the patient is myopic, then they may have had a retinal detachment or retinal tear that has resulted in a torn retinal blood vessel. Such patients require *urgent* referral.

If the patient is already known to have diabetic retinopathy then the most likely diagnosis is vitreous haemorrhage, secondary to proliferative disease. This is by no means certain, however, as diabetics may lose vision for many different reasons, including a retinal detachment. If the diagnosis is virtually certain – for example, the patient has had multiple previous episodes and has sustained a further attack of painless visual loss – then there is less urgency about the referral. Such patients may be managed conservatively and attend their routine outpatient follow up appointment if this is within the next few weeks. By that time, some of the blood may have settled enough to allow laser treatment.

If the patient is a known diabetic but is not under follow up at the hospital, they should be referred *urgently*.

What will the hospital do?

□ It is important for the hospital to ensure that there is

no retinal detachment by ultrasound scanning of the globe.

Once this has been ascertained, the further management depends upon the cause. The most likely cause is rupture of some of the new vessels associated with diabetic proliferative retinopathy. If the patient has had previous pan-retinal argon laser treatment, the decision might be to wait for the haemorrhage to resolve. Alternatively, early surgery may be indicated, namely a vitrectromy to remove the blood, thereby restoring vision and allowing laser treatment to be given.

Laser treatment requires the retina to be visible, and thus some resolution of the haemorrhage.

What do I need to do?

□ If the patient has diabetic retinopathy then they have probably developed proliferative disease with neovascularisation of the retina. Their diabetic control needs addressing and optimising.

What to tell the patient

□ They have had a bleed that is related to the abnormal retinal blood vessels caused by their diabetes. They need further laser treatment to remove the remaining ischaemic retina. If the vision does not improve, they may need an operation to clear out the blood.

Problems that may arise, and how to deal with them

□ Further haemorrhage is a concern.

CHOROIDAL MELANOCYTIC LESIONS

□ Also: choroidal naevus; indeterminate melanocytic lesion; benign choroidal naevus; suspicious choroidal naevus.

What's going on?

□ The retinal pigment epithelium that lies underneath the retina is composed of pigmented cells. Excessive melanin in these cells will result in a localised naevus. Most naevi are completely benign, but some have malignant potential.

If I examine the patient, what will I find?

□ A pigmented lesion of variable size within the retinal pigment epithelial layer beneath the retina (figure 24.3).

What if I've diagnosed it?

□ Refer *routinely*.

What will the hospital do?

□ The lesion will be assessed, photographed and probably scanned by ultrasound. Elevated lesions are a concern, as are orange pigment (lipofuscin) on the surface of the lesion or the presence of a retinal detachment around the pigmented area. The presence of drusen on the surface is an indication that the lesion is probably benign.

If the lesion is completely flat, the patient will probably be discharged. If the lesion is elevated and suspicious, the patient may be followed up on a six-monthly or yearly basis.

If there is a real concern that the pigmented lesion is a malignant melanoma, the patient will be referred to an ocular oncology centre.

A diagnosis of an indeterminate melanocytic lesion means that after assessment the exact nature of the lesion is still uncertain.

What to tell the patient

□ They have the ocular equivalent of a mole on their skin, which is unlikely to grow or become malignant but is worth keeping under observation, either by their optician or the hospital eye service.

RETINAL DETACHMENT

What's going on?

□ There is retinal tear, allowing fluid from the vitreous cavity to flow under the retina and peel it off. The vision goes down in this area and, if the detachment progresses to lift off the macula, the central vision and thus visual acuity is markedly reduced. The retina needs to be stuck back down.

If I examine the patient, what will I find?

□ You may be able to see the raised, 'ruffled' appearance of the retina (figure 27.5).

What if I've diagnosed it?

□ If you are confident you can see a retinal detachment, refer *urgently*.

If the patient is suffering from flashes and/or floaters refer them to their optician for assessment. If the patient has risk factors for retinal detachment such as a previous retinal detachment or tear, high myopia or has had previous cataract surgery they should be referred to the hospital *soon*.

What will the hospital do?

□ Treatment will involve either an internal repair by means of a vitrectomy with cryotherapy to seal the break in the retina or an external approach with a scleral buckling (indentation) procedure.

What to tell the patient

□ Visual prognosis is better if the macula remains attached. If the macula has been detached for a considerable period of time, the chance for visual recovery is minimal.

Problems that may arise, and how to deal with them

□ Such patients are at risk of a further detachment in the operated eye and in the other eye. Vigilance for symptoms of retinal detachment should be advised.

Paediatric ophthalmology

AMBLYOPIA

What's going on?

□ This is what is known as a 'lazy eye'. The brain relies on visual input in the first five years of life to lay down the visual pathways for normal vision. If the brain is deprived of normal focused vision in one or both eyes in early life, it ignores that eye and vision does not develop to its full potential. This is irreversible after approximately five to eight years of age (depending on type), but if the problem is alleviated, vision may be restored to its full potential.

Many adults have a long-standing lazy eye, in which vision may vary from 6/9 to counting fingers.

If I examine the patient, what will I find?

□ By definition the findings will be normal. However, the patient may have a squint.

What if I've diagnosed it?

□ Amblyopia is a diagnosis of exclusion. Adults with unexplained visual loss from childhood with no evidence of any pathology will have amblyopia. If the patient is not certain that the vision has been poor from childhood or they feel that there has been a further deterioration in vision, they should be assessed by the ophthalmology service *routinely*. When there is a concern about a child's vision in one or both eyes they should be referred *soon via letter* for formal assessment and potential treatment.

What will the hospital do?

□ Organic pathology will be excluded and a full orthoptic assessment carried out to look for a squint. In children, spectacles may be prescribed, and occlusion (patching) treatment may be started on a full- or part-time basis to encourage use of the lazy eye. Subsequently, squint surgery may be considered.

What do I need to do?

□ If the child is prescribed spectacles or patching, it is vital that the parents are advised about the importance of compliance. Saying that it is difficult to make an uncooperative child wear spectacles or a patch is an understatement!

Problems that may arise, and how to deal with them

□ Patching treatment can be difficult because children don't like it, and lack of compliance can hamper progress. It is important to emphasise the window of opportunity in childhood to restore vision, and the need for regular follow up.

RETINOPATHY OF PREMATURITY (ROP)

What's going on?

□ The neonatal eye is not fully developed. Normally, the retina grows out, sweeping over the retinal pigment epithelium (RPE) from the optic disc to the periphery. This growth is stimulated by ischaemia of the bare patches of RPE. If the baby is premature and is given high concentrations of supplementary oxygen the RPE cells are not ischaemic and thus fail to stimulate the retina to grow. When the supplementary oxygen is removed, the RPE cells are suddenly rendered profoundly hypoxic. In attempting to 'catch up', they overstimulate retinal growth, causing new vessels to grow and fibrovascular membranes to form. This condition is called retinopathy of prematurity (ROP) and, if untreated, can be blinding.

If I examine the patient, what will I find?

□ The view may be hazy, the disc hyperaemic and the blood vessels tortuous and dilated. In the periphery will be a patch of pale retina with no blood vessels on the surface (although this is very peripheral and you are unlikely to see it).

What will the hospital do?

□ Babies who are under 32 weeks' gestation or weigh less than 1500 g at birth are screened for the presence of ROP. Different centres use different criteria for screening.

The ischaemic area of retinal pigment epithelium is usually killed off by laser therapy under general anaesthesia.

What to tell the patient

□ If treated early enough, the prognosis for long-term normal vision is generally good, although less so for very premature babies.

Problems that may arise, and how to deal with them

□ Premature babies are at increased risk of other ocular problems, including refractive error (usually myopia) and squint. If you notice these, then referral *routine via letter* is appropriate.

Trauma

TRAUMATIC MYDRIASIS

What's going on?

□ A blunt injury to the eye has ruptured the pupil sphincter muscle. The pupil will not be able to react properly to light and will remain larger than that of the other eye at all levels of illumination (anisocoria). It will, however, still react briskly to light but will not be able to constrict as much as the normal eye. Vision may be slightly down.

If I examine the patient, what will I find?

□ One pupil will be larger than the other, but there will be no RAPD detected on swinging flashlight testing. If you look very closely using the ophthalmoscope as a magnifying glass, you may see some irregularity of the pupil margin related to the position of the rupture.

What if I've diagnosed it?

□ If there are no other features, such as hyphaema or ocular pain, and vision is good, the patient should be referred to the hospital eye service *soon via letter*.

What will the hospital do?

□ A thorough assessment will be done of the front and back of the eye to ensure no other damage has occurred.

What do I need to do?

□ The patient should be told to minimise the risk of further injury. If the injury was sports-related, the patient should be advised about protective measures such as wearing goggles.

What to tell the patient

□ They have had a permanent injury that will not resolve. They may suffer from photophobia and glare caused by too much light entering their eye through their dilated pupil.

CHEMICAL INJURY

What's going on?

□ Strong acids or alkalis can cause severe damage to the eye. Alkalis are much worse than acid at causing corneal burns. The patient may lose all of their corneal epithelium but, more worryingly, may also lose the progenitor cells at the limbus that supplies the epithelial cells and allow healing. The degree of limbal cell loss tends to dictate how much damage has been done. Without an epithelium, the cornea will scar and opacify. The intraocular pressure may go up and the eye may become inflamed.

Household cleaners and chemicals are unlikely to cause significant injury, unlike oven and drain cleaners. Industrial acids and alkalis are potentially very dangerous. Wet plaster or cement can enter the eye and be sequestered into the fornices, continually bathing the eye in damaging alkali.

If I examine the patient, what will I find?

□ The eye will be red. The cornea may be cloudy. The normal fine vessels that run up to the periphery of the cornea may be missing, due to the limbal burn.

What if I've diagnosed it?

□ WASH OUT THE EYE WITH WHATEVER IS AVAILABLE. Ideally, use sterile water but in significant injuries use tap water. Get rid of any solid particulate, as this will continue to dissolve in the tears, bathing the eye in alkali and causing progressive damage. Do not refer until the eye has been bathed continually for at least fifteen minutes. Then refer *immediately* if there is a significant acid or alkali injury.

What will the hospital do?

□ Irrigate immediately and then treat as appropriate.

Problems that may arise, and how to deal with them

□ Following a severe chemical burn, the patient is at risk of ocular surface problems, dry eye, cataract and glaucoma. They are likely to have regular follow up at the eye clinic.

HYPHAEMA

What's going on?

□ This is the result of rupture of a blood vessel on the iris caused by trauma, which then bleeds into the anterior chamber. Usually the vision goes blurry immediately but gradually improves as the blood settles to the bottom of the anterior chamber, forming the hyphaema. The blood cells may occlude the trabecular meshwork, causing the pressure to go up. Bed rest is required to prevent the worrying complication of secondary bleeding. Once the initial clot falls off, at approximately three to five days, there is a danger of further bleeding. This is usually much more severe than the original bleed and can lead to sight-threatening raised intraocular pressure and blood staining of the cornea.

If I examine the patient, what will I find?

□ There will be blood in the bottom of the anterior chamber (figure 29.1). The degree of blood will be variable and may even fill the whole anterior chamber, giving the eye a black appearance – this is called an 'eight ball hyphaema'.

What if I've diagnosed it?

□ Refer *urgently*.

What will the hospital do?

□ The pressure will be checked and the eye examined for other anterior or posterior segment injury. The pupil may or may not be dilated. If the patient is a child, they may be admitted to ensure complete bed rest.

What do I need to do?

□ Encourage the patient to have strict bed rest if that is what has been advised. They really shouldn't be in your surgery at all.

Problems that may arise, and how to deal with them

□ If the vision deteriorates suddenly after the initial blurring has resolved, the patient should be re-referred to the hospital, as they may have had another bleed.

ANGLE RECESSION

What's going on?

□ A blunt injury to the eye has caused a pressure wave to rip open the drainage angle of the eye. The rip heals, leaving scarring that impedes aqueous outflow. If the extent of the recession is great, the patient may develop glaucoma months or years later.

If I examine the patient, what will I find?

□ You may see signs of the previous injury, but equally you may see no obvious abnormality.

What will the hospital do?

□ If the recession involves most of the angle, then the patient may be followed up at regular intervals to detect the onset of glaucoma. If the injury is minimal, the patient is usually discharged but advised to see their optician for regular pressure checks.

What do I need to do?

□ If the patient is not followed up at hospital, they should be examined regularly by an optician for the onset of glaucoma.

What to tell the patient

□ They have sustained damage that increases their risk of developing glaucoma.

ORBITAL WALL FRACTURE

What's going on?

□ Severe sudden pressure on the globe causes a massive increase in pressure within the orbit. This pressure causes fracture of one or more of the bony orbital walls, with prolapse of orbital tissue into the adjacent sinuses. Enophthalmos occurs, and there will be some restriction of ocular movement, particularly looking up and down.

If I examine the patient, what will I find?

□ Oculomotility will be restricted, particularly when the patient attempts to look up or down. The patient's cheek may be numb, owing to compromise of the infraorbital nerve. The eye may appear retracted. There may be surgical emphysema (air under the skin).

What if I've diagnosed it?

□ Refer the patient to a maxillofacial surgeon and ophthalmologist for assessment *soon*.

What will the hospital do?

□ Imaging will be used to assess the extent of injury and surgery planned as appropriate.

What do I need to do?

□ Warn the patient against blowing their nose, as this will force air, and possibly infective organisms, into the orbit.

Problems that may arise, and how to deal with them

□ If the orbit suddenly becomes red and painful, the patient may have developed infective orbital cellulitis (*see* Chapter 23), requiring intravenous antibiotics.

SYMPATHETIC OPHTHALMIA

What's going on?

□ This is rare. The eye is in the privileged position of being separated from the body's immune system by the tight blood-retinal barrier. When this barrier is broken by trauma or even surgery, the retinal antigens are exposed to the immune system and the body becomes sensitised. Weeks, months or even years after an eye injury or surgery, the body can react against the other, normal eye, causing severe, potentially blinding inflammation. After severe blinding ocular injury, removal of the damaged eye within two weeks is thought to protect against this disastrous complication.

If I examine the patient, what will I find?

□ The eye with no history of injury will be red and inflamed. The redness will be around the limbus because the inflammation is inside the eye. Vision may be reduced.

What if I've diagnosed it?

□ This is a sight-threatening problem that may affect the patient's only good eye, the other having been injured. Refer *urgently*.

What will the hospital do?

□ High-dose topical and systemic steroids will be required to stop the inflammatory process. Some patients require formal systemic immunosuppression.

3 | Referrals to you for appropriate management

I have no doubt that you are frequently faced with letters from optometrists who have seen something in the back of the eye or have a concern about a patient's visual field or intraocular pressures. These letters explain the findings in great detail and ask you to follow up. You have to make a decision about patient care without all the pertinent information and occasionally without completely understanding what you are being told.

If there is a recommendation to refer to the hospital eye service, you may not know how urgent this is. Even if the optician specifically asks for an urgent referral, does that mean now by phone, by ambulance to eye casualty or via urgent referral letter by fax or phone? I hope this section will help you to decide how to deal with patients referred to you for 'appropriate management'. The referral terms used here are identical to those used in Chapter 2.

Glaucoma-related

Your patient has high pressure

□ The key to managing these patients is to be able to differentiate angle-closure glaucoma from chronic open-angle glaucoma.

If the patient has angle-closure glaucoma, they are usually symptomatic with a red eye, pain, nausea, a cloudy cornea, a mid-dilated fixed pupil and pressure usually in excess of 40 mmHg. The optometrist will usually document a shallow anterior chamber or narrow angles and should have measured the pressure. Feel the eyes – if the pressure is markedly raised, the affected eye will feel like a cricket ball; compare it to the other eye or to your own. Sometimes the episode of angle closure will have been precipitated by instillation of dilating drops. Such patients should be referred *immediately* to hospital as an emergency.

If the patient has open-angle glaucoma, the pressure is usually in the region of 24 mmHg to 32 mmHg. The optician will have commented on the optic disc, and if there is a significant cup associated with the raised pressure, the patient probably has glaucoma. The eye is comfortable and the patient is usually asymptomatic. There may or may not be a visual field defect. Raised intraocular pressure causes damage over several months and so the urgency of referral is minimal. Such patients do require referral to the hospital eye services, but they can be referred through the usual channels. If the pressure is closer to 40 mmHg and the optic disc is described as markedly cupped, then an *urgent referral via letter* is warranted, as here the progression of glaucoma can be quite quick. The sooner the patient is seen and started on treatment, the better.

Your patient has a suspicious optic disc

□ A suspicious optic disc is one with a high degree of optic disc cupping. Generally if the cup-to-disc ratio is more than 0·5 – i.e. the vertical dimensions of the cup are more than half the total top-to-bottom distance of the disc – then there may be some degree of pathological cupping. Another cause for concern is asymmetry between the optic discs of the right and left eye. Usually the discs are relatively symmetrical. If there is a discrepancy between the cup–disc ratios of the eyes, then the eye with the larger cup may have glaucoma.

If the pressure is measured as normal and the disc is suspicious, the patient may have normal-tension glaucoma. Such patients require *routine referral* for assessment.

A haemorrhage at the optic disc can be a sign of progression of glaucomatous damage and warrants *routine referral* in itself.

Your patient is already on treatment for glaucoma but the pressure is still high

□ Glaucoma damage occurs over several months to years. Short-term fluctuations in pressure are not uncommon: indeed there is some daily change in intraocular pressure (IOP). Optometrists tend to measure IOP using air puff tonometry, which tends to overestimate pressure. As a general rule, if the patient is already on treatment and has pressure in excess of 30 mmHg, it is worth contacting the hospital and expediting their appointment for review. If the pressure is less than 30 mmHg and the patient's glaucoma is not severe, then they can usually wait for their next follow up.

Your patient has a visual field defect

□ Usually the optometrist is basing their opinion on automated perimetry. They should send you a copy of the visual field printout. Look to see if it is neurological (e.g. a hemianopia obeying the midline in each eye) or glaucomatous (usually arcuate – arcing around the centre of the plot). Make sure there is no obvious cause for the defect, e.g. a previous occipital infarct or a retinal scar. If the optician is querying glaucoma then there should be supporting features such as raised IOP and optic disc changes. Patients should generally be referred *routinely*. If the patient has a bitemporal hemianopia, referral should be *soon via letter* as they may have a pituitary compression.

Your patient has shallow anterior chambers

□ The key question here is whether the patient is at risk of angle-closure glaucoma. Shallow anterior chambers are not uncommon and tend to occur in very long-sighted individuals, particularly those of East Asian ethnic origin.

Patients may be having episodes of intermittent angle closure without realising it. A typical history is intermittent eye ache associated with some blurring of vision occurring at night (when illumination is low and the pupil dilated). These episodes are relieved by bright light (causing pupil constriction and reversal of the angle blockage).

If the optometrist thinks the anterior chamber is so shallow that the angles are at risk of occluding, the patient should be referred for formal assessment. The referral may be *routine* but the patient should be warned about the signs and symptoms of acute angle-closure glaucoma (red, firm, painful eye, blurry vision, nausea). If they develop these symptoms, they should attend the emergency eye service *immediately/ urgently*.

Your patient had a high-pressure rise after the optometrist dilated their pupils

□ The concern is angle-closure glaucoma. If the pressure rose above 30 mmHg and failed to return to normal, the patient should be referred *immediately/ urgently*. The pressure may go up transiently after dilating drops and return to normal after a short while.

Cornea-related

Your patient has a corneal ulcer

□ Is the eye red? If not, there is unlikely to be an infective corneal ulcer.

Stain the eye with fluorescein. If it stains, there is an ulcer. If the eye is white and the cornea does not stain, the white opacity in the cornea is likely to be related to an old scar.

If the patient does have a corneal ulcer they should be referred *urgently*.

Your patient has keratoconus

Refer *routinely*.

Your patient has a corneal dystrophy

□ Refer *routinely*. If the dystrophy is described as epithelial in origin and the patient is experiencing a foreign-body sensation, they may benefit from topical lubricant drops (artificial tears) until they are reviewed in hospital.

Your patient has a corneal opacity/scar

□ Patients are often diagnosed as having a corneal opacity, and the optometrist may be concerned that the patient has a corneal ulcer. If the eye is red and painful, the patient should be referred *urgently* to the hospital eye service. Try to avoid giving antibiotic drops unless ophthalmology review will be delayed. Topical antibiotics may affect the pick-up rate of the hospital's corneal microbiology scrapes.

If the eye is white and the patient asymptomatic, there is unlikely to be any infection.

Ask the patient if they have had a previous eye injury that would explain the scar.

If the patient is asymptomatic and the eye is not red, then you have the option of simply observing the patient. If they develop symptoms such as blurring of vision, it is worth referring them *routinely*. If the eye subsequently becomes red, treat it as a corneal ulcer until proven otherwise.

Oculoplastics-related

Your patient has a ptosis

□ Check pupil sizes and eliminate Horner's syndrome.
   Check history for symptoms of myasthenia gravis.
   Refer *routinely*.

Your patient has an entropion

□ Check the cornea and ensure that it is healthy. If there is redness or evidence of fluorescein staining, give lubricant drops.
   If lashes are abrading the cornea, tape the lower lid down to the cheek as a temporising measure.
   Refer *routinely* if the cornea is healthy.

Your patient has an ectropion

□ Give thick lubricant drops to protect the cornea as exposure keratopathy is a risk.
   Refer *routinely* if the cornea is healthy.

Strabismus-related

Your patient has a squint

□ If the squint is due to a nerve palsy then the patient should be referred *soon* for assessment, particularly if the patient is not hypertensive or diabetic. If the patient has a third nerve palsy with a dilated pupil, they should be referred *immediately*.
   If the patient has a long-standing squint and is motivated for surgery, they should be referred *routinely*.
   If the squint is relatively recent and the patient is symptomatic for diplopia, they should be referred *soon via letter*.
   A child should be referred *soon via letter* directly to the orthoptic service if possible. A baby with a squint is at risk of developing amblyopia (a lazy eye) and should be referred early.

Your patient has a latent squint (phoria)

□ Latent squints are common. Assess how troubled the patient is. Community optometrists can fit prisms to spectacles to help with latent squints. If the community optometrist is unable to control the patient's symptoms, refer *routinely*.

Paediatrics-related

This baby has a cataract

□ Check the red reflexes, comparing both sides. These are often hard to see in dark-skinned babies. If the baby has a white pupillary reflex there is something seriously wrong – refer *urgently*.
   In neonates, a clear visual axis is vital for the development of normal vision. If the baby has a cataract, the risk of long-term visual morbidity is high and the patient should be referred *urgently via letter*.
   If the baby has already developed nystagmus, there is an urgent need for paediatric ophthalmology review.

This baby has a squint

□ It is important to find out whether the parents have noticed the squint. The risk of amblyopia is high if the squint is long-standing and constant in nature.
   Examine the corneal reflexes to see if the baby does indeed have a squint. Ignore the amount of sclera showing – concentrate on the light reflex on the cornea. Prominent folds of skin at the inner canthus can fool the examiner into thinking that the baby has a convergent squint. It is probably best to refer all such babies, as only an assessment by an orthoptist will determine for certain that ocular alignment is normal.
   Such babies should be referred *soon via letter*, either to the paediatric ophthalmologist or direct to the orthoptic services, if this route of referral is available to you.

Vitreoretinal-related

Your patient has flashes and/or floaters

□ This is difficult. Flashes and floaters are common and rarely indicate significant pathology. The key question is whether the patient has a retinal tear or hole, or retinal detachment. Optometrists are usually good at examining the fundus. The decision to refer and the urgency of the referral should be guided by the confidence of the optometrist in making the diagnosis of, or excluding the presence of, significant pathology.
   If the optometrist is confident that the patient has an isolated posterior vitreous detachment and no retinal

breaks, there is no need to refer. The patient should be warned about the symptoms of retinal detachment – sudden new hail of floaters, an increase in flashes or a solid curtain across the peripheral vision – and advised to attend their ophthalmology service immediately if they get any of these.

If the optometrist has seen a retinal detachment or a retinal tear or hole, the patient should be referred *urgently*.

If the optometrist had a good look at the retina and could not see any pathology, but still feels that referral is warranted for assessment, the patient should be referred *routinely/soon via letter*.

If patients have risk factors such as pseudophakia, aphakia, a previous history of retinal detachment or high myopia, then the suspicion of pathology should be greater.

If the optometrist has seen 'pigment in the vitreous' or evidence of a vitreous haemorrhage, the patient has a retinal tear until proven otherwise and should thus be referred *urgently/soon*.

I have seen a retinal detachment

□ Refer *urgently*.

I have seen a retinoschisis

□ This is a retinal cyst and not a detachment. It is a hard diagnosis to make and so the optometrist may require confirmation from the ophthalmology department. Refer *routinely*. Warn patients about the symptoms of retinal detachment – see above.

I suspect a macular hole

□ If the patient has had the macula hole for many years, a good visual outcome is unlikely. If the patient is motivated for surgery, they should be referred *soon via letter/routine*.

I have seen an atrophic patch/scar in the retina

□ If the scar is inactive, there is no need to refer. Scars are common and some are of an unknown origin. Old toxoplasmosis scars are extremely common and require no treatment or investigation. A scar in isolation does not require referral, unless there is the suspicion of an active progressive process. Old toxoplasmosis scars can reactivate but this will be associated with other symptoms, such as blurred vision.

I suspect retinitis

□ Active retinitis is sight threatening if the underlying cause is not discovered and treated urgently. Refer *urgently/soon*.

Medical retina

Your patient has dry age-related macular degeneration (AMD)

□ No need to refer. Warn the patient that they are at risk of developing wet AMD and that this may cause them to lose a significant amount of central vision. They should check the vision in each eye on a daily basis and, more importantly, check for the presence of distortion. Either give the patient an Amsler chart (a large black grid) or tell the patient to look at straight lines such as those on a window frame. If the lines are obviously not straight the patient may have wet AMD and should go back to their optician for assessment as soon as possible. Alternatively, you may refer the patient urgently to the local photodynamic therapy service for possible treatment.

Your patient has wet age-related macular degeneration

□ Refer *soon/urgently via letter*. If you have access to a fast-track photodynamic therapy screening service, refer via this route.

I suspect your patient has central serous retinopathy

□ Refer *soon via letter*.

Your patient has a swollen disc

□ Is the vision reduced? If so, consider an ischaemic optic neuropathy or an optic neuritis. Does the patient have GCA? – check ESR and CRP. If the vision is not reduced, then either this is pseudo-disc swelling (the appearance of disc swelling without true disc swelling) or the patient has papilloedema and requires urgent investigation for raised intracranial pressure. If the disc swelling is unilateral and vision normal, refer the patient *urgently via letter* to the hospital eye service. If the vision is reduced and the disc swollen, refer *urgently*. If the disc swelling is bilateral and the vision normal (papilloedema), refer to a physician to exclude raised intracranial pressure secondary to a space-occupying lesion. If the physician is unsure whether the discs are indeed swollen, they may refer directly to the ophthalmologist.

Your patient has vascular changes

□ Vascular changes are common in older people and arteriolar attenuation virtually universal. Visualisation of arterial changes, such as arteriolar narrowing, and arteriovenous changes require a blood pressure check and treatment if appropriate.

If the blood pressure is normal and the patient has marked vascular changes, refer *routinely* for assessment.

If the venous vasculature is abnormally dilated and tortuous, the patient should be referred *soon via letter* as they may be at risk of developing a venous occlusion.

Your patient has a haemorrhage in the macula

□ If this is small, the patient should be assessed for hypertension and diabetes.

If the haemorrhage is larger and associated with visual loss, the concern is that the patient has suffered a branch retinal vein occlusion or has wet AMD.

Refer *urgently via letter/soon via letter.*

Your patient has haemorrhages in all quadrants/one quadrant of the retina

□ If in one quadrant, the patient probably has a branch retinal vein occlusion. If in all four quadrants along with visual loss, the patient has had a central retinal vein occlusion. In both cases, refer *urgently via letter/ soon via letter.*

If the patient has haemorrhages in all four quadrants without vision loss, check for diabetes and refer according to the diabetic retinopathy guidelines.

Cataract

Your patient has a cataract

□ Is the patient symptomatic? Is their life restricted by their visual morbidity? Is the patient motivated for surgery? If the answer is yes to all of the above, refer *routinely.*

Your patient has posterior capsular opacification

□ Refer *routinely* for YAG laser posterior capsulotomy.

Diabetes

Your patient has new vessels at the disc or elsewhere

□ This patient is at risk of vitreous haemorrhage and significant visual loss – refer *urgently via letter.*

Your patient has macular oedema

□ Refer *soon via letter.*

Your patient has a diabetic maculopathy

□ The need to refer depends upon the severity. Isolated microaneurysms do not need referral, but should be reassessed regularly by the optometrist. Patients with macular exudates or haemorrhages that are severe or close to the fovea should be referred *soon via letter.*

Your patient has background diabetic changes

□ No need to refer. Regular optometrist review needed.

4 | Operations – how, why and what goes wrong

It is useful to know the types of procedures and operations done by the ophthalmology department. Understanding what goes on will help you counsel your patients about what to expect and explain their likely postoperative course.

It will also help you decide whether to refer the patient, as you will be able to give the patient a reasonable idea of what will happen to them and the likely prognosis.

Complications are a concern in any surgical speciality, but patients are often particularly upset when that complication affects their eyes, especially if their vision might be compromised. Here is an outline of the most common and worrying complications that your patients may face under our care, which I hope will help you counsel these patients effectively.

Phacoemulsification of cataract

This is the modern gold standard technique for removing a cataract. A small incision is made in the cornea, a special ultrasonic (phacoemulsification) probe is placed into the eye and the cataract emulsified and removed. An intraocular lens is folded and placed through the incision into the bag that held the natural cataractous lens (figures 18.4a and b, and 18.5).

Postoperatively, patients are usually prescribed a topical antibiotic and steroid combination for approximately four weeks.

COMPLICATIONS

Posterior capsule rupture

□ The capsule that surrounds the natural lens is left in place to support the new synthetic lens. Any weakness in this capsule can cause it to rupture and the vitreous to prolapse forwards. This vitreous is cleared away with an anterior vitrectomy.

More worryingly, sometimes there is no longer any support for the synthetic intraocular lens (IOL) in the capsular bag, which means the lens must be placed in the sulcus that is anterior to the capsular bag but behind the iris. This is not usually a problem and the patient can achieve good vision.

If the front of the capsule is also compromised, however, the patient may be left without a lens (aphakia) or have to have a lens placed anterior to the iris (an anterior chamber IOL). Anterior chamber IOLs can cause problems with the corneal endothelium, and the vision may not be as good as if the lens were placed behind the iris. Sometimes a sutured lens is placed behind the iris using sutures in the sclera.

Loss of lens fragment

□ If the posterior capsule ruptures before the cataract has been removed, part of it may fall into the vitreous cavity. If left in place, it will cause problems such as excessive inflammation and pressure rise. The fragment usually has to be removed with another operation – a vitrectomy and removal of lens fragments. These eyes are usually quite inflamed for longer and the vision may not be optimal.

Excessive postoperative uveitis

□ The eye is always inflamed after a cataract operation. Some patients develop excessive inflammation and require more than the usual four-times-a-day steroid drops. It is always a concern that this excessive inflammation may be the start of an infective endophthalmitis.

Cystoid macular oedema

□ This is not uncommon after cataract surgery, particularly if the procedure was complicated. The blood-retinal barrier in the macula breaks down and macular oedema develops, with consequent blurring of vision. The condition classically occurs about a week after surgery. Some cases resolve spontaneously, but others require treatment in the form of topical NSAIDs, oral acetazolamide, periocular or even intraocular steroid injections. Rarely, the condition fails to resolve and the patient is left with long-standing blurred vision. Patients are at risk of developing the same problem if they have cataract surgery to the other eye.

Endophthalmitis

□ This is an ophthalmic emergency that requires immediate treatment, but is fortunately rare. The eye is red and painful, and the vision blurred. A vitreous tap is done to remove a sample for microbiological microscopy and culture. Antibiotics are injected intravitreally (into the vitreous cavity) to try to control the infection. Sometimes a vitrectomy is done in order to clear a heavy infective load. Some clinicians also advocate a short course of systemic steroids to control inflammation. Visual prognosis in established infection tends to be poor. A red painful eye with blurred vision after any intraocular surgery should be referred *immediately*.

Suprachoroidal haemorrhage

□ This complication is rarer now in the days of small-incision surgery. A haemorrhage occurs in the layer between the choroid and the sclera. The blood accumulates in the wall of the eye and increases the intraocular pressure dramatically. When the eye is open, the ocular contents try to work their way out of the wound. If the haemorrhage is large, vision can be lost completely and permanently.

Posterior capsule opacification

□ This is not really a complication. It develops because epithelial cells remain in the old lens capsule and continue to grow. They spread across the posterior capsule behind the new intraocular lens and lead to blurry vision. A YAG laser capsulotomy usually clears the visual axis by burning a hole in the new layer (figure 18.6).

Extracapsular cataract extraction

This method of cataract extraction has been largely superseded by phacoemulsification. It requires a larger incision involving almost one-third of the corneal periphery with the subsequent need for corneal sutures (figure 18.3). Patients are also left with a greater degree of astigmatism (irregularity of the corneal surface).

This technique is still used for some forms of hard cataract or when there was a problem with the phacoemulsification procedure.

Complications are as for phacoemulsification above.

Vitrectomy

This is the removal of the vitreous jelly with a special cutter (vitrector). It is often done in cases of vitreous haemorrhage or retinal detachment.

In patients with diabetes, a vitrectomy is often coupled with endolaser of the ischaemic retina, in the hope of reversing or preventing neovascularisation.

In the treatment of retinal detachment, vitrectomy is accompanied by cryotherapy (freeze/thaw cycles) to seal the retinal breaks and allow flattening of the detached retina. Expansile gas is often left inside the eye to help push the retina flat. The gas is reabsorbed over several weeks. Initially, the patient cannot see through the gas, but vision returns once the gas disappears and the eye fills with clear transudate.

Patients with gas in the eye should not travel by air.

COMPLICATIONS

Retinal detachment

□ The vitrectomy procedure itself may precipitate a retinal detachment.

Secondary intraocular lens implant

□ If the patient was left without a lens (aphakia) at their first operation, then they will require a contact lens or thick spectacles. They may elect to have an intraocular lens placed into the eye as a secondary procedure.

Corneal grafting

Pathology that compromises the cornea's clarity or integrity may be treated by a corneal graft, also called a penetrating keratoplasty (figure 19.5). Graft material comes from a bank of donated tissue. The original cornea is cut away and the new cornea sutured in place. The sutures inevitably cause some irregularity and astigmatism. The sutures may have to be removed once the cornea has healed (usually after at least a year), or other procedures may be required to minimise the astigmatism. Topical steroids are usually given for an extended period.

COMPLICATIONS

Rejection

□ Graft rejection is a significant concern months or even decades after the procedure. An eye with a corneal graft that becomes red should be assessed very quickly by the ophthalmology department (*urgent*). Early intervention with intensive topical or even systemic steroids may reverse the rejection and save the cornea.

Loose sutures

□ The many sutures holding the graft in place are prone to loosen over time (figure 19.7). They will give a foreign-body sensation but, more worryingly, may cause rejection or infection of the graft. They should be removed immediately by the hospital eye service. If this occurs in the early postoperative period, the stitches may need replacing.

Retinal detachment repair

Retinal detachments may be repaired by vitrectomy (see above), cryobuckle or pneumatic retinopexy.

Pneumatic retinopexy involves injecting a gas into the vitreous cavity. The gas is light and floats upwards to exert pressure on a superiorly located detachment in order to flatten it. Cryotherapy is also applied to the retinal break to seal it. The patient usually has to keep their head in a specific position to allow the floating gas to press upon the appropriate area.

Cryobuckle is an external repair, as opposed to the internal repair of the vitrectomy procedure. Cryotherapy is applied to the sclera in the area of the retinal break to seal it by inducing a scar in the choroid, which involves the retina. As no internal pressure can be placed on the retina in order to flatten it, an external force is applied. Plastic or sponge material (explant or buckle) is sutured to the outer surface of the eye to indent the sclera.

COMPLICATIONS

Unfortunately, detachment may recur and require a further operation.

Ptosis repair

This procedure is usually carried out under local anaesthetic. An incision is made in the upper lid and the disinserted levator muscle is re-attached to the upper lid's tarsal plate. It is important that the height and contour of the lid is assessed per-operatively to ensure adequate postoperative appearance and function.

COMPLICATIONS

If the lid is left too high postoperatively, the eye will not close fully (lagophthalmos) and the cornea will be at risk of exposure keratopathy. If the lagophthalmos is marked, the patient may require another operation. Lubricants may be required to protect the cornea.

YAG laser therapy

The laser is applied via a slit lamp. After topical anaesthetic, a contact lens is placed on the eye and the laser applied.

The YAG laser creates a focused burst of energy that creates a momentary shock wave, blowing tissue away.

It is primarily used for posterior capsulotomy procedures to clear a gap in any posterior capsular opacification seen after cataract surgery. It is also used to 'punch' a hole in the iris for a peripheral iridotomy in shallow-angle glaucoma.

Argon laser therapy

The laser therapy is applied via a slit lamp. After topical anaesthetic, a contact lens is placed on the eye and the laser applied.

The argon laser is used in retinal laser treatment, and creates thermal burns in the retinal pigment epithelial layer with secondary effects on the retina.

In cases of focal laser therapy to aid the sealing of leaking vessels, the procedure takes about 10 minutes and is relatively pain free.

If pan-retinal photocoagulation is required – e.g. for a proliferative diabetic retinopathy – the patient will need more than 2000 burns. This can be painful, and so treatment is usually given over several sittings. Advise your patients to take analgesia before they arrive for treatment.

COMPLICATIONS

Foveal burn. This is a delicate procedure. If the patient looks into the laser light at the moment the ophthalmologist fires a shot, the patient can sustain a foveal burn with a marked permanent reduction in vision.

Laser refractive eye surgery

The aim is to change the curvature of the cornea and thus affect its focusing power, allowing the patient to see in the distance without spectacles. It is used more often to correct short sight than long sight.

There are many different forms of laser refractive surgery:

PHOTOREFRACTIVE KERATECTOMY (PRK)

The superficial corneal epithelium is scraped off and the laser applied to modify the curvature of the cornea. The corneal epithelium then heals over by itself. This procedure can be painful in the early postoperative period, as the patient effectively has a total corneal abrasion. Vision will not improve until the cornea has healed completely.

LASIK (LASER-ASSISTED IN SITU KERATOMILEUSIS)

This is the most common form of laser refractive surgery. The surgeon uses a special, fine automated blade to cut a flap half through the thickness of the cornea. This flap is then lifted up and the laser used under the surface to change the shape of the cornea. The flap is then laid down and adheres by itself without the need for stitches (figures 7.10 a–d). Patient comfort is not usually a problem, and the vision is often much improved by the following morning.

LASEK (LASER EPITHELIAL KERATOMILE)

This is similar to LASIK, but rather than making a cut in the cornea, the whole sheet of epithelium is lifted off using alcohol, and laser applied to the underside to alter the shape. The above procedures are carried out under topical anaesthesia.

COMPLICATIONS

These are effectively cosmetic procedures and so complications, particularly if sight threatening, are particularly upsetting for the patient.

Dry eye

□ This is quite common, and usually self-limiting.

Per-operative button holing

□ In the LASIK procedure, the cut may go too deep and into the eye, or may be too superficial, not forming a complete flap. If this is recognised, the procedure is usually abandoned. The situation is not usually disastrous, however, and the procedure may still be done successfully at a later date.

Haze

□ After laser treatment, the cornea may heal but not retain total clarity. The patient might be left with some residual haze and, therefore, reduced vision.

Infection

□ Infection can be disastrous. It usually occurs in the interface beneath the flap, and can be caused by organisms of different virulence. The condition is commonly called diffuse lamellar keratitis (DLK). If the organism is of low virulence, the infection may be treated successfully but may leave the vision hazy.

Flap dislocation

□ Because the LASIK flap is not sutured into place, this will always be a weak area, although the flap usually sticks down well. Injury, such as being poked in the eye, may cause the flap to lift off and wrinkle. The flap can often be 'floated' back into place, however.

Background and basics

5 | Basic anatomy

The eye is very similar to a camera. Its function is to allow light to fall on the photosensitive retina with the subsequent production of impulses that are carried to the visual cortex of the brain and interpreted as images. Thus sight is achieved.

The eye is a mobile globe that lies within the bony orbit of the skull, mostly filled with a clear jelly called the vitreous. This vitreous jelly is made up of a network of fine collagen fibrils supporting a gel of hyaluronate molecules. It is avascular, contains very few cells and is virtually transparent to allow the unimpeded transmission of light to the retina.

Overall clinical anatomy and the major landmarks are shown in figure 5.1.

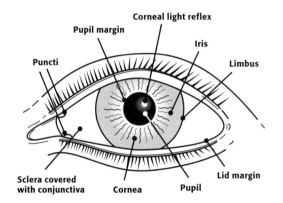

FIGURE 5.1 **Front view of the eye.**

Sclera

The outer coat of the globe is a white collagenous tissue called the sclera. The sclera is reflective, preventing unwanted light entering the eye, and is also tough enough to protect the ocular contents from inadvertent damage. Unfortunately, consisting primarily of collagen, it is susceptible to systemic disorders that attack collagen elsewhere in the body. At its anterior aspect, it changes nature dramatically to form a clear window for the entry of light. This transparent area is the cornea.

Cornea

In order to allow light into the eye, a specialised area of collagen that has adapted to be completely clear forms the front of the sclera. The circumferential line marking the margin between white sclera and the clear cornea is a transition zone called the limbus. The collagen forming the cornea is specially arranged to allow light to pass through with the minimum of interference. In order to maintain its clarity the cornea is avascular, obtaining nutrients from the atmosphere and the tear film, or from diffusion from the clear nutrient fluid in the anterior segment of the eye (the aqueous). As well as transmitting light into the eye, the cornea also has a vital function in bending (refracting) the incoming light in order to bring it into focus on the retina. Without this focusing mechanism, it would be impossible to see.

The cornea consists largely of a middle stromal layer, which is covered by a superficial stratified squamous corneal epithelium made up of several layers of cells (figure 5.2). On the inner surface of the cornea lies an important single layer of endothelial cells, the corneal endothelium.

The cornea retains its clarity by maintaining a relative state of dehydration. This dehydration is facilitated by the endothelial cells actively pumping water out of

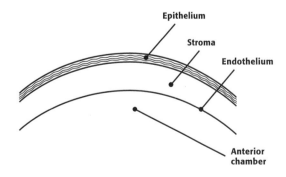

FIGURE 5.2 **Cross-section of the cornea showing the superficial epithelial layer with underlying stroma. The epithelium is approximately five cells thick while the endothelium is only one layer thick.**

the corneal substance. Unfortunately these cells cannot replicate, and over the years many are irreversibly lost. This is not usually a problem in most eyes, but if the density of endothelial cells falls below a certain critical value, the pump sometimes fails and the cornea becomes too wet, thickens and loses clarity (corneal oedema), with subsequent loss of vision (figure 19.4).

The cornea is convex, bulging forward. Behind it lies the lens, suspended centrally by its zonular fibres (see below). The area between the back of the cornea and the anterior of the lens is the anterior chamber, which is filled with clear aqueous (figure 5.3).

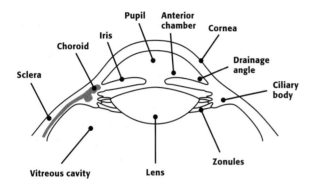

FIGURE 5.3 **A cross-section of the anterior segment showing the relationship between the cornea, the iris, the lens and the ciliary body. The lens is suspended from the ciliary body by the fine zonules.**

Uvea

The middle coat of the eye, called the uvea, is made up of connective tissue filled with numerous blood vessels and pigmented cells. It is the layer beneath the sclera and separates sclera from the inner layers of the eye. The uvea emerges at the front of the eye and projects into the anterior segment as the iris.

Iris

The iris is part of the uvea and has developed as a diaphragm or sphincter to control the amount of light entering the eye. It is darkly pigmented on its inner/rear surface but has variable pigment on its anterior surface, which is why people's eyes are different colours. Those with a large amount of pigment on their irises have dark brown eyes, while those with little pigment have blue eyes. The circular orifice in the centre of the iris is the pupil, and within the pupil margin is a rim of muscle. When this muscle contracts, the pupil becomes smaller (constricts or mioses) and when it relaxes the pupil enlarges (known as mydriasis). Just behind the iris at its peripheries (and thus

hidden from view) the uvea bulges to form a specialised organ called the ciliary body.

Ciliary body and aqueous

Behind the edges of the iris within the eye there is a circumferential thickened, specialised area of the uvea called the ciliary body. The ciliary body produces the clear aqueous fluid that circulates around the anterior segment of the eye, maintaining the eye's shape by means of internal pressure and helping light to travel unimpeded. The aqueous also provides vital oxygen and nutrients to avascular structures such as the lens and cornea. The muscular part of the ciliary body is called the ciliary muscle. Attached to this muscle are hundreds of thin fine ligaments (called zonules or zonular fibres) that fix on the edge of the lens and hold it in place behind the iris.

Lens

The lens is a clear avascular structure with a double convex shape, i.e. like a 'Smartie' or magnifying glass. It is formed of cells that become highly specialised by losing their nuclei and becoming filled with clear molecules called crystallins. In the centre of the lens is the nucleus and surrounding that is the cortex. Both are clear so, until one or the other becomes cloudy (thus forming a cataract), they cannot generally be distinguished from each other.

Around the lens is a thin capsule into which the zonule fibres (see above) insert and attach. The young lens is elastic and highly malleable. Movement of the ciliary muscle results in a pull on the zonules and thus on the lens, changing its shape. This, in turn, alters the anterior and posterior curvature of the lens, thus changing its focusing power. This mechanism of changing focus and increasing the lens power is a key factor in the process of accommodation (*see* Chapter 7, The focusing mechanism of the eye [refraction]).

Choroid

Further back than the iris and ciliary body, the uvea takes the form of a highly pigmented layer called the choroid. The choroid is extremely vascular (in fact, it is the most vascular organ in the body) and lies within the sandwich of the outer sclera and the inner retina.

Lids

The globe lies within the bony orbit for protection.

Anteriorly, the globe must be free of bone in order to allow light to enter. The eyelids protect the front of the eye.

The upper and lower lids have loosely adherent skin anteriorly, to allow them to move; muscle in the middle layer, to pull the lids open or squeeze them closed; and an inner layer of fibrous tissue (called the tarsal plate) to maintain their shape and add a firm protective sheet. Lining the inner surface of the lids is a specialised epithelium called the conjunctiva. The conjunctiva runs superiorly and inferiorly, where it folds back to form the superior and inferior fornices, respectively. From the fornices, the conjunctiva is reflected back to line the surface of the globe and eventually merge with the cornea at the limbus on the front of the eye.

Blinking removes foreign material from the corneal surface and coats the front of the cornea with much-needed lubricating tears. The superficial layers of the cornea obtain their nutrients and oxygen from the tear film, whereas the deeper layers have to rely on the aqueous fluid inside the eye.

Tears and lacrimal drainage apparatus

The cornea and conjunctiva must be kept moist to stay healthy. The lacrimal gland, together with numerous minor salivary glands, produces tears. Tear production is divided into two types: baseline and stimulated. Baseline secretion occurs continually throughout the day and night, while stimulated secretion occurs in response to a trigger and results in a bolus of tears. This trigger can be emotion or corneal irritation.

Tears drain into the lacrimal puncti – two small ori-

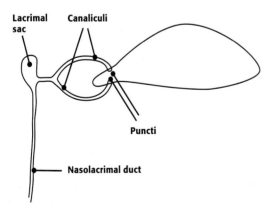

FIGURE 5.4 **The nasolacrimal system drains from the upper and lower puncti on the medial aspect of the upper and lower lids. They drain into the upper and lower canaliculus, then into a common canaliculus and then into the lacrimal sac. From the lacrimal sac tears drain down the nasolacrimal duct to empty into the nose.**

fices placed medially on the lid margins, one on the lower surface of the upper lid and one on the upper surface of the lower lid (figure 5.4). These puncti drain into ducts (called canaliculi) that run medially/nasally to enter the lacrimal sac. From there, tears drain down the nasolacrimal ducts into the nasal cavity.

Anterior chamber

The anterior chamber is the space behind the convex dome of the cornea and in front of the iris and lens. It is continually filled with clear aqueous fluid produced by the ciliary body. This aqueous fluid flows out of the eye via the trabecular meshwork, a sieve-like structure lying in the angle between the inner surface of the peripheral cornea and the very periphery of the iris.

When the cornea is very convex, the distance between the back of the cornea and the lens is great and the anterior chamber is described as deep (figure 5.5a). When the cornea is less convex (i.e. flatter) the distance to the lens is smaller and the anterior chamber is described as shallow (figure 5.5b).

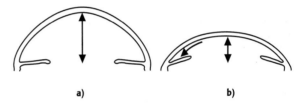

a)   b)

FIGURES 5.5a and b **a) A deep anterior chamber (double-ended arrow). Note the drainage angle is wide open, facilitating drainage of aqueous fluid. b) A shallow anterior chamber (double-ended arrow). Note the drainage angle is much narrower (single-ended arrow).**

Ocular muscles

The eyes must move in order to align themselves with the object under observation. To facilitate this, numerous muscles attached to the sclera rotate the globe. There are six muscles – four recti muscles and two oblique. The medial, lateral, superior and inferior recti muscles come from the bone at the back of the orbit and project forward to insert into the sclera, approximately 6 mm behind the limbus on the medial, lateral, superior and inferior aspects of the globe, respectively (figure 5.6). The inferior and superior obliques have slightly more complex courses. As their name suggests, they run obliquely and attach into the sclera at an angle. The superior oblique is particularly unusual in that its tendon runs through a specialised pulley called the trochlea. (*See* Chapter 12 for more information.)

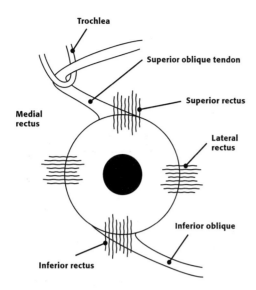

FIGURE 5.6 The four recti muscles attach to the sclera approximately 5–6mm back from the limbus. The superior oblique runs through the trochlea pulley and reverses direction to attach to sclera. The inferior oblique attaches at an angle directly on to the sclera.

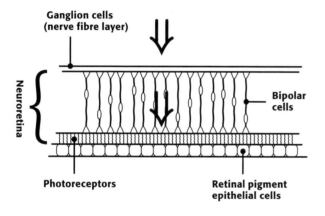

FIGURE 5.7 Cross-section of retina. The light enters (big arrows) the eye and passes through the whole thickness of the clear retina before it hits the photoreceptors.

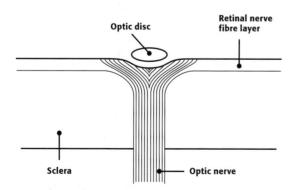

FIGURE 5.8 Cross-section of the eye where the optic nerve exits the eye. The nerve fibres running in the nerve fibre layer turn by 90° to exit the eye through the sclera and form the optic nerve.

Blood supply

The blood supply to the eye comes from the ophthalmic artery, a branch of the internal carotid artery. The anterior and posterior ciliary arteries supply the outer coatings of the eye and the anterior segment. The choroid is the most vascular structure of the body, as it consists mainly of a network of blood vessels. The choroidal plexus of vessels also supplies the adjacent retinal pigment epithelium (see below) and the outer third of the neuroretina (including the photoreceptors). The inner two-thirds of the neuroretina are supplied by branches of the central retinal artery (CRA). The CRA is a branch of the ophthalmic artery and enters the eye with the optic nerve and central retinal vein (CRV). At the optic nerve head, the CRA splits into four major vessels: the superotemporal, superonasal, inferonasal and inferotemporal retinal arteries. Venous drainage of the retina is via the retinal veins, which run adjacent to the retinal arteries back towards the optic nerve head, where they combine to form the CRV.

Retina

The inner layer of the eye is the retina, the neurosensory part. The retina is a continuation of the optic nerve and thus a part of the central nervous system (the only part we can see directly!). It is responsible for detecting incoming light and changing these photons of energy into nervous impulses for transmission to, and analysis by, the optical centres of the brain. The retina is formed of two main layers: a pigmented layer tightly stuck to the choroid (called the retinal pigment epithelium or RPE), and the neurosensory retina, which lies on top of this pigmented layer and incorporates all of the photoreceptors needed for light detection and sight (figure 5.7).

The structure of the retina is unusual, as the photoreceptors lie deep to the bulk of the neurosensory retina. The light has to pass through the clear neuroretina before it reaches the photoreceptors. When we look into the eye, we cannot see the retina unless there is some pathology. We see right through the sensory retina and observe the orange reflection of the pigmentary retina (the RPE).

A biochemical reaction takes place in the photoreceptors, and the neural impulse generated passes back into the neurosensory retina via a series of intermediate nerve cells (bipolar cells), eventually reaching the ganglion cells. The axons of the ganglion cells run towards the optic nerve and form the innermost layer of the retina (the nerve fibre layer). All of the ganglion cell axons sweep towards the optic nerve head from all parts of the retina, and these form the neurones of the optic nerve (figure 5.8). This is a simplification of the true retinal structure, as there are many other cells at work that modify and enhance the function and output of the photoreceptors.

The optic nerve

The nerve fibres from the retina run towards the optic nerve head. There they dip back to exit the globe via a gap in the sclera called the lamina cribrosa. As they run posteriorly, they become enclosed in a dural sheath and form the optic nerve. At the optic nerve head (and anterior visible portion of the nerve), the nerve fibres have to change direction by 90°, i.e. they move from the plane of the retina to run perpendicularly backwards in the nerve. As they turn the corner to enter the nerve, they form a slight depression within the centre of the nerve head. This depression is called the optic disc cup. A mild degree of cupping is normal, but in some pathological conditions where some of these nerve fibres are lost (particularly in glaucoma), this cup may get bigger. The optic nerve runs directly backwards within the cone formed by the bodies of the four recti muscles and exits the orbit via the optic canal. After a short journey through the skull, it enters the brain and joins its opposite number in the optic chiasm.

The optic chiasm

The optic chiasm lies within the anterior portion of the middle cranial fossa. It is formed by the meeting of the right and left optic nerves. Within the optic chiasm, there is a selective right-to-left, left-to-right exchange of optic nerve neurones (figure 5.9). Neurones originally projecting from the temporal side of the retina (thus representing the patient's nasal visual fields) continue directly back on the same side of the brain. Neurones that originate from the nasal retina of each eye, thus representing the patient's temporal field of vision in that eye, cross over (decussate) to run on the other side of the brain.

This decussation is vital in order that the corresponding images from each eye reach the same place in the visual cortex. An object in the patient's left visual field (i.e. just to their left as they look straight ahead) projects to an area of retina on the nasal side of the left eye and the temporal side of the right eye (figure 5.10). In order for the brain to see this image

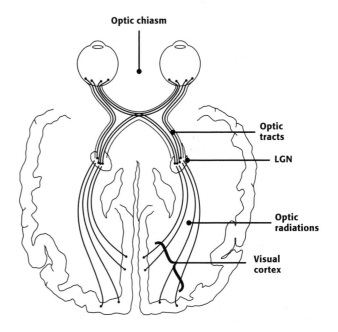

FIGURE 5.9 The visual pathway from the retina back to the optic chiasm. Here the nasal fibres decussate running to the lateral geniculate nucleus (LGN) with the contralateral temporal fibres in the optic tract. From the LGN they run back in the optic radiations to the occipital (visual) cortex.

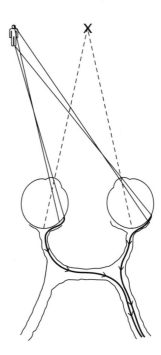

FIGURE 5.10 When fixating a point in the distance (X) an object in the patient's visual field is projected to corresponding areas on the retina of both eyes. Impulses from these areas of retina run back and run in close proximity to each other after the chiasm, eventually joining each other at the visual cortex.

as one, both of these retinal areas should eventually send impulses to the same part of the visual cortex. This retinal image from the temporal part of the right eye is sent back via the optic nerve to the optic chiasm, where it projects directly back to the right visual cortex in the occipital lobe. The corresponding image from the left eye in the nasal retina is sent back via the optic nerve to the optic chiasm, where the fibres cross over to join those from the right eye in projecting to the right visual cortex. The visual cortex is thus receiving corresponding inputs from each eye and can put the two images together.

Optic tracts

From the optic chiasm, the neurones run posteriorly in the optic tracts to the lateral geniculate nucleus (LGN). Within the LGN, the neurones synapse and then proceed via the optic radiations to the visual cortices. Once the impulses reach the visual cortex in the occipital lobes, they are analysed and interpreted as sight.

6 | Basic physiology/how the eye works

The eye is a highly specialised organ developed to convert photons (packets) of light energy into nervous impulses that are transmitted to the brain and interpreted as colours and shapes.

Central vision and peripheral vision are facilitated by two separate areas in the retina. Fine detailed vision is supplied by the specialised central area called the macula. The macula lies at the posterior pole of the eye and is responsible for the central 30° of vision. The macula is used to see detail and for reading. The field of vision depends on the peripheral retina, which lies outside the vascular arcades that delineate the macula (figure 6.1). The peripheral retina is used to see things at the edges of vision, e.g. to avoid bumping into furniture when the individual is walking around and to dodge objects thrown from the side.

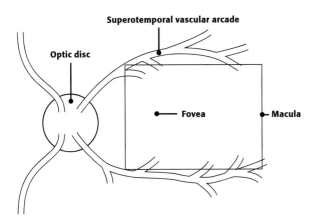

FIGURE 6.1 **The macula lies between the superotemporal and inferotemporal vascular arcades temporal/lateral to the optic disc. At the centre of the macula lies the fovea.**

When someone looks at an object, their eyes are orientated so that the light from that object enters the centre of the cornea and the pupil to land on the macula (this is called the visual axis). The refractive apparatus of the eye then brings this light into focus (*see* Chapter 7, The focusing mechanism of the eye [refraction]).

The light energy lands on the photoreceptors of the retina and creates a highly specialised biochemical reaction. This biochemical reaction causes an electrical impulse to pass from the photoreceptor to the ganglion cells of the retina and from there to the neurones of the optic nerve. The reaction depends on photosensitive proteins or photopigments, based upon the structure of the vitamin A molecule.

There are two types of photoreceptors: rods and cones, which are structurally and functionally very different. The rods are responsible for black and white vision in the peripheral retina, while the cones are responsible for fine detail and colour vision within the macula.

Central vision/the macula

The macula contains cones that are gradually replaced by rods towards its edges. The greatest concentration of cones lies in the very centre of the macula, in a tiny area called the fovea. Here cones project to only one neurone each, thus each is effectively generating one pixel of the total image. Because of the high cone density in this area, resolution and perception of fine shape is at its greatest here, which means that the image/vision obtained and transmitted to the brain is most detailed.

As you read these words, the light reflected from the white paper around each letter is focused on to your fovea and your cones are sending impulses to your brain. The areas in black (the words) reflect no light, and so the corresponding cones remain unstimulated and you see black – the letter itself. As letters become smaller, so the areas where there is blackness (i.e. no light being reflected) become smaller, until only one cone is not being stimulated and the cones either side of it are sensing light. If the blackness (the letter) gets smaller still, none of the cones are spared light and so we cannot see that blackness or letter. This is the limit of our resolution and dictates how much detail we can see.

There are three subtypes of cone, to detect the three primary colours of light – red, green and blue. Each colour represents light of a particular wavelength. These specialised cones react preferentially to photons of light energy at these wavelengths. When presented with mixtures of colours (e.g. purple) these photoreceptors are stimulated to differing degrees and the relative proportion of light picked up by the three types of receptor will dictate what colour is 'seen' by the brain.

Peripheral vision/the peripheral retina

The peripheral visual field extends out from each eye. Normally we can see more than 90° temporally; 60° nasally and superiorly (blocked nasally by the nose and superiorly by the supraorbital ridge, respectively); and 70° inferiorly. The greatest sensitivity is centrally (the macula, see above) and this sensitivity (resolution) decreases progressively as we move into the peripheral retina.

The peripheral retina gives us rough images of our surroundings. Looking straight ahead we can see the central image very clearly, but while still staring ahead we have an impression of objects in our peripheral field of vision. They are not distinct: we can see their colour and general shape, but the image is far from clear. Certainly, if we try to read anything using our peripheral vision, we can see letters there but cannot possibly read them.

The peripheral retina is dominated by rod photoreceptors. Rods are larger than cones and used mainly to detect light in darkness. In the dark, the cones are worthless and the eye must rely on the rods to see. The photoreceptor pigments in the rods do not react to specific wavelengths, but to light in general, hence we cannot distinguish colours in the dark.

Structure of the retina

The structure of the retina is unusual in that the photoreceptors lie deep to the bulk of the neurosensory retina (figure 5.7). The light has to pass through the body of the neuroretina before it reaches the photoreceptors. Thus the neuroretina must be completely clear to maintain normal vision. When we look into the eye, we cannot see the retina unless there is some pathology there. We see right through the sensory retina to the orange reflection of the pigmentary retina (RPE). The biochemical reaction takes place in the photoreceptors. The neural impulse generated here passes back through the neurosensory retina via a series of intermediate nerve cells (called bipolar cells) and eventually reaches the ganglion cells. The axons of the ganglion cells run towards the optic nerve and form the innermost layer of the retina, called the nerve fibre layer (NFL). The ganglion cell axons sweep towards the optic nerve head from all parts of the retina and form the neurones of the optic nerve. There are many other cells that act to modify and enhance the function and output of the photoreceptors.

The visual pathway

All the axons of the ganglion cells go to form the optic nerve. The impulses carried in that nerve run through the optic chiasm where some decussate (*see* Chapter 5, Basic anatomy). From there, the impulses run towards the back of the brain via the lateral geniculate nucleus and the optic tracts and radiations. When impulses reach the visual centres of the occipital cortex (this takes milliseconds), they are analysed and converted to images. There are many areas of brain adjacent to the visual centre that act to modify and fine-tune those images.

7 | The focusing mechanism of the eye (refraction)

The eye is specifically developed to allow us to see. In order to do this, the retina contains millions of photoreceptors that detect photons of light energy by means of specialised biochemical pathways. This process generates nerve impulses that travel via the optic nerve to the brain, and then to the visual centres in the occipital cortex, where they are interpreted as sight.

In order for us to be able to see around us, the light from our surroundings must be focused clearly on the retina. This focusing is called refraction. As with when using a hand-held magnifying glass, if we do not focus the image properly by moving the glass backwards and forwards, then we find that image is blurry and indistinct. Those of us who wear glasses are well aware of the poor image obtained if the light is not focused correctly.

The main function of the front of the eye is to allow in controlled amounts of light and then to focus this light effectively on the retina. This is done through the basic principles of physics that govern the way light behaves as it passes through different substances.

Light travels at the 'speed of light' (!) through a vacuum, fractionally slower through air and slower still through water or solids such as glass. The exact speed depends on the refractive index (similar to the density), of the material through which it is moving. The higher the refractive index, the slower the speed.

When a light wave moves from one material to another that has a higher refractive index, it is slowed down. If it enters that material at an angle, however, then it does not slow down uniformly. The segment of light wave that hits the new material first is slowed down first, before the segment behind it. This results in the light bending in its course (figure 7.1).

The eye uses this phenomenon at two main points in order to bend all incoming light, so that it is then focused on the retina and optimised for photoreceptor detection.

The most important interface is at the cornea. The cornea's refractive index is greater than that of the air

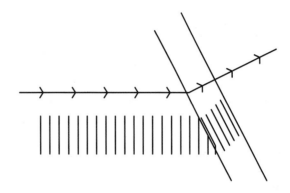

FIGURE 7.1 **As the light rays enter the material of higher refractive index (e.g. cornea or glass) they are bent because their upper segment is slowed down before the lower segment. The direction of the light ray is thus changed (refracted).**

and so, at its curved anterior surface, light is bent in towards the fovea. The degree to which the light is bent depends on the degree of curvature, and thus the steepness, of the cornea. A steep cornea will focus the light more than a flat cornea (figures 7.2 a and 7.2 b). Most of the eye's focusing power depends on this characteristic. Light waves coming in from objects at different distances will require different degrees of bending or refraction before they hit the fovea. The cornea cannot change shape, however, and is thus unable to fine-tune the focusing to deal with different distances of view. This responsibility is left to the lens. The lens regulates the eye's refractive power, allowing it to focus light from near, middle-distance and distant objects on to the retina. The lens is able to change shape, thus allowing its focusing power to vary.

The lens is suspended by the zonular ligaments (zonules) that exert radial tension, i.e. pull it. If the lens were free of this pull, it would become fat and thus increase its focusing power (a thicker magnifying glass). The zonules are attached peripherally to the circular ciliary muscle. When this circular muscle contracts, the zonules become lax and the lens becomes thicker (figure 7.3). When this muscle is relaxed, the zonules become taut and the lens flattens, with corre-

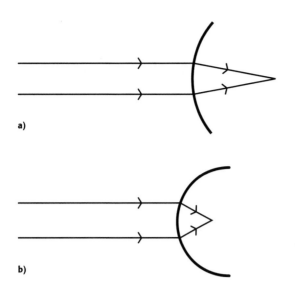

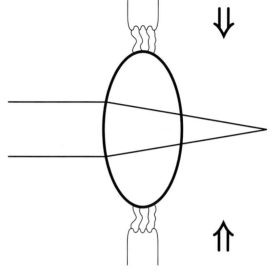

FIGURES 7.2 a and b a) A shallow corneal curvature results in less bending (refraction) of the light than does a steep cornea. b) Light is brought into focus much closer with a steeper cornea.

FIGURE 7.3 As the ciliary body contracts (remember it's a circular, sphincter-type muscle) the tension on the zonules is released and the natural springiness of the lens causes it to fatten and thus increase its power.

sponding reduction in lens power (figure 7.4).

Light from a distant target is effectively coming in straight (by convention, all light from a distance of more than 6 m is considered to be coming in straight, i.e. as if from infinity). A person fortunate enough to be able to focus this incoming light directly on to the retina with their lens at its flattest (i.e. full tension on the zonules because the ciliary muscle is relaxed and pulling on them) is described as emmetropic (they do not need spectacles for clear distance viewing) (figure 7.5). If, however, the light is not focused correctly, the patient is ametropic and requires some degree of refractive correction (usually contact lenses or spectacles) to see properly.

If the refractive power of the eye is too great (i.e. excessive focusing) light from an object in the distance (therefore straight) becomes focused too early in front of the retina in the vitreous cavity (figure 7.6). When this patient looks at an object closer than 6 m, however, because the light from that object is actually spreading out as it gets closer to the eye and is thus divergent, that light *can* be brought into focus on the retina (figure 7.6). This patient cannot see clearly in the distance but can see objects close to them. They are thus short-sighted (can see at short distances and read without spectacles) or myopic.

The converse happens in long-sighted (hypermetropic) people. The focusing power of the eye is too weak (figure 7.7 a) so light entering the eye from a distance can only be brought into focus by the active focusing mechanism of the eye using the lens to bend

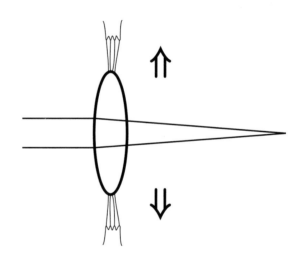

FIGURE 7.4 As the ciliary body relaxes, the zonules pull on the periphery of the lens causing it to flatten and decrease its refracting power.

in the light to a maximum (figure 7.7 b). When the incoming light is divergent (i.e. from an object close by), the eye does not have the power to bring this light into focus on the retina, as the lens has already used up all its focusing power in allowing the patient to see clearly in the distance (figure 7.7 b). Thus the patient can see clearly in the distance (long-sighted) but cannot see things close by.

When an emmetropic patient moves their focus from an object in the distance to one close by, they have to increase the power of their lens. This is done through a contraction of the ciliary muscle. Remem-

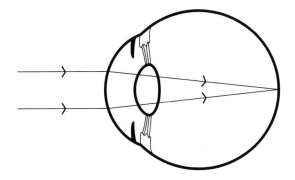

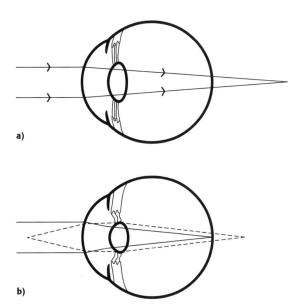

FIGURE 7.5 An individual who sees clearly without spectacles is able to focus the light on the back of their retina when their lens is completely relaxed and at its weakest power. They have all their lenses' focusing power in reserve for looking at objects close up.

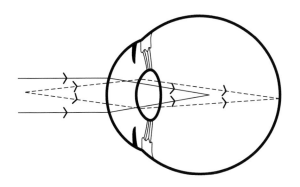

FIGURE 7.6 A short-sighted eye. Light from a distant object (solid line) is refracted too much by the effects of the cornea and it thus comes into focus in front of the retina and cannot be seen clearly. When an object is close by, the light from it diverges (dashed line). This diverging light needs the excessive focusing of the cornea to allow it to be seen clearly and thus short-sighted people can see objects clearly at a short distance.

FIGURES 7.7 a and b a) The long-sighted eye is underpowered. Light rays from the distance are not focused enough and so the patient cannot see clearly. b) Hypermetropic eyes can see by using their lens to add refractive power and focus the light from distant targets (solid line) on the retina. When objects come closer (dashed line) the eye cannot see it clearly as it has already used up its lens power to see in the distance.

ber that the ciliary muscle is a circumferential muscle, similar to a sphincter muscle. When it contracts, the ring becomes smaller and paradoxically the tension on the zonules is relaxed. This, in turn, takes the tension off the lens, allowing it to thicken and increase in power because of its natural springiness (figure 7.3). It is thus more capable of converging incoming light.

Astigmatism

The descriptions of the above mechanisms assume that the cornea is perfectly spherical, but in most people the cornea is shaped more like a rugby ball. When light in one plane, say vertical, hits the oval cornea it is focused according to the steepness of curvature of this vertical aspect. Light in the plane perpendicular to this (i.e. the horizontal) hits the cornea and is focused according to the steepness of that plane. The

powers of each of these corneal focusing mechanisms may be totally different. Thus the two planes of light may be altered in two different ways and they will subsequently not both focus at the same point (figure 7.8). While one of these rays may fall on to the retina, the other will fall too far forward or too far back. This is called astigmatism and will result in degradation of vision, because half of the light energy is lost through inappropriate focusing.

Management of refractive errors

If the eye is either long- or short-sighted, the incoming light and thus image are focused behind or in front of the retina respectively. To correct these discrepancies, lenses are placed in front of the eyes to change the direction of the incoming light, making it more divergent or convergent.

Spectacle correction

In myopic (short-sighted) patients the power of the eye is too great, so to weaken this (decrease its converging power) and allow the focal plane to move deeper on to the retina, concave lenses are placed in front of the eye to diverge the light. These are called minus lenses, as they move the light rays further apart. Thus a typical

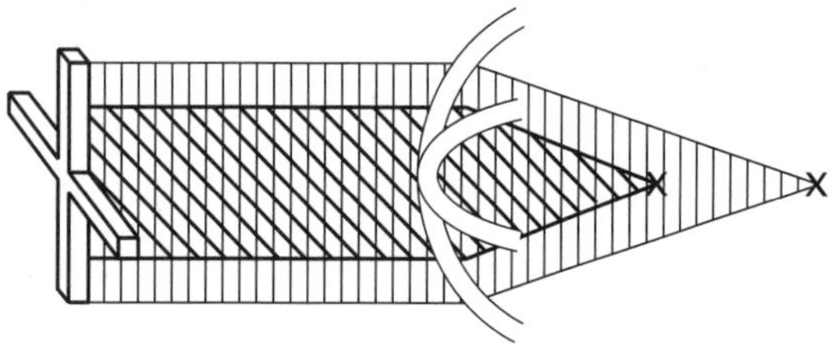

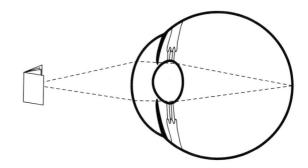

FIGURE 7.8 Astigmatic eyes have corneas that are rugby ball-shaped. Vertical light rays (the vertical lines) are focused by the vertical part of the lens. The horizontal light rays (the diagonal lines) are focused by the stronger horizontal part of the lens. The two sets of rays are focused in two different places. Thus even if the vertical rays are focused on the retina, half the image (the diagonal rays) is out of focus and blurry.

mildly myopic patient would wear a –2 spectacle correction for the right eye and a –1·5 for their left eye. A highly myopic patient might wear –7 lenses for both eyes.

In hypermetropic (long-sighted) patients, the power of the eye is too weak. To improve its converging power, therefore, and allow the focal plane to move more anteriorly on to the retina, convex lenses are placed in front of the eye to converge the light. These are called plus lenses. Thus a hypermetropic patient might wear a +2 lens for the right eye and a +2·75 lens for the left eye.

If you struggle to remember which is concave and which is convex (as I did at first), concave (minus) lenses have a cave on their surface, i.e. it dips in and is hollowed out. Convex (plus) lenses are the typical magnifying glass lenses.

When astigmatism is present, a special lens is placed in front of the eye that focuses/refracts the two planes of light to differing degrees, thereby compensating for a cornea with two different degrees of curvature. For example, in a hypermetropic (long-sighted) patient with astigmatism, the lens might converge the light in the vertical plane more than it converges the light in the horizontal plane.

The shape of the cornea varies and the meridians of different powers may not lie exactly horizontal and vertical, i.e. the rugby ball may not be completely on its side but slightly tilted. The power in each plane is described according to the axis measured in degrees on which it lies when compared with the other power meridian, i.e. the tilt of the rugby ball. Thus the hypermetropic patient referred to above may wear a +2 lens for the right eye but with an astigmatism correction of +1·5 at 85° to the vertical. This tells us that the cornea is not totally spherical but oval, and, furthermore, that the oval is not completely on its side but tilted by 85°.

Presbyopia

When we are young, our lenses are extremely elastic. When the tension is taken off the zonules, the lens springs into its thickest shape and its power increases to maximum. When an individual reads something close up, their eyes have to bend the light to a greater degree because the incoming light from the near object of regard is already spreading out (diverging). The circular ciliary muscle contracts in towards the lens taking the tension off the zonules and allowing the lens to spring thicker and increase in convergent power. This process is called accommodation, and allows us to go from looking in the distance to looking at something close by (figure 7.9).

As we get older, our lenses become less elastic and lose some of their ability to change shape. The lenses are no longer able to increase their power sufficiently and thus, when the patient tries to read 'close up', the image remains blurred, despite maximal accommodative effort. This process occurs almost universally from the age of about 45 years, and is called presbyopia.

Close one eye, hold one finger up at arm's length and stare at it. Bring the finger slowly closer to your eye. As the finger approaches, your ciliary body is progressively contracting and releasing the tension on the lens (remember that this is the opposite to what you would expect – usually when something contracts it pulls, but in this case the circular (sphincter-type) muscle gets smaller). Your lens is getting thicker, increasing its power to allow you to focus on the finger that is getting closer and closer. When your finger is about 15 cm from your eye, you will notice the image goes

FIGURE 7.9 When an eye goes from looking in the distance to near, the lens thickens and the focusing power increases to focus on the new, closer target.

blurred. This is because your lens has become as fat and powerful as it possibly can. You are at the limit of your accommodation and cannot see clearly any closer because the light coming from your finger is no longer brought into focus on the retina. As you get older, your lens becomes less elastic and is unable to become quite as thick, so the distance from your eye at which your finger becomes blurred will increase. Presbyopic patients' lenses are so inelastic that even when they hold a book as far away from themselves as possible their lenses cannot accommodate enough to bring the letters into focus and thus their reading vision is blurred.

To overcome this, when presbyopic patients look at a nearby object, they use small plus lenses (+1 to +3) that add the missing focusing power, originally supplied by their native lens thickening during accommodation. This is called 'reading add' and may be in the form of separate reading spectacles or may be incorporated into their ordinary spectacles in the form of bifocal or varifocal glasses.

Contact lenses

Contact lenses are becoming more and more popular for correcting the refractive mechanism of the eye. They consist of thin lenses that lie directly on the cornea and alter the contour of its front surface, allowing correct focusing.

Patients tend to use contact lenses to avoid the inconvenience and cosmetic appearance of spectacles.

As you may recall, the cornea takes a large proportion of its nutrients from tears and the atmosphere, because it is avascular. Even the most biocompatible and advanced contact lens materials deprive the cornea of some of these nutrients. Contact lenses put the cornea at risk of hypoxia that may manifest in the growth of blood vessels into the peripheral cornea and problems with the healing of its superficial cells.

Many different materials are used to make modern contact lenses. Some are harder than others. Harder lenses are usually used to correct high refractive errors or large degrees of astigmatism. Gas-permeable lenses are designed to allow oxygen, tears and nutrients to pass through them, with the aim of keeping the underlying cornea healthy. Daily and monthly disposable lenses are now available.

Contact lenses also put patients at risk of corneal infections and ulcers. They compromise the normal defence mechanisms of the eye and interfere with the circulation of the tear film, preventing normal blinking from clearing foreign particles and microbial contaminants from the surface of the cornea. In addition, bacterial pathogens may stick to the contact lens and, by having a foreign material to act as a nidus, may grow and eventually invade the cornea, causing sight-threatening infections.

The key to safe contact lens wear is hygiene and avoiding overwear. Strict cleanliness when handling and disinfecting lenses is essential.

Surgical correction of refractive errors

Many patients do not want the inconvenience associated with contact lenses and look for a permanent solution.

Surgical correction of refractive errors is becoming more and more popular. It usually involves changing the shape of the cornea in order to affect the way it refracts light, allowing it to bring light into focus directly on to the macula.

Initially, this was done by making incisions in the cornea to change its curvature, a procedure called radial keratotomy.

Now with the development of a laser precise enough to shave off minute amounts of corneal tissue (excimer laser), laser refractive surgery is increasingly used. An early technique involved scraping off the corneal epithelium and applying the laser to the underlying corneal stroma, with the aim of changing corneal curvature and thus the refractive power of the eye. This procedure is called photorefractive keratectomy (PRK) and is still used. The corneal epithelium then grows back over the surface but, until this is complete, patients are in a lot of discomfort. The process is also complicated sometimes by haze clouding the vision due to exaggerated epithelial healing.

A newer technique called laser in situ keratomileusis (LASIK) is now widely practised. This involves slicing through the middle of the corneal stroma with a fine blade (a microkeratome), lifting up the flap and applying the laser to the underlying stroma to change the shape of the cornea. The flap is then laid back down and sticks into place (figures 7.10a–d). The patient recovers quickly and the procedure is carried out under topical/drop anaesthesia.

So far results appear very good, but only time will tell whether the outcomes are universally good in the long-term.

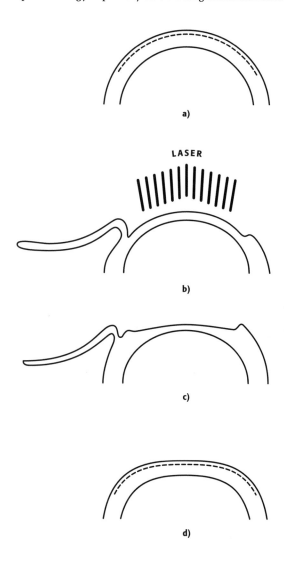

LASER

FIGURES 7.10 a–d a) An incomplete slice is made horizontally through the cornea (dashed line). b) A flap of cornea is folded back and laser applied to the stroma underneath to remove a specified thickness of it. c) This leaves a flatter profile of the cornea. d) The flap is replaced and sticks on by itself. The cornea is now much flatter and thus has less refractive power.

Examination techniques

8 | Examination techniques in the GP surgery

Although in an ideal world every examination would be done 'by the book', in practice short cuts and mini-examinations are inevitable in the busy surgery. As long as the key features of any pathology are elicited, and the examination is safe, abridged examination techniques are adequate.

Not every ophthalmic assessment requires the use of an ophthalmoscope. A good examination can be done with simple tools that are easily to hand.

Ideal kit

- An ophthalmoscope – rechargeable (make sure it is continually charged).
- A bright light source – a pen torch or a Maglight.
- A method of testing vision – ideally a Snellen chart, placed 6m from the patient.
- A magnifying lens – any form of magnifier will do. The ophthalmoscope with a plus lens dialled up can be used.
- Some fluorescein-impregnated strips – once placed in contact with the tears, the fluorescein spreads and covers the ocular surface, highlighting any areas of deficient epithelium. A cobalt blue light will help detect staining.
- A drop of local anaesthetic – any anaesthetic will do, e.g. amethocaine or benoxinate. Boxes of single-use Minims are easily purchased.
- Dilating drops – short-acting drops such as tropicamide are ideal.

Assessing visual acuity

Ideally, a Snellen chart should be used but any form of reading or vision-based test will suffice. Snellen acuity is handy for assessing objectively the degree of visual loss and charting change in acuity over time. However, simple reading print is sufficient for a gross comparative estimation of vision. If a patient who could read small print in the newspaper with both eyes the day before can now only read the headlines with one of their eyes, they have lost vision.

With the chart at 6m, the smallest line that the patient can read represents their vision. If they read the 24 line, their vision is 6/24 (six–24 or six over 24). If they cannot read any line but can count fingers, their vision is 'count fingers'. Test their vision when they are wearing their most recent distance spectacles. Try also to get them to look through a pinhole (simply punch a small hole in a piece of paper) to see if their vision can improve. The pinhole acuity will mimic their best possible vision. If their vision does improve, it may mean that they need new spectacles and should see their optician.

Assessing visual field

Sit in front of the patient and close one of your eyes. The patient should close their opposite eye and stare straight at your open eye. Use an object like a hatpin or the tip of a biro and bring the small object in from the periphery. Test one eye at a time and ensure the patient keeps staring straight into your eye. When the patient sees the object, they will tell you – it should be the same moment you see it too. Bring the object all the way in until they – and you – are staring straight at it. Keep encouraging the patient to tell you if they lose sight of it at any stage. If the object disappears at any stage, the patient has a localised visual field defect.

Always remember the visual field defects you are trying to elicit or exclude.

Defects in one eye represent pathology anterior to the chiasm, i.e. optic nerves or retina. Visual field loss not crossing the vertical midline in both eyes points to pathology behind the chiasm. Visual field loss in an arc around the central vision is characteristic of glaucoma. A defect respecting the vertical midline in each eye, i.e. loss of one side or the other, is a hemianopia (*see* Chapter 2), which may be bitemporal or homonymous (matching).

A central field defect will represent some form of macular disease or optic nerve pathology – get the patient to look at your face one eye at a time – 'any bits missing?'

Assessing pupil reactions

See if the pupils are the same size. A slight discrepancy is acceptable and occurs in 20% of the normal population. As long as the pupils react normally and the ratio of pupil sizes remains the same in all light conditions, the most likely diagnosis is essential anisocoria (*see* Chapter 2).

Change the lighting in the room and see what happens to the pupil sizes. You may uncover a pathological difference in pupil sizes.

Shine a light source on each eye. Both pupils should constrict equally when the light is shone into either of them. The degree of constriction depends on how bright the light is and, more importantly, on how bright the brain sees this light. In optic nerve damage the transmission of light is impaired along the nerve and the brain 'sees' lights as duller.

Shining a light into an eye with optic nerve disease will elicit a slower pupil response than shining it into the fellow healthy eye. Start with the light on one eye causing both pupils to constrict. Move the light over to the other eye. While it is in transit across the nose neither eye gets illumination and both pupils begin to dilate back to their baseline size. When the light reaches the other eye both pupils constrict again as long as that eye is normal. In the abnormal situation when the light is moved over to an eye with a relative afferent pupillary defect (RAPD) the pupil continues to dilate rather than constricting again. That eye sees a duller light due to the nerve pathology and does not think it has to constrict again in response to it.

Ophthalmoscopy

Make sure the battery is fully charged and the pupil dilated with one drop of tropicamide 1%.

There is often concern about dilating a patient's pupils in case they develop angle-closure glaucoma. This is a risk, but it is minimal. The need for adequate examination overrides this risk if you are careful. If the patient is emmetropic or myopic, their chances of having a shallow anterior chamber and thus a risk of angle closure are slim. Look at the patient from the side, and you should see that their cornea is dome-shaped. Very long-sighted people are at a greater risk of developing angle closure. Counsel the patient adequately and refer them immediately to the hospital eye service if their eye becomes red or their vision goes blurry. Patients should not drive until the drop has worn off.

Dim the light slightly. Ask the patient to look at a specific point on the wall. Rotate the lens dial on the ophthalmoscope to zero and look through it. Look for the red reflex. Get down to the same level as the patient and approach them from approximately 15° to one side of straight. Follow the red reflex in. Eventually you should see the retinal vessels or the disc. Do not stop. Move in until you are about 2 cm from the eye. The closer you are, the bigger your field of view.

Move the dial for the lenses until the image is clear. Rotate the dial five clicks one way and if your view has not cleared, stop and go back five clicks the other way (taking you back to zero). Now go five clicks further and it is to be hoped that at some stage the image will clear. Most fundi can be seen adequately with ophthalmoscope lenses at between +5 and –5.

Look at the disc and the vessels. Move laterally from the disc to look at the macula or, even better, ask the patient to look directly into the light. To see the peripheries of the retina, look straight into the eye and ask the patient to look up and out (superotemporal quadrant), up and in (superonasal quadrant), down and out (inferotemporal quadrant), and down and in (inferonasal quadrant).

Fluorescein staining

In order to detect any damage to the ocular surface and particularly the corneal epithelium, it is important to stain the eye. Fluorescein strips are readily available and easy to use. Ask the patient to look up and place the tip of the strip into the inferior conjunctival fornix. The patient's own tears will soak into the strip and release yellow fluorescein on to the eye. Asking the patient to blink a few times will spread the fluorescein over the eye. It is usually better to administer an anaesthetic drop to the eye first.

The normal corneal epithelium will resist the fluorescein, but the stain will highlight the bare corneal stroma in any patches that are missing, and thus damaged. This fluorescein staining is best seen with a blue light and will show up green.

Sometimes patients say they are in so much pain that they cannot open their eyes. This points to a corneal pathology. In order to examine the eye you will need to put in a drop of local anaesthetic. It may be a struggle, but the patient will be thankful for the temporary relief of their symptoms. Once the cornea is anaesthetised, you will be able to examine it and stain it.

Everting upper lid

It is important to look under the top lid to assess whether there is a foreign body and to look for abnormal conjunctiva.

Ask the patient to look down and grasp their upper eyelashes. Place a cotton bud or similar thin stick on to the lid at the level of the upper border of the tarsal plate. Pull the lid by the lashes up and over the bud. This will allow you to see the under-surface.

Eye movements

Are the eyes straight?

Shine a light at the patient and look at the corneal reflexes (where the light reflects on to the cornea). Are they symmetrical?

Ask the patient to keep their head still and to look directly at your light. Do they see one or two lights? If they see two, they have a baseline deviation in ocular alignment – *see* Chapter 13, Cover testing.

Ask the patient to follow your light with their eyes only – tell them that you will assume they see only one light unless they tell you otherwise.

Move your light into all the primary positions of gaze.

If they do see double, are the two images one above the other or side by side? Vertical diplopia is caused by a vertical muscle problem, horizontal diplopia by a problem with the medial or lateral rectus.

9 | Ophthalmoscopy

Ophthalmoscopy is the technique whereby the fundus is visualised through the pupil. It is usually carried out through a pharmacologically dilated pupil, although limited views can be obtained through undilated pupils.

The ophthalmoscope uses lenses and a light source to visualise (predominately) the posterior segment (back) of the eye. The ophthalmoscope incorporates many different powers of lenses to overcome refractive errors in the patient's eyes. If the patient is emmetropic (i.e. does not require spectacles), then any incoming light will automatically be focused upon the retina. When the examiner looks into these eyes with the ophthalmoscope, the image will be clear, even without the use of the built-in lenses (assuming the examiner is also emmetropic). If the patient's focusing apparatus is not perfect, then the light bouncing off the retina will not be focused and the image the examiner sees will be blurred. Lenses will therefore be needed to bring this image into focus.

There are many types of ophthalmoscope, but they all work in essentially the same way. They may be battery operated or rechargeable. The light source/bulb is housed in the body of the ophthalmoscope, and the light bounces off a mirror into the patient's eye. The reflected image is seen through the lenses. Because the examiner is seeing the retina directly through the pupil, this piece of equipment is called a direct ophthalmoscope.

Ophthalmologists often use special lenses to obtain virtual or projected three-dimensional views of the retina, either at the slit lamp or with a head-mounted apparatus – this is called indirect ophthalmoscopy.

Ophthalmoscopes usually have a small dial on the front to change the light emitted from the shape of a large circle to a small circle or a slit; or to a green (red-free) light. The uses of these settings are explained below.

Direct ophthalmoscopy gives a highly magnified assessment of the retina, but allows only a small field of view.

Examination technique

Introduce yourself.

Seat the patient and ask them to look at ('fix on') a specific point in the distance (select a light switch or equivalent on the wall of the examination room as this stops their eyes from wandering).

The patient should ideally be dilated.

Check the ophthalmoscope – ensure:

- The light is on and bright
- The light is pointing the right way (away from you!)
- You have selected the correct light setting (usually the large circle of light to give you the best chance of getting a decent view), and
- That the dial/lenses are on zero.

If you have a refractive error and are not wearing contact lenses, you can dial up your own refractive error on the ophthalmoscope's lenses before you begin.

Get down to the patient's eye level and maintain a distance of approximately 1 m.

Use your right eye and right hand to examine the patient's right eye and your left eye/left hand to examine the left eye.

Look through the ophthalmoscope and shine the light into the patient's eyes from a distance – observe the red reflex. If there is no obstruction to the reflection of the light from the retina, you will see a bright red shine (like the red eye seen on photos). If the patient has a cataract, the bright red background will be blocked by black, spoke-like opacities. If there is opacity in the vitreous or an extremely dense cataract, the red reflex will be globally dull. Compare the red reflexes between eyes to ensure that a reduced red reflex is indeed pathological.

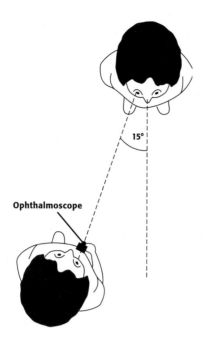

15°

Ophthalmoscope

FIGURE 9.1 **The examiner should approach the patient from approximately 15° from straight to allow them to see the optic disc.**

Afro-Caribbean and Asian patients tend to have a natural dark red reflex, due to large amounts of pigment in their retinal pigment epithelial (RPE) layer (the layer of cells under the clear retina), so it is important to compare the two eyes before diagnosing an abnormality.

Approach the patient at eye level and at approximately 15° to one side (figure 9.1). This should bring your view immediately on to the optic disc.

Keep looking at the red reflex all the way in and take your time. If you lose the red reflex, move the ophthalmoscope vertically or horizontally until you regain it. Do not be afraid of backing away and starting again.

When you are approximately two inches away, an image should come into focus. You should be looking at the optic disc or you should see one of the major retinal blood vessels. A common mistake is for the examiner to stop the moment they see the retina. At this range your field of view is too small. Continue to approach the patient – the closer the better – until you achieve maximum field of view.

If you are not looking at the optic disc, follow the blood vessels as they get larger and you should come on to the disc.

(NB. The disc will usually fill nearly all of your view when you are looking straight at it (figure 9.2). This is a common source of confusion, as novices expect the disc to sit neatly in the centre of the view, as shown in text books.)

Look carefully at the disc. If you have a good view, then the media will be clear and should be commented on. (The media is a general term describing the clarity of the vitreous cavity.) If the view is out of focus, move the dial a few clicks up to see if the image clears. If not, move the dial in the opposite direction back to zero and then on by a few more clicks. Most patients you examine will have a small refractive error, which means you will not have to move the dial too far from zero. If you move the dial too much, you will move into the high lenses and your view will become less and less clear. If this happens, it is best to stop, put the dial back to zero and try again. If you still cannot achieve a clear view, then methodically go up to higher plus and minus lens powers. Check the patient's spectacles – if you have to go up to very high lens powers, they should be wearing really thick spectacles.

(NB. Positive lenses are represented by black numbers, while negative lenses have red or green numbers.)

If you struggle, ask the examiner if the patient is long- or short-sighted as this will give you a clue as to what lenses you should be using. The examiner will not tell you if they don't want to.

If the patient is long-sighted (hypermetropic) then you will probably need to use the plus lenses on the ophthalmoscope (black) in order to get a clear fundal image. If the patient is short-sighted (myopic), you will need minus lenses (green or red).

If the patient has a massive refractive error and you cannot overcome it with the ophthalmoscope, try examining the patient when they are wearing their distance spectacles. Their own lenses will do the focusing for you.

When assessing a disc, it is important to comment on or document three features: the colour, contour and margins.

Colour □ a normal healthy disc is yellow-pink. A pale optic disc is whiter. Compare it with the colour of the optic disc in the other – it is to be hoped, healthy – eye.

Contour □ here it is important to assess the cup–disc ratio. A normal disc is fairly flat. In certain conditions, particularly glaucoma, however, the centre of the disc becomes deeper than the surrounding disc, i.e. a cup forms. Compare the vertical distance between the top and bottom of the cup to the total vertical diameter of the disc. This will give you the (vertical) cup–disc ratio. A normal disc has no cup. However, a small (physiological) cup is a normal variant and simply represents the dipping into the optic nerve of the radially orientated nerve fibre layer. With the direct ophthalmoscope, you only obtain a two-dimensional image, thus making it difficult to assess the three-dimensional cup effectively. Observe where the retinal blood vessels bend to dip over the brim and down the sides of the cup, as this should give you the required clues as to its position (figure 9.3).

Margins □ essentially the question here is whether there is any disc swelling. If the disc is swollen, the margins will be indistinct and the nerve fibres will be visible as linear, radially projecting 'glistenings', due to their engorgement (figure 9.4).

Now look at the arteries and veins, and comment on their calibre. The veins should be slightly larger than the arteries (artery:vein ratio = 2:3). Counterintuitively, the retinal vein at the optic disc may be pulsating, not the artery – this is normal.

If the arteries are markedly smaller than the veins, there is arteriolar attenuation (thinned arterial system, usually caused by ageing or hypertensive changes). Follow the vessels away from the disc, keeping to the superotemporal, inferotemporal, superonasal and inferonasal arcades. The arcades are the main trunks of the retinal arteries and veins running together (figure 6.1).

In order to view the peripheral retina, ask the patient to look up and out, and look straight into their eye. This will ensure you are looking at the superotemporal retina. Ask the patient to look up and in so that you can see the superonasal retina, and so on.

In order to view the anterior segment – i.e. the cornea, anterior chamber and the iris – dial up +8 to +10 on the ophthalmoscope and use it as a magnifying glass. To obtain a clear view you must be within about an inch of the patient. This will give you a magnified view of the front of the eye. Look at the tip of your finger first to ensure you have dialled up the correct lens and to get an idea of how close you need to be to see a clear image.

Look first at the lid margins and the eyelashes. Then assess the conjunctiva – hold the lower lid down and ask the patient to look up, down, left and right. Now look at the cornea – it should be clear, bright and shiny. It can be useful to use the slit light to assess the anterior chamber; this will give you a cross-section view of the three-dimensional anatomy and the relation of the cornea, iris and lens.

The large circular light is used for most dilated fundus examinations. The smaller circle may be used when examining patients who are excessively photophobic or if the pupil cannot be dilated. The green (red-free) light is used to examine the blood vessels, as it will be reflected from the red vessels, which will appear black, thereby helping visualisation.

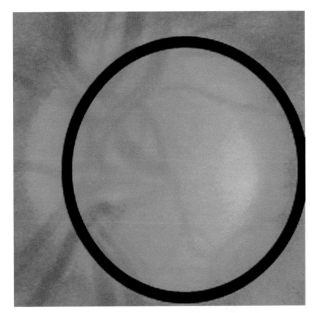

FIGURE 9.2 **View obtained through ophthalmoscope of optic disc. The black circle outlines exactly what is seen. The whole optic disc is rarely visualised as a whole.**

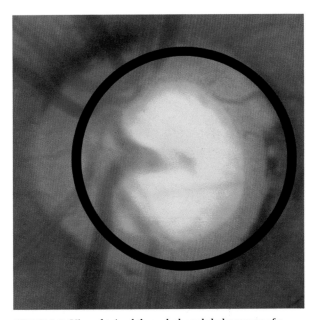

FIGURE 9.3 **View obtained through the ophthalmoscope of a cupped optic disc. The vessels can be seen dipping over the edge of the cup. The presence of a pigment ring around the optic disc is a normal finding.**

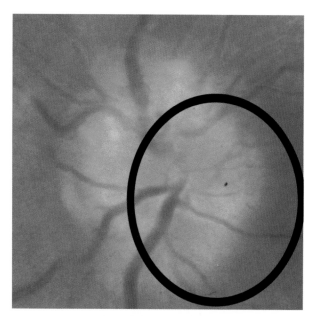

FIGURE 9.4 View obtained through the ophthalmoscope of a swollen optic disc. Compared with figures 9.2 and 9.3 you can see that the disc margin is indistinct and the blood vessels are not as clear because they are engulfed by swollen nerve fibres.

10 | Visual fields

The visual field is the total area we are able to see when we look straight ahead. When we look directly ahead and focus on an object, we are bringing that object on to our visual axis, and the light from it is passing through the centre of our cornea, the centre of the lens and the centre of the vitreous cavity to the centre of the macula (the fovea). We are using our fovea to see the exact detail. As you read these words, the light from the letters and words is hitting your fovea and macula. The macula is dominated by densely packed cone photoreceptors that are responsible for fine and colour vision, and it is responsible for your central 30° of vision.

You can obviously see more than 30° when you look straight ahead. If you test your own vision by moving your hand around you will see that you can actually see your hand, albeit not entirely clearly, over a large area. This area of view is called your field of vision or visual field.

The peripheral visual field is 'seen' by the peripheral retina (i.e. the area of retina outside the macula). This area of retina has no cone photoreceptors, but contains rod photoreceptors. Rods are less densely distributed and do not detect colour to the same degree as cone receptors. As rod receptors are the predominant type of receptor responsible for night vision, in low light we tend to see in black and white.

The visual field is often described as a 'hill of vision'. If you draw a three-dimensional plot of retinal sensitivity (i.e. the ability of the retina to detect fine detail) against the distance from your visual axis (effectively the distance from the fovea), the highest point (the most sensitive part of the retina) will be in the very centre (the 'peak of the hill'), and this sensitivity will rapidly reduce as you move further away, being very low when the plot reaches the far retinal peripheries, where only the widely spaced rods are active.

If you stare straight ahead and place some writing into your peripheral vision, you will note that you can see that words are there, but they will be impossible to read. The retina in this area just is not sensitive enough to allow you to pick out the letters and words. If you now move your eyes to look at the words, thus bringing them to the top of your hill of vision, they become clear.

The normal visual field of one eye extends approximately 90° temporally (out), 60° nasally (in) and superiorly (blocked nasally by the nose and superiorly by the supra-orbital ridge), and 70° inferiorly.

In order clinically to assess a patient's visual field, we can use an automated or semi-automated test such as the Goldmann or Humphreys visual field machines (*see* Chapter 21, Glaucoma) or we can place objects into different parts of the patient's field of vision and ask if they can see them.

Examination technique

Introduce yourself.

Ensure adequate light in the room.

Ask the patient if they wear distance spectacles.

If they do, ask them if they can see reasonably well without them.

If they have a high refractive error and struggle to see without their spectacles, then they should wear these spectacles for the test.

It should be mentioned to the examiner at this point that the glasses may cause some artefact in the peripheral visual field, due to the frame of the spectacles getting in the way and also to an edge effect from their lens (lenses do not focus light properly at their edges – hence you only get a clear image when you look through the centre of a magnifying glass).

Sit directly in front of the patient about 1m away and at the same eye level.

As a screening method, ask the patient to look directly at your nose and ask them if there are any 'bits missing', 'black patches' or 'blurred areas'. This will detect gross binocular (both eyes open) central visual field problems.

Now repeat the test with one eye at a time. Ask the patient to cover one eye with the palm of their hand (right hand for right eye and left hand for left). It is important that the patient use their palm as sometimes they attempt to look through their fingers. This is particularly the case if the patient is trying, consciously or subconsciously, to deny they have a visual problem.

Ask the patient to stare at your nose again and ask them about any abnormalities obscuring your face. If they volunteer that there is a central 'blob' or 'blur' blocking their view of the centre of your face, then they probably have some form of central scotoma (visual field defect), most likely due to a macular pathology. If they say that half of your face is missing, they probably have some form of hemianopia (see below).

For a formal visual field assessment, you should use red and white hatpins. However, testing with fingers should be acceptable, as long as it is stipulated and understood that this is a further screening test and does not give entirely accurate results.

Finger testing

Ask the patient to cover their left eye with the palm of their left hand and you should close your opposite eye (i.e. the patient closes their left eye and you close your right).

Ask the patient to stare at your left eye.

Now you are eye to eye and your visual field should match that of the patient if their vision is normal. You will now be able to compare the patient's visual field to your normal visual field and detect any abnormalities. A common error is to ask the patient to look at your nose. This is incorrect, as your visual fields no longer overlap – the patient is looking slightly down and in towards your nose.

Waggle a bent index finger directly between your eye and the patient's eye approximately halfway between you. Ask the patient if they can see it. This will show the patient what to look for during the visual field assessment and also ensures that they have sufficient vision to co-operate during the examination.

Tell the patient that you will be bringing your finger in from the peripheries of their vision and that you want them to say 'yes' when they see the finger appearing.

Now bring in your finger from the superotemporal (upper outer) quadrant. You should see it coming in and, at the same time or shortly after, the patient should see it too. Once the patient sees the finger, continue to bring it in towards the centre of your (and the patient's) vision. Ask the patient if it disappears at any

stage. Once the finger is in the centre of vision, document the relative position of the most peripheral field (when the patient first saw the finger) and whether there were any visual field defects (any areas where your finger disappeared).

Repeat this process in the inferotemporal (lower outer) quadrant, then the inferonasal (lower inner) quadrant and finally the superonasal (upper inner) quadrant.

Use your left hand to examine the temporal field of the patient's right eye and the nasal field of the patient's left eye. Use your right hand for the temporal field of the left eye and the nasal field of the right eye. This will stop you having to cross over your arm awkwardly.

Using hatpins

This technique is far more accurate and ensures consistent visual field assessments.

Hatpins are available from many shops. If it proves difficult to obtain the red and white ones required for this technique, then buy hatpins of any colour and paint them with red and white nail varnish.

The process is identical to that above, but you use hatpins instead of fingers.

Begin with the white hatpin. Place it in the central vision to ensure the patient can see it and then explain that you are going to bring the pinhead in from their peripheral vision and you want them to tell you when they first see it. Continue to move the pin towards the central vision and ask the patient to tell you if it disappears. If it does disappear, move the pin horizontally and vertically until it reappears, thus mapping the precise size and shape of their visual field defect.

Now use the red hatpin. Place it in the central vision to ensure the patient can see it. Ask them what colour it is and then explain that you are going to bring the pinhead in from their peripheral vision as before, and again they should tell you when they first see it. Also, explain to the patient that when they first see the red pin, it will appear black. (Try it yourself, it really does look black. Remember the rods are responsible for peripheral visual field and they cannot see colour.) Ask the patient to tell you when they first see the pin, but continue to move it towards the central vision and ask the patient when it first appears red. At this point you will know that the pin has crossed into the macula and you will have an idea of the macular field of vision.

Continue bringing the pin in until it lies in the centre of both your vision and that of the patient (i.e. you are both staring straight at it), all the while asking the patient if it disappears at any stage.

If it does disappear, plot any visual field defect within the macula by moving the hatpin around the area of visual field loss.

Assessing the blind spot

The blind spot represents the area of the fundus where the optic disc resides (see figure 10.1). In this area, there is no retina and thus no photoreceptors to detect light. The blind spot is an example of a negative scotoma. We cannot see anything at all within the blind spot (making it an absolute scotoma) but we are not conscious of this. The brain fills in this area of our perception, and our vision in that area appears continuous until we place a small object (such as the hatpin) within it. If this were a positive scotoma (see below) we would see a blank or black patch in our vision and we would be aware of it.

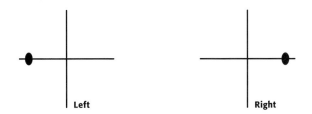

FIGURE 10.1 **Diagrammatic representation of normal visual fields. The blacked out areas represent the blind spots. To imagine what the patient can see, close your right eye and look directly at the middle of the cross-wires on the right diagram. The black areas are scotomas.**

In order to assess the blind spot, we need a red hatpin as the blind spot lies just within the central 30° of vision and thus just within the macula. 'Wagging' fingers are far too large for this task.

Place the red hatpin halfway between you and the patient at approximately 15° to the line drawn directly between your eye and that of the patient (figure 10.2). This should place the pin into your blind spot and that of the patient. If it is not immediately in the correct position, move it slightly horizontally and vertically until the patient says the pin has disappeared. Once the pin is within the blind spot, map it out – it should be the same size as yours.

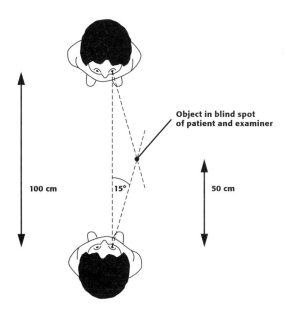

FIGURE 10.2 **To examine the blind spot the examiner should be 1 m from the patient and place a hatpin 50 cm away from them at approximately 15° out.**

Pathology

Localised scotoma

Positive versus negative scotomas

A localised scotoma is a patch of visual field that is lost or reduced in sensitivity. It may be positive, where the patient notices it and sees a blank, blurred or blocked patch in their vision, or it may be negative, where the patient does not notice any defect in their vision at all. Important examples of a negative scotoma are the physiological negative scotoma of the optic disc (the blind spot) and glaucomatous field loss. Patients may lose enormous areas of their visual field and not notice any field loss.

If you examine your own visual field once again you will note that you do not notice any margin or edge to your vision where the field ends. There is no black line where your vision ceases: it just seems to fade away to nothing. If the field of vision gradually constricts, the patient will not be conscious of this creeping loss until all of the peripheral vision has been compromised and the central vision is finally affected.

Absolute versus relative scotomas

Scotomas may be absolute or relative. Within an absolute scotoma, the patient sees nothing within the area of the visual field loss, regardless of how bright the stimulus or object placed into it. In a relative scotoma, retinal sensitivity is reduced, but if the stimulus is large enough or bright enough it will be seen. The blind spot is an example of an absolute scotoma, as however bright an object is placed into the blind spot, the individual cannot possibly see it. Glaucomatous visual field defects begin as relative scotomas but gradually become absolute as the damage progresses.

Localised central/macula scotomas may be related to optic nerve disease, age-related macular degeneration, localised macular haemorrhage beneath or in front of the retina, or other forms of macular disease. Such scotomas tend to be positive, and may be relative or absolute, depending on the damage.

Fully formed retinal scars produce absolute localised scotomas corresponding directly to the area of the scar, as the photoreceptors within this area are lost and no stimulus, however bright, can be seen.

Hemianopia

A hemianopia means that the patient has lost one half of their visual field in both eyes. Patients either lose the nasal or temporal half of their visual field respecting the vertical meridian (i.e. not crossing a vertical line down the centre of the vision in each eye).

Homonymous hemianopia

Patients with a homonymous hemianopia have lost corresponding segments of their visual field in each eye (the field defect is homonymous or 'matching'). If the patient has a right homonymous hemianopia, they have lost their temporal visual field in their right eye and their nasal visual field in their left eye. When they

are looking straight ahead they cannot see anything to the right (figure 10.3). The converse is true for a left homonymous hemianopia.

Locating potential lesions that may cause this phenomenon is easy when you consider the anatomy of the visual pathway. With a right homonymous hemianopia, the patient has lost their right temporal and left nasal field of vision. Light from the right temporal visual field hits the right nasal retina, whereas light from the left nasal visual field hits the left temporal retina. In patients with a right homonymous hemianopia, the light impulses from these two areas of retina are either not reaching the brain or not being processed by the visual cortex.

By tracing the path of the neurones projecting from these areas of retina, we may work out where the pathology lies (figure 10.4). The fibres from the left temporal retina run into the optic nerve, back to the optic chiasm and back to the ipsilateral optic tracts and radiations, finally arriving at the left visual cortex within the left occipital lobe of the brain. The fibres

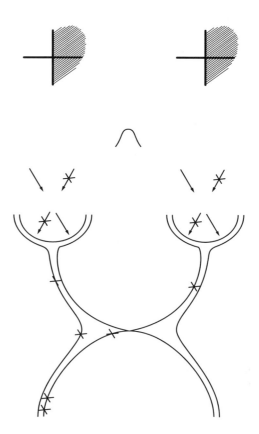

FIGURE 10.4 If the patient has a right homonymous hemianopia they are not seeing light approaching their eyes from the right. This light lands on the nasal retina of the right eye and the temporal retina of the left eye. The impulses from these areas are not reaching the brain. By tracing their paths backwards we can see that they only run together behind the optic chiasm and thus the lesion must be localised there.

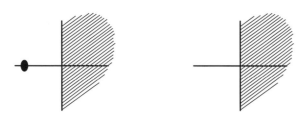

FIGURE 10.3 Diagrammatic representation of a right homonymous hemianopia. When looking out of the left eye the patient cannot see anything to the right of the vertical midline (they still have their normal blind spot). When looking out of the right eye they cannot see anything to the right.

from the right nasal retina run back into the optic nerve and when they reach the optic chiasm, they decussate (cross over to the other side of the brain) and run in the contralateral optic tract to arrive at the visual cortex of the left occipital lobe.

After the optic chiasm, these two groups of neurones travel in close proximity, so a lesion causing a right homonymous hemianopia must lie within the left optic tract or radiation, or involve the left visual cortex itself.

In a homonymous hemianopia, the loss of visual field does not have to involve all the hemifield (all of one side). Degree of visual field loss will vary, depending on how large an area of brain the lesion involves. Small localised lesions may produce smaller homonymous hemianopic defects. Furthermore, the area or pattern of field loss does not have to be identical between each eye, as explained below.

Within the visual cortex, the brain must analyse the data from the corresponding retinal areas of the two eyes in order to create a composite image of what is being seen. In order to facilitate the analysis of the two images, the paired impulses from each eye must arrive at the visual cortex in exactly the same part of the brain. If the corresponding images arrived at opposite sides of the brain, or even if they arrived at the occipital cortex 1cm apart, integration would be difficult. From the optic chiasm to the visual cortex within the optic tracts and radiations, this close proximity between the neurones from the two eyes is not necessary. The further back towards the visual cortex the impulses go, the closer the corresponding segments from each eye run.

Lesions of the visual cortex (commonly due to a cerebrovascular accident) will result in homonymous hemianopias that are identical in shape between the two eyes (figure 10.5). This is called a congruous visual field defect, and occurs because identical pairs of reti-

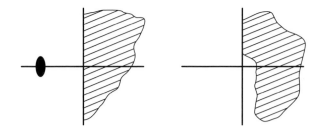

FIGURE 10.6 **The degree of visual field loss in each eye is different but is still all off to one side and not crossing the vertical midline. This is an incongruous homonymous hemianopic defect.**

nal impulses are lost. If a lesion affects the optic tracts or optic radiations (i.e. further forward where the corresponding neurones from each eye are not necessarily running next to each other), then the pattern of visual field loss may not be identical between each eye (an incongruous hemianopic visual field defect; *see* figure 10.6). The more posterior (close to the visual cortex) the pathological lesion is, the more congruous or symmetrical the visual field defects will be.

Bitemporal hemianopia

Patients with a bitemporal hemianopia have a visual defect affecting half their field in both eyes as before, but in this case the field defect is not homonymous (same side), but bitemporal (figure 10.7). A bitemporal hemianopia occurs when a patient loses both temporal visual fields. They can only see centrally, and can be said to have a form of tunnel vision, although in true tunnel vision all the peripheral visual field is lost, and the patient has only a small central 'island' of vision.

Once more we can work out the site of the lesion by thinking about the anatomy. The patient has lost their temporal visual fields in both eyes. The light from these areas falls upon the nasal retina of each eye. Impulses run back through the optic nerve and

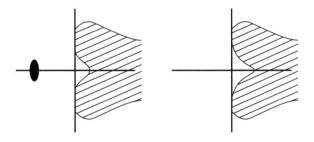

FIGURE 10.5 **An incomplete right homonymous hemianopia. Not all the vision to the right of the vertical midline has been lost and both traces are identical in size and shape. This is a congruous visual field defect. Note that it does not cross the vertical midline.**

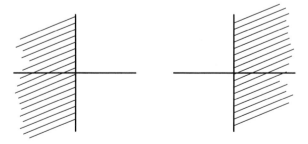

FIGURE 10.7 **A bitemporal hemianopia. The patient cannot see anything to the left of the midline in their left eye and to the right of the midline in their right eye.**

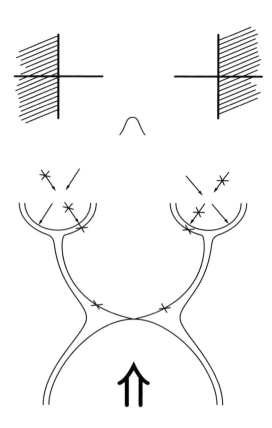

FIGURE 10.8 **If the patient has a bitemporal hemianopia they are not seeing light approaching their eyes from the right in their right eye and from the left in their left eye. This light lands on the nasal retina of both eyes. The impulses from these areas are not reaching the brain. By tracing their paths backwards we can see that they only run together at the optic chiasm, otherwise they are on opposite sides of the brain.**

then cross over in the optic chiasm. From there, they run back on opposite sides of the brain (far away from each other) to the visual cortex.

Lesions of the optic chiasm (the only place where the fibres from the nasal retinas of both eyes run together) result in bitemporal hemianopia (figure 10.8). The commonest cause is compression of the optic chiasm by a pituitary tumour. Patients with a bitemporal hemianopia require neuro-imaging to determine the presence and nature of a space-occupying lesion.

11 | Pupil reactions

The pupil reaction is a physiological response to ensure that an appropriate amount of light enters the eye. Just as in photography, if too much light enters the camera, the image is too bright and full of glare. In response to excessive light, the normal pupil constricts (miosis) to prevent too much light hitting the retina. Conversely, when the retina is unable to detect enough light for sight, the pupil dilates (mydriasis) to let more light in.

The eye and brain can be considered to have an inherent light meter to judge how large the pupil should be. The input to this light meter is from the photoreceptors and retinal fibres that project into the optic nerve.

The pupil response fibres take a slightly different route from the fibres that project to the visual cortex for vision (figure 11.1). Fibres from the temporal retina, i.e. the nasal field of vision, project into the optic nerve and run back to the optic chiasm. From there they run back ipsilaterally within the brain, but leave the visual fibres before they reach the lateral geniculate nucleus (LGN). They then run to a region called the pre-tectal nucleus near the superior colliculus, where the impulse splits and runs to both the right and left Edinger-Westphal nuclei (EWN), in other words, bilaterally.

The EWN is the parasympathetic segment of the third (oculomotor) nerve, and effectively acts as the light sensor. From there, the impulses travel back to the pupillomotor fibres via the third nerve and ciliary ganglion to dictate the pupil size (figure 11.1). The light meter analogy is a simplification but I hope it helps to explain the concept.

Pupil response fibres from the nasal retina of each eye (i.e. temporal field of vision) travel back to the chiasm via the optic nerve and then decussate to travel back towards the contralateral pre-tectal nucleus with the temporal pupil response fibres of the other eye.

The EWN stimulates both pupils equally. Thus there is a direct pupil reflex affecting the eye being stimulated and an equal consensual reflex on the other eye. Light entering both eyes contributes to the eventual pupil size, but the pupils react according to the greatest illumination seen by either eye, so if one eye is covered, the size of both pupils will be dictated by the uncovered eye.

Motor stimulation to the pupillary sphincter muscle is from two main sources, the parasympathetic and sympathetic nervous systems.

Parasympathetic pupillomotor fibres originate in the EWN and run with the oculomotor nerve. They synapse in the ciliary ganglion before reaching the pupil and supplying the pupil sphincter to cause pupil constriction (miosis). Lesions of the parasympathetic supply to the pupil will result in deficient pupil constriction and thus a dilated pupil.

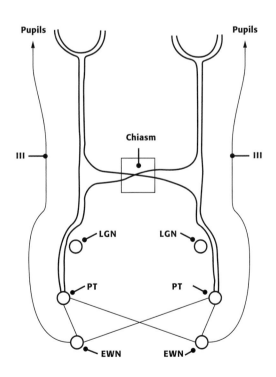

FIGURE 11.1 **The pupil reflex. PT = pre-tectal nucleus. LGN = lateral geniculate nucleus. EWN = Edinger-Westphal nucleus. III = third nerve.**

Sympathetic supply to the pupil is from the sympathetic plexus of nerves. Sympathetic innervation runs a complex course originating from the posterior hypothalamus. Neurones run through the brainstem and out of the spinal cord into the paravertebral sympathetic chain. From there, they run up to the superior cervical ganglion and then into the plexus of nerves surrounding the internal carotid artery. After entering the skull, they run through the cavernous sinus and enter the orbit via the superior orbital fissure. They finally reach the pupil via the long ciliary nerves. Sympathetic innervation causes pupil dilatation (mydriasis). Lesions will result in pathological pupil constriction.

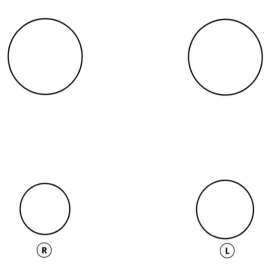

FIGURE 11.2 **The pupils are slightly different sizes. In the light and dark the ratio of the pupil sizes remains the same.**

Examination technique

Observation

Observation is the key initial step in examining the pupils. Look closely at both eyes. Ask the examiner to increase the light of the room to maximum. Both pupils should be equal in size, relatively small and round. If there is a difference in the size, the patient has anisocoria. Look for irregularity in shape, as a distorted pupil margin/shape may indicate a congenital abnormality, inflammation or previous trauma or surgery.

Twenty per cent of the population have essential anisocoria: their pupil sizes are slightly different. This is a normal finding and of no clinical significance as long as pupil reactions are normal (see below). The diameters of the pupils are normally within 1 mm of each other.

Now ask the examiner to turn down the light to a level at which you can just still see the pupils. The pupils should again be identical in size, but now slightly larger.

If the patient had a slight discrepancy between pupil sizes in full light, this difference should remain in dim light. If this is the case, the patient has essential anisocoria, as above. If the difference in pupil sizes alters with a change in the ambient light, one of the pupils is abnormal.

For example, if in bright light you notice that the patient's left pupil is 1 mm larger than the right, you can confidently say the patient has an anisocoria. Now you need to determine whether this is essential (normal/physiological) or pathological. Decrease the light. Both pupils should dilate slightly. If the left pupil is still 1 mm larger than the right and subsequent pupil reaction testing is normal, the patient probably has

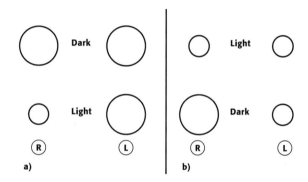

FIGURES 11.3 a and b **a) In the dark the pupil sizes are only slightly different; however, in the light the difference is marked. The abnormal pupil is the one that has failed to constrict normally. b) In the light the pupil sizes appear identical; however, in the dark one of the pupils fails to dilate normally and the discrepancy is marked.**

essential anisocoria (figure 11.2). If when the illumination is increased, you notice that the left pupil is now 4mm larger than the right, you know there is a pathological anisocoria (figure 11.3a). Here the left pupil is probably abnormal, as it failed to constrict despite the increase in light. In figure 11.3b the left pupil is abnormal as it fails to dilate in the dark.

Direct pupil reflex

Have the light in the room sufficiently dim to ensure that both pupils are reasonably dilated but that you can still see them adequately.

Shine your torch into one eye from below. Make sure you shine the light directly into the eye and observe it all the time. The pupil should constrict rapidly. If it does, the patient has an intact direct pupil light reflex.

Now shine the light into the same eye, but this time observe the other eye. The other eye should also constrict briskly when the light is shone into its fellow. If it does, the patient has an intact consensual pupil light reflex.

Swinging flashlight test

If both eyes are normal (see figure 11.4) then when a light is shone into one eye, the light meter will detect the bright light and both pupils will constrict (miose) to, for example, 2 mm. As the light source moves across to the other eye, it passes over the nasal bridge and during that time is not shining into either eye. The light meter is receiving no stimulation except that from the background illumination, and both pupils thus begin to dilate to baseline, e.g. 4 mm. When the light finally reaches the other eye, the bright light is again detected and both pupils constrict again to 2 mm. This is the principle of the swinging flashlight test. Abnormal findings and their implications are discussed below.

If the light reaction is abnormal or absent, then it is worth assessing the near response. When faced with an object of regard that is close up, the eyes must be brought into a position to focus upon it. The eyes converge (move in) to ensure that both foveas are pointing at the same thing. Accommodation occurs, whereby the power of the patient's lens changes in order to increase the refractive power of the eye, and the pupils constrict (miose).

In order to test for the pupil reaction (miosis) stimulated by accommodation, ask the patient to look into the distance and then ask them to focus upon an object one foot in front of them. Ideally, this should be a fine-detailed object or some writing that requires the patient actively to accommodate in order to read it. A pen torch or other light source is less than ideal as the patient does not need to accommodate fully to bring this into focus, unlike when reading print. A normal response is pupil constriction. Some conditions may result in loss of the light reaction, but maintenance of the accommodative reaction (see Chapter 7). If the light reaction is normal, there is usually no need to test for accommodative miosis.

Pathology

Relative afferent pupillary defect

If the optic nerve is damaged or if the retina is so badly damaged as to make it completely ineffective, then when a bright light is shone into the affected eye, its light meter 'sees' a dull light. This is either because the light impulses are not passing through the compromised optic nerve or because the retina is so damaged that it cannot detect the light, and the pupil responds accordingly.

If, for example, the patient described above has optic nerve disease of the left eye and a normal right eye, then when a light is shone into the good right eye, both pupils will constrict to 2 mm as before (an intact direct and consensual reflex). When the same light is shone into the bad eye, the EWN light meter 'sees' a duller light, 'assumes' the pupil does not have to be fully miosed, and so causes both pupils to constrict to only 3 mm (a correct response for the light intensity that the light meter 'believes' is there).

Thus, during a swinging flashlight test, the course of events is as follows (figure 11.5):

i)   Light shone into good eye: both pupils constrict to 2 mm

ii) Light moving across nose: both pupils begin to dilate, heading for 4 mm (baseline – the appropriate size of pupils for the ambient light in the room)

iii) Light reaches bad eye: EWN 'sees' duller light and 'thinks' the pupils should be at 3½ mm – thus *both* pupils *continue to dilate* rather than constricting again to 2 mm as would occur if this eye were normal.

This patient demonstrates a left relative afferent pupillary defect (RAPD).

RAPD is a sign of optic nerve disease or marked diffuse/extensive retinal disease. Problems such as cataracts or vitreous haemorrhage do not usually cause an RAPD. This is because although these pathologies scatter and distort the light so much that vision is impossible, the total light entering the eye eventually hits the retina, thus stimulating the light meter to the appropriate level.

Another sign of optic nerve disease is a phenomenon called red desaturation. The eye with optic nerve disease sees colours as washed out. If you show the patient a red object, they will notice that the red appears duller to their damaged eye. The reason for this is similar to that for RAPD. The red impulses transmitted from the macula by its neurones are impeded and degraded by passing through the damaged optic nerve. The brain thus sees the object as less red.

If the patient has an optic nerve lesion, they will have either a total or relative afferent pupillary defect.

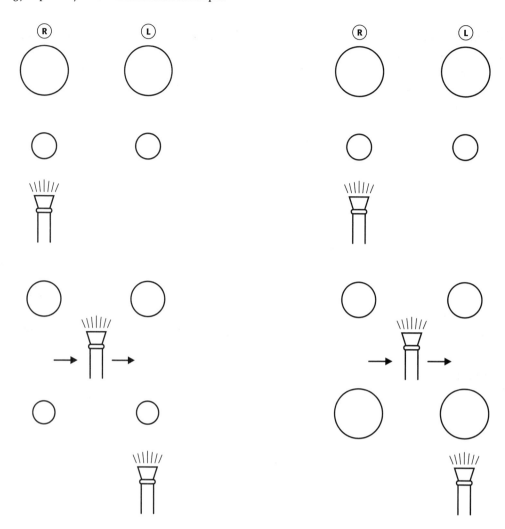

FIGURE 11.4 When no light is shone on the eyes the pupils adopt sizes appropriate for the room illumination. The light is shone into the right pupil causing a symmetrical direct and consensual reflex – both pupils constrict. The light is then moved over the nose. Both pupils begin to dilate as they are receiving only the room illumination. Once the light reaches the left eye both pupils constrict normally.

FIGURE 11.5 There is a normal right direct and consensual reflex. While the light is travelling over the nose both pupils begin to dilate as they are only receiving the room illumination. When the light gets to the left eye the pupils do not constrict again but continue to dilate. This is a left afferent pupillary defect.

If the optic nerve is totally transected, the patient will have a blind eye and thus a total afferent pupillary defect. In this case, shining the light into the blind eye will cause no consensual or direct reflex, but shining the light into the unaffected eye will result in a normal direct and consensual reflex. *Both pupils will be the same size.* An afferent defect is only relative because there is still a reflex present that may be compared with the other eye, and it is only by this comparison that it may be detected.

Holmes-Adie pupil

A Holmes-Adie pupil is a form of acquired internal ophthalmoplegia. It is thought to result from a viral attack on the ciliary ganglion that damages the efferent (motor) parasympathetic pathway to the pupil. It commonly affects young to middle-aged adults and may present as blurred vision. The pupil becomes tonically dilated, reacting poorly to light and accommodation. Indeed, accommodative power may be significantly reduced and patients may struggle to focus on near objects. The other pupil is usually normal, and so the abnormal pupil will be the dilated one. This condition may be bilateral, however.

Horner's syndrome

Horner's syndrome is a congenital or acquired condition caused by an interruption of the sympathetic nervous supply to the eye. As already described, the sympathetic supply comes via the spine, ascends in the neck running close to the carotid vessels, and from there to the eye. Pathology may interrupt this supply in the spine, in the thorax or in the neck, resulting in a constricted pupil among other features. The nerve plexus runs in close proximity to the apical pleura of the lung and thus a neoplasm of the lung apices (called a Pancoast tumour) may result in an ipsilateral Horner's syndrome.

Horner's syndrome results in a mild 1–2mm ptosis (droopy upper eyelid), miosis of the pupil (small pupil), anhidrosis (loss of sympathetic innervation to one half of the face, resulting in decreased sweating) and apparent enophthalmos (the droopy upper lid and slight elevation of the lower lid make the eye appear recessed).

In acquired cases, it is important to investigate the patient for a neoplastic lesion compressing or invading the sympathetic pathway.

Argyll Robertson pupil

Classically, this condition is associated with syphilitic (luetic) disease affecting the pupillomotor pathways. The patient will have poor or absent light reflexes but maintain near/accommodative induced pupil constriction. This phenomenon is called light-near dissociation.

NB. Be careful not to mention syphilis in front of the patient. It is best to refer to luetic disease to avoid offence.

Traumatic mydriasis

After injury or surgery, the pupil may be distorted and if the pupil sphincter muscle has been damaged, it cannot react normally. Non-penetrating injury may result in subtotal sphincter muscle rupture, secondary to a concussion wave of energy being transmitted throughout the ocular structures. The pupil will be slightly dilated (traumatic mydriasis) and its reactions, particularly constriction, will be impaired. Sometimes a traumatic mydriasis will resolve but it is often permanent and may cause problems with glare and blurring of vision, due to too much light entering the eye.

12 | Ocular movements

In order to ensure that the brain receives complementary images from each eye for integration and formulation into 'vision', the eyes must be pointing in the same direction. This maintenance of alignment is vital to avoid visual discrepancy between the eyes and, therefore, diplopia (double vision). Children can ignore the image from one eye when confronted with dissimilar images, but adults do not have this ability.

A complex neural mechanism ensures that the eyes move together in a symmetrical manner. When the right eye moves to the right to look at an object in the patient's right field of vision, the left eye also moves to the right to exactly the same degree in order to supply an identical complementary image to the brain. The movement of both eyes to fix on an object originally within the peripheral visual field (i.e. to look at something to the side) is called a saccade.

This process is controlled through the cranial nerve nuclei of the oculomotor nerves and their various interconnections with other parts of the midbrain and the cerebellum. Impulses from the oculomotor centres in the midbrain are sent via the third, fourth and sixth cranial nerves to cause precise movements of both eyes during saccades.

If there is a defect within the neural oculomotor control system – e.g. as a result of a problem affecting the cranial nerve nuclei, the nerves themselves or the ocular muscles – the eyes will be unable to move correctly. This will manifest as a deviated eye or defective eye movement.

The commonest oculomotor problem that will be encountered (particularly in examinations or assessments) will be a cranial nerve palsy.

Three cranial nerves supply eye movement:

- Oculomotor nerve (third) – supplies all the recti muscles except the lateral rectus (hence superior, inferior and medial recti), the inferior oblique and the levator palpabrae muscle
- Trochlear nerve (fourth) – supplies the superior oblique muscle
- Abducent nerve (sixth) – supplies the lateral rectus.

To simplify, the abducent nerve causes the eye to abduct (look out), while the trochlear nerve causes the eye to look down and in (towards the tip of the nose).

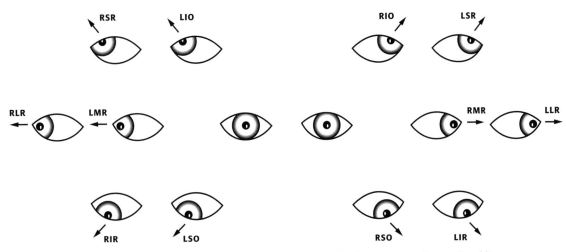

FIGURE 12.1 **The eye movements and the major extraocular muscles responsible for them.** RSO = right superior oblique, RIO = right inferior oblique, RSR = right superior rectus, RIR = right inferior rectus, RMR = right medial rectus, RLR = right lateral rectus. LSO = left superior oblique, LIO = left inferior oblique, LSR = left superior rectus, LIR = left inferior rectus, LMR = left medial rectus, LLR = left lateral rectus.

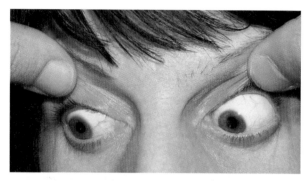

FIGURE 12.2 The orbits are pyramidal and pointing slightly outwards. With the eyes pointing straight they are actually medially rotated in relation to the orbits. Thus the vertical recti do not cause straight up and down ocular movements.

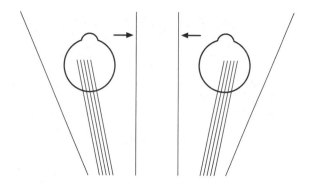

FIGURE 12.3 A patient with a left fourth nerve palsy. The discrepancy of eye movements is not clear until the corneal light reflexes in the pupil are compared. The left eye is failing to move down and in enough thus the corneal light reflex is close to the pupil margin on the left whereas in the normal right eye it is more central.

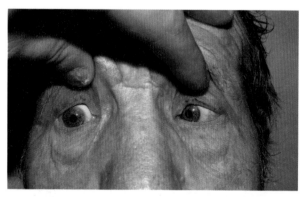

FIGURE 12.4 Patient with a right sixth nerve palsy. The patient is attempting to look right; however, the right eye is failing to match the left due to weakness of the abducent nerve. The corneal reflexes are asymmetrical with the right reflex resting at the pupil margin while the left is midway onto the iris.

The third nerve supplies all other eye movements.

Each extraocular muscle may be thought of as primarily moving the eye in one particular direction (figure 12.1):

- Medial rectus: adducts the eye (moves eye in)
- Lateral rectus: abducts the eye (moves eye out)
- Superior rectus: moves eye up and out
- Inferior rectus: moves eye down and out
- Superior oblique: moves eye down and in
- Inferior oblique: moves eye up and in.

Note that the superior and inferior recti do not move the eye directly up or down, as you might expect. This is because, although these muscles insert into the top and bottom of the globe, the eye is actually always turned in slightly when looking straight ahead. The orbit forms a pyramid pointing backwards and medially. In order for the vertical recti muscles to have a purely vertical effect, the globe has to line up with the apex of the pyramid, i.e. the eye has to be abducted slightly. When the eye is in primary position (looking straight ahead), it is not aligned with the axis of the orbit and is thus effectively adducted, giving the vertical recti a different total effect (figure 12.2).

If one of the oculomotor nerves is weak or inactive, the patient will experience diplopia, because the affected eye will be unable to activate the denervated muscle and will thus be unable to maintain itself in the appropriate position. Depending on the degree of nerve palsy, the patient's eyes may not be straight when they are trying to look straight ahead. If this is the case, they will have a squint and see double all the time. Remember, however, that children may not see double as they are able to suppress the image from one eye. Also, if one eye is blind or has very poor vision, the patient will obviously not see two images.

In some cases, particularly where the nerve palsy is incomplete, the patient may be able to keep their eyes straight when they look ahead but experience double vision when the eyes are moved in a particular direction. When the abnormal eye moves into the position where the affected muscle is supposed to be doing most of the work, the problem will be worse, as that eye cannot match the other good eye. The patient will experience more diplopia (i.e. the two images will be much more noticeable and further apart) when they look in the direction of action of the weakened muscle.

Fourth nerve palsy

Patients with trochlear nerve palsies will notice their diplopia when they look down and inwards (figure

12.3). For example, a patient with a right trochlear nerve palsy (weakening the right superior oblique) will experience double vision when they look down and to the left, thus moving their affected eye to look towards the tip of their nose (the primary muscle action of the right superior oblique).

Sixth nerve palsy

Patients with an abducent nerve palsy will have their most acute problems when they look to the affected side (figure 12.4). A patient with a left abducent nerve palsy (weakening the left lateral rectus) will experience diplopia when looking to the left, forcing their affected eye to abduct (the primary muscle action of the left lateral rectus).

Third nerve palsy

A third nerve palsy has a much more dramatic effect on ocular motility because of the number of muscles affected. An eye with a total third nerve palsy will be left 'down and out'. The eye will be abducted because of the unopposed effect of the still functioning lateral rectus, and depressed because of the effect of the functional superior oblique. The superior oblique is trying to push the eye down and in, but cannot achieve this without the help of the non-functioning medial rectus, thus is only able to push it down. Remember that the third nerve also supplies the levator muscle, and thus a complete third nerve palsy will also result in a complete ptosis (figures 12.5 a–c).

The parasympathetic pupillomotor nerve fibres (the nerves responsible for autonomic constriction of the pupil) also run with the third nerve, and thus the pupil may also be affected. It is important to remember that a lesion of the third nerve does not always involve the pupil.

The pupillomotor fibres that supply pupil movement run around the outside of the third nerve and receive their blood supply from its surrounding meningeal sheath. The rest of the nerve receives its blood supply from the vasa nervorum (small arteriole running within the centre of the nerve itself). Pathology such as that seen in a hypertensive or diabetic mononeuropathy will affect the blood supply to the nerve by compromising its vasa nervorum. It will thus disrupt the oculomotor nerve fibres (those to the extraocular muscles and levator palpabrae) causing a 'down and out' eye with a ptosis but, importantly, the pupil fibres will be spared and pupil reactions will be normal, as they will still receive their blood sup-

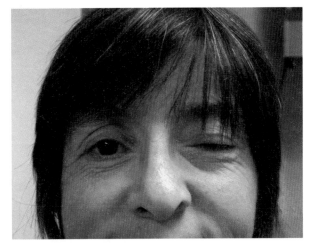

a)

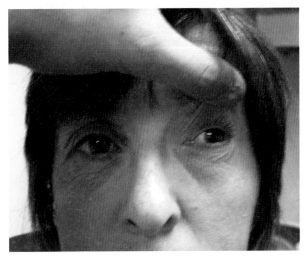

b)

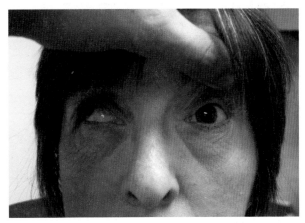

c)

FIGURES 12.5 a–c a) Patient has a complete left ptosis. Both pupils are pharmacologically dilated. b) On lifting the left lid we see that the left eye is slightly down and abducted due to weakness of all the extraocular muscles except the lateral rectus and superior oblique. c) On attempted right and up gaze we can see that the left eye fails to adduct and elevate due to loss of medial and superior rectus power.

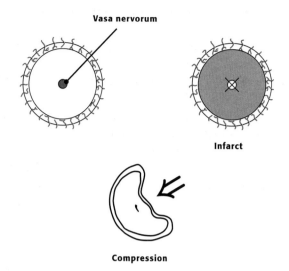

FIGURE 12.6 **Cross-section of the third cranial nerve. The vasa nervorum runs down the centre of the nerve. When this vessel is compromised the surrounding pupil fibres can still function as they get their blood supply from the surrounding pial plexus. A compressive lesion squeezes the whole nerve and causes loss of both the motor and pupil fibres.**

ply from the oculomotor nerve's meningeal sheath.

If the lesion of the third nerve is complete and the pupil is dilated because of the loss of the parasympathetic pupillomotor fibres (leaving unopposed effect of the sympathetic nervous system), this indicates that the underlying aetiology is not simply a mononeuropathy. It is more likely that there is a compressive lesion affecting the oculomotor nerve, squeezing the pupillomotor fibres directly as they run around the outside of the nerve (figure 12.6). Tumours may compress the nerve. However, the most worrying aetiology of a pupil-involving third nerve palsy is an aneurysm of the posterior communicating artery, a potentially life-threatening condition. These patients require urgent neuro-imaging and possibly neurosurgical intervention.

For the examination or assessment

Introduce yourself.

Ensure adequate lighting in the room.

Offer to do a cover test (*see* Chapter 13, Cover testing). This will allow you to assess the baseline position of the eyes when they are looking straight ahead (primary position) and detect the presence of any manifest squint.

Sit in front of the patient.

Ideally, the patient should take off their spectacles as they may experience edge artefact from their lenses or an effect from their frames, causing problems when you are assessing the position of the eyes and any diplopia in extreme positions of gaze.

Shine a pen torch or similar light source at the patient.

Ask the patient if their vision is reasonable in both eyes and if they can see the light.

Ask the patient how many lights they see. If they see two lights, they have some degree of ocular misalignment when looking straight ahead, due either to a squint or nerve palsy. If this is the case, offer to do another cover test to determine the nature of the squint. If the patient has a completely blind eye, they will obviously not experience double vision, hence the need to ask about their vision.

Now you must assess the eye movements in each position of gaze: straight to the right; straight to the left; up and right; up and left; down and right; and down and left. By moving the eyes into each of these positions, you are effectively isolating each individual muscle for each eye. Asking the patient to look straight up and straight down reveals little, as these movements are governed by many muscles, not just the vertical recti (see above).

Ask the patient to keep their head still and follow the light source with their eyes only.

It is important to keep on encouraging the patient to follow the light with their eyes only and to keep their head still throughout the examination.

Tell the patient that you will assume they are seeing only one light unless they say otherwise. Encourage them to report any double vision (two lights seen).

Now move the light source into each position of gaze, carefully watching the eye movements and observing the corneal light reflexes (they should be symmetrical between each eye).

Some teachers advise an 'H' pattern, while others advise a star configuration for assessing the eye movements. Either is effective, but I prefer a star configuration, which returns to the centre before assessing movement in each direction of gaze. In the 'H' configuration, the patient looks laterally and then moves their gaze up and down from that point.

Pause a moment at each extreme of gaze and watch the eyes for any abnormal movements, such as nystagmus. Ask the patient if they are getting any double vision in these positions, as subtle lesions will only be detected if they are far into the defective muscle's most important direction of action.

If the patient does report double vision (two lights), stop a moment and look at the corneal reflexes. Discrepancy between the symmetry of the corneal reflexes will demonstrate that the eyes are not in the same positions. Ask the patient whether the two lights they see are side by side or one above the other. If the lights are side by side, this indicates that there is a defect with one of the horizontal muscles (the medial or lateral recti). If the lights are one above the other, it indicates a problem with a vertical muscle (the superior rectus, inferior rectus or one of the obliques).

Next, ask the patient how far apart the two lights are. Then move the light further into the direction of gaze.

The lights should move further apart as the eyes move further into the weakened muscle's territory, because the defective muscle will be struggling even more.

If the patient experiences diplopia in right gaze, they either have a problem with the function of their right lateral rectus or their left medial rectus. The likelihood of an isolated medial rectus problem is slight, whereas the abducent nerve supplies only the lateral rectus and therefore is the likely culprit.

If the patient experiences diplopia most when your torch is down and to their left, the likely problem lies within the right superior oblique muscle and thus the right trochlear nerve. The problem will be exacerbated when the patient tries to look towards their nose with their right eye – the major action of the affected muscle.

If one eye is 'down and out' (apparently looking down and abducted) or demonstrates marked limitation of elevation and adduction, the likely diagnosis is a third nerve palsy. You must look for and comment upon the presence of a ptosis and whether or not the pupil is normal ('pupil-sparing' or 'pupil-involving'). The patient's diplopia will be present in virtually all positions of gaze, but will be particularly severe when the patient looks up and away from the side of their palsy.

Although the trochlear and abducent nerves are most likely to be affected by a mononeuropathy resulting in demonstrable oculomotility defects, any pattern is possible and a thorough examination should be undertaken to identify precisely where the defect lies.

Identify where the patient experiences most diplopia and whether this is vertical or horizontal in nature. This should allow you to narrow down the list of likely muscles responsible. Patients with previous trauma or thyroid eye disease may have bizarre patterns of restriction that do not fit into any specific pattern. It is thus important to describe where the problem lies and which muscles may be involved before making a specific diagnosis.

13 | Cover testing

Cover testing is the examination used to detect an ocular misalignment or squint. It involves covering one of the patient's eyes with an occluder or similar object that obscures or completely blurs the vision in that eye.

The eyes are maintained straight (both pointing in the same direction) by numerous cerebral pathways. These pathways rely on reasonable vision in each eye to check that the eye is in the right position and make fine adjustments.

If the eyes are not straight, the patient's brain will see two different images that it cannot fully integrate, so the patient will see double. Because of their immature visual system, children are able to ignore an image from one eye and so may not experience double vision.

Squints may occur because of nerve palsies, so if a cover test detects a defect, it is vital to check ocular motility as well. This may not be easy in children. The degree of ocular misalignment due to a nerve palsy or muscle problem will vary according to the direction in which the eyes are pointing. If the eyes are looking in the opposite direction from the main action of a weak muscle, they may be perfectly aligned. When they look the other way, however, forcing the compromised muscle to work, the deviation becomes obvious.

Pure squints are due to mis-wiring of the ocular alignment mechanisms and show as a constant deviation between the eyes, regardless of which way the patient is looking. If the eye movements are checked one eye at a time, no muscle or nerve weakness will be found.

Squints may be vertical or horizontal, but most seen in the assessments will be horizontal. A cover test will demonstrate a vertical squint by stimulating vertical eye movements when the covers are placed or removed.

For the examination or assessment

Introduce yourself to the patient.

Ensure adequate lighting so you can see the eyes clearly.

Ensure you have a pen torch or similar light source, and that it is not too bright.

Ensure you have a suitable occluder. Any object that blocks vision will be adequate but it must be small and firm. A special opaque occluder or the occluder used for visual acuity testing is ideal.

Begin by shining the light into the patient's eyes at a distance of approximately one-third of a metre and ask the patient to look directly at it. It is often helpful to hold the light source as close to your eyes as possible but pointing at the patient (e.g. just above your right ear). This ensures that the corneal reflections are shining brightly back at you.

If the patient wears spectacles, the test should be done both with and without them. It should also be done with the patient looking at a distant target (6m) and at a near one. In practice, close assessment should be sufficient for the examination; however, mentioning the need for distance assessment as well will gain you extra points.

NB. You may be asked why you should do the cover test for both distance and near vision. The answer is that some squints vary with distance. Some patients have no squint at all when looking at an object 6m away, but develop a marked squint when they look at your pen torch one-third of a metre away.

Ask the patient if they see one or two lights. If they see one, and assuming they have useful vision in both eyes, they are unlikely to have a squint in the primary position of gaze (staring straight ahead). If the patient is a child or has had the squint for a long time, they might be able to ignore the image from one eye and thus not experience diplopia.

Note the corneal reflexes and comment upon them. If the eyes are straight, the corneal reflexes will be symmetrical, i.e. the light reflected from the corneal surface will be reflected from exactly the same point on the cornea in each eye (figure 13.1).

If the reflexes are not symmetrical, the patient has some degree of ocular misalignment or squint.

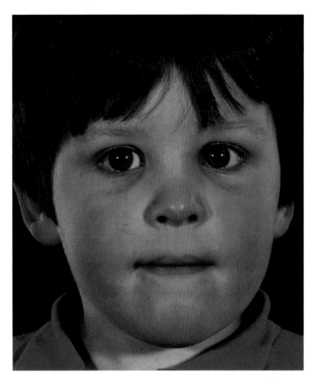

FIGURE 13.1 **This boy has the appearance of a convergent squint due to the folds of skin near his nose (epicanthic folds) obstructing the sclera. The corneal reflexes are however symmetrical and thus his eyes are actually straight (he has no squint). (Courtesy of Mr R.M. Gregson.)**

If one of the eyes is obviously turned in or out, the patient has a squint in the primary position of gaze. A squint that is present with both eyes open is called a manifest squint or a tropia.

Even if a patient has a squint, they will still be able to see with both eyes, assuming that they have good vision in both.

When eyes point in different directions, the brain must choose one to use for vision, so it can align that eye and allow the light from objects under regard to fall on to that eye's macula.

This eye is called the fixing eye, while the other, which is left to deviate, is the deviating eye. Which eye the brain chooses depends upon which eye is dominant and which has the better vision.

If the fixing eye is covered while the patient is looking at an object – e.g. your light source – the brain is forced to switch to the other eye to see with. The deviating eye will now swing to take up fixation and look directly at the torch (straighten up). This is the basis of the cover test.

Example

If the patient has a convergent squint (one eye turning in) and is asked to look at your torch, you will notice

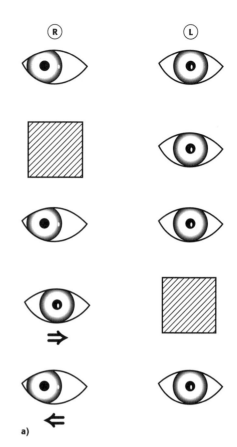

FIGURES 13.2 a and b **a) Cover test for exotropia. Assessment of the corneal reflexes will show some asymmetry. The right eye is divergent. If the right eye is covered there will be no movement as the left eye is already straight and 'fixating'. When the left eye is covered the right eye moves inward to take up fixation, as the left eye can no longer see. This inward movement confirms that the right eye was out. The patient has a right divergent squint. If the left eye is dominant, when the cover is removed the right eye will move back to its squinting position. b) Cover test for esotropia. Assessment of the corneal reflexes will show some asymmetry. The left eye appears convergent. If the left eye is covered there will be no movement as the right eye is already straight and 'fixating'. When the right eye is covered the left eye moves outwards to take up fixation, as the right eye can no longer see. This outward movement confirms that the left eye was in. The patient has a left convergent squint. If the right eye is dominant, when the cover is removed the left eye will move back to its squinting position.**

that one eye (say, the right) is looking straight with its corneal reflection right in the middle of the cornea, while the left eye is turned in. The right eye is the fixing eye, while the left is the deviating eye. In this deviating eye, the corneal light reflex will not be central but will be on the temporal/lateral aspect of the cornea. The brain may have chosen to fix with the right eye because it is the dominant eye (everyone has one eye they prefer – it's usually the eye they use for taking photos) or because vision is better than that in the left eye.

Now if you cover the right eye, the patient will still

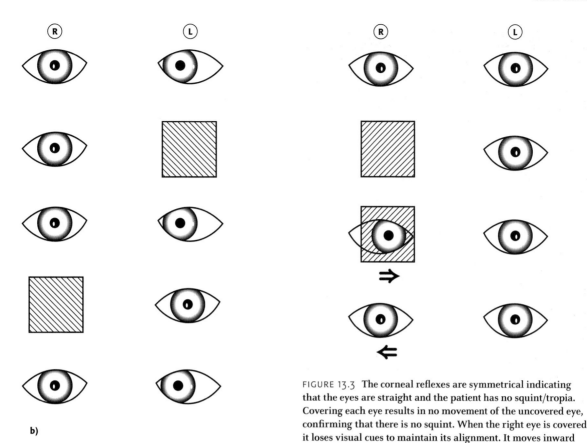

b)

FIGURE 13.3 The corneal reflexes are symmetrical indicating that the eyes are straight and the patient has no squint/tropia. Covering each eye results in no movement of the uncovered eye, confirming that there is no squint. When the right eye is covered it loses visual cues to maintain its alignment. It moves inward under the cover. The moment the cover is removed from the right eye the eye swings quickly back outward to become straight again. This is a latent convergent squint.

be trying to look at your torch but cannot use the right eye. The brain goes for the second-best option of using the left eye, which moves outwards to fix (look straight at) the light.

Cover test

Ensure the patient is looking directly at the target light source (see figures 13.2a and b).

Cover the patient's right eye with the occluder while carefully watching the patient's left eye.

If there is no movement of the left eye, it is normal and is fixing your target.

If the left eye moves nasally (in) to look at your target and take up fixation, it must have been too far out, i.e. divergent. In this case the patient has a left divergent squint, or exotropia.

If the left eye moves temporally/laterally (out) to take up fixation, this indicates that it was too far in, i.e. convergent. The patient therefore has a left convergent squint, or esotropia.

Repeat the test for the left eye. With the left eye covered, watch the right carefully and note if it moves.

The cover test will detect any manifest squint. In order to test for a latent squint you should use the cover–uncover test (see below).

A latent squint, or heterophoria, is one that is only present when the brain is not able to use sight to fine-tune the position of an eye and maintain its straight alignment. Nearly everyone has some degree of latent squint, and this is usually of no clinical significance unless it starts to become manifest. A latent squint becomes a problem if the affected eye loses its sight for some reason, as the brain cannot keep the eye straight without the cues of sight.

Cover–uncover test

Begin with the cover test as above.

Assuming that both eyes are straight and that you have found no evidence of manifest squint or tropia, you now wish to look for a latent squint or a phoria (see figure 13.3).

Cover one eye and then while uncovering it observe that eye very carefully as it emerges from behind the occluder.

With the eye covered, the brain cannot use vision to align it. The eye therefore goes into its baseline default position, which is often a little convergent or divergent.

When the cover is removed, the brain recognises that that eye is not correctly aligned, and compensates appropriately and rapidly by straightening it.

If the eye that has been covered moves medially in order to straighten and look at your light, the patient has a latent divergent squint (*exo*phoria). If the eye that has been covered moves laterally when uncovered, the patient has a latent convergent squint (*eso*phoria).

Swinging cover test

By moving the occluder back and forth between the eyes, you interfere with the brain's ability to co-ordinate eye position. Any movement of the eyes that you see will be the result of a combination of the manifest squint and any latent squint. Do not do this too many times as it can be quite disorientating for the patient. Try it on yourself or your colleagues.

14 | Visual acuity

The measurement of visual acuity is the assessment of the resolving power of the patient's optical system. To read a character, the individual must be able to see where the lines of that character are drawn and, to do this, they must be able to see the dark lines of the 'arms' and 'body' of the letter against the white background. As the character becomes smaller, so the gap between the dark lines and the white background becomes smaller. When the letter is so small that the eyes cannot distinguish the dark of the letter and the white of the background, the individual has reached the limit of their resolution. The size of the character, and thus the smallest type size that the person can resolve (read), represents that individual's visual acuity.

Standard visual acuity testing uses an illuminated white chart on which black characters of decreasing size are placed at specified distances. The most widely used chart is the Snellen, but there are others. The LogMAR (log of the minimal angle of resolution) chart is becoming more popular. This relies more on linear calculations to determine the character sizes, allowing the visual acuity values to be used more accurately in statistical analyses and research. The log of the minimal angle of resolution refers to the minimal angle between the arms of the letters to allow resolution as described above. A LogMAR chart has the same number of characters on each line, while the Snellen has one large character on the top line, two smaller characters on the second line, and so on.

Both the Snellen and LogMAR rely on the patient recognising the character and being able to read it aloud. There are charts with different-sized pictures for children who cannot yet read. The child either names what they see or points to a corresponding picture when it is offered to them on another card.

Adults who cannot read can use what are known as illiterate E charts. On these, the letter 'E' is printed repeatedly but is orientated differently, e.g. back to front or with the three 'arms' pointing up or down.

The patient may indicate in which direction the 'E' is pointing. Another type of chart shows different-sized circles, each with a gap in it, and the patient has to identify in which quadrant the gap lies. In all the above tests, the patient continues to look at smaller targets until they fail to identify them. That is then taken as the patient's visual acuity.

With the Snellen chart, patients are positioned 6m away. They then read down the chart (see below) as far as possible. The lowest character read gives the visual acuity. If the patient can only read the top character (known as the '60' line) then their vision is documented as 6/60 (six-over-60 or simply six-60). This means that all the smaller letters are unreadable. The '60' line is so called because an individual with normal sight can read this top character at a distance of 60m.

If the patient can read the characters on the '24' line but fails to identify letters on the '18' line below, their vision is 6/24 (six-twenty four). A person with normal vision is able to read this character size at 24m. Normal vision is achieved when the patient reads the '6' line, which means their vision is 6/6 (six-six). Of course, some people can read even smaller print on the chart at 6m, achieving 6/5 (six-five) or 6/4 (six-four) vision (reading the '5' and '4' lines, respectively). An individual who can read the 6/4 line is reading what a 'normal' person can read only when within 4m of the chart.

Different units are used in some other countries. If the distances are measured in feet, the chart is placed at 20ft. Thus, normal vision is 20/20 (twenty-twenty), which is the same as 6/6. Six-12 equates to 20/40 and so on.

Sometimes the patient can read the whole of one line and only two characters of the next line. In this case, vision is documented as '+2'. If the patient can read the whole of the '12' line but only two characters of the '9' line, then their vision is 6/12 +2 (six-12 plus two). Equally, if they can read nearly all the '9' line but get one of the letters wrong, their vision is documented as 6/9 –1 (six-nine minus one). This may appear an unnecessary distinction, but it is helpful when monitoring a patient for any deterioration in vision.

If a patient cannot see any of the letters clearly enough to identify them (i.e. their vision is worse than 6/60), a portable chart may be brought closer than 6m or the patient moved closer until they can read the top '60' letter. If the patient can see the top letter when the chart is at 2m, vision is documented as 2/60 (two-over-60 or two-60). If the patient can only see the letter when it is 1m away, the visual acuity is 1/60 (one-60).

If the patient still fails to identify the top letter on the Snellen chart at a distance of 1m, the vision may be assessed by asking the patient to try to count fingers. Hold up some fingers at approximately 2ft away and ask the patient to count them. If they succeed, their vision is described as 'counting fingers (CF) at 2ft'.

If the patient cannot see well enough to count fingers at a distance of 1ft from the eye, the assessment can be based on whether they can see hand movements.

If the patient is able to detect a hand when it is waved directly in front of their eye, their vision is 'hand motion' (HM). If they cannot see even this, shine a bright light directly into the eye, ensuring the other eye is well covered, and ask the patient to say when the light is shining at them. If they can correctly identify when the light is shone, the vision in that eye is 'perception of light' (PL). If they cannot detect any light, their vision is 'no perception of light' (NPL).

Pinhole acuity is assessed by asking the patient to look at the chart through a pinhole. A pinhole is a small hole in an occluder, which obviates the need for refraction. The patient's eye usually brings the incoming light into focus on the retina (*see* Chapter 7) by bending incoming light rays at the cornea and the lens. The pinhole allows only one ray of light to enter the eye from the target or, in the case of visual acuity testing, the character on the chart. As that ray of light runs directly through the centre of the cornea and the lens, directly to the fovea, it requires no bending (refraction or focusing) in order to be seen clearly.

The patient therefore needs no spectacles to see clearly through the pinhole. Furthermore, if the patient is able to see better through the pinhole than with their spectacles, this may mean that they need a new prescription for their glasses. Sometimes, despite better pinhole acuity it is impossible to improve the spectacles, but it is always worth re-refracting and checking again to make sure. If the patient

has a 'corrected' visual acuity of 6/12 and a 'pinhole' acuity of 6/6, their spectacle prescription probably needs updating.

Examination

Introduce yourself to the patient.

Ensure that there is adequate light in the room and that the chart is illuminated.

Place the patient 6m from the chart.

NB. Often the rooms used for assessing visual acuity are less than 6m long, in which case mirrors can be used instead. For example, if the room is 4m long, a mirror is placed at the opposite end of the room to the chart. The patient faces the mirror, 2m away from it with their back to the chart. As the patient is 2m from the mirror, and the mirror is 4m from the chart, the total viewing distance is 6m.

Ensure the patient is comfortable and has a clear view of the chart.

Ask them to remove any spectacles.

Block the vision from the patient's left eye with an occluder. Ask them to read down the chart until they reach the smallest character that they can see clearly.

Assess and document the visual acuity as described above. This is the patient's 'unaided' visual acuity with the right eye.

Repeat for the left eye and document.

Now ask the patient to put on their spectacles, if they wear them. Ensure that the spectacles are the patient's distance, not reading, glasses.

Repeat the visual acuity assessments, occluding one eye at a time. This is the patient's 'corrected' visual acuity.

If the patient's corrected visual acuity is 6/4 in each eye then there is no need to proceed further. Otherwise, it is worth using the pinhole to obtain a 'pinhole' acuity (see above).

It is possible to test reading vision with special books containing text of different sizes. Patients wear their reading spectacles and hold the book themselves at a distance that is comfortable for them. They then try to read the text, and the smallest print read correctly is documented as their reading vision. The sizes of the characters are categorised according to traditional printing standards, using the 'N' scale. Thus a patient with good reading vision may be able to read N5, while someone with a macular problem may only be able to read N24.

Ophthalmic conditions

15 | Red eye

An eye is red because the vessels of the conjunctiva, limbus or sclera become engorged with blood as a result of some inflammatory stimulus. The vessels dilate and become 'injected', giving the eye a red appearance. Red eyes are commonly seen in general practice and in accident and emergency departments. Every medical practitioner is almost certain to see a patient with a red eye and be expected to deal with it, or at least to come up with a list, albeit short, of possible diagnoses. There are many causes of red eye, but they are easily distinguished by taking a careful history and carrying out basic examination.

Assessment

Take a history:
- When did the symptoms start?
- Any injury?
- Any history of drilling, grinding or welding?
- Any previous episodes?
- Any previous ocular history?
- Is the vision affected?
- Any photophobia?
- Any recent eye operations?

Examine:
- Check visual acuity. If the redness is unilateral, compare the vision between the eyes. A Snellen chart may not be available but you can use any reading print.
- Check pupil reactions.
- Look at the eye in all positions of gaze.
- Try to identify where the redness is:
  - Is it more pronounced in the fornix than around the limbus? Is there pus? If so, this points to a conjunctivitis rather than an intraocular or corneal problem.
  - Is it more around the limbus (ciliary injection) than in the fornix? If so, this points more to a keratitis, iritis or angle-closure glaucoma (figure 15.1).

- Use the direct ophthalmoscope to look at a magnified image of the front of the eye.
  - Look for the irregular pupil and keratic precipitates of iritis (figure 15.2).
  - Look for the fixed, mid-dilated pupil and cloudy cornea of angle-closure glaucoma (figure 15.3).
  - Look for the creamy corneal opacities and hypopyon (collection of whitish pus at the bottom of the anterior chamber inside the eye) of an infective keratitis (figure 15.4).
- Put some topical anaesthetic and fluorescein on the eye and look closely (preferably with the aid of a cobalt blue light) for any staining indicative of a break in the corneal epithelium – which might be a keratitis/infective ulcer or a corneal abrasion.

There are three common serious causes of red eye that require identification and treatment: iritis, keratitis and angle-closure glaucoma. Angle-closure glaucoma is described at length in Chapter 21. The key clinical features of iritis and keratitis are described here. There are many other causes of red eye that are beyond the scope of this book, but the more common serious causes are described below and a more clinically orientated description of red eye is found in Chapter 1.

Iritis

Iritis is a common inflammation of the iris.

Symptoms

A patient with iritis feels pain when their pupil constricts in response to light. This is because the iris sphincter forms the pupil and the inflamed iris tissue is being forced to move. This phenomenon is called photophobia. As the whole eye will be inflamed, the patient may also experience an ache or foreign-body sensation.

The inflamed iris vessels leak protein and inflamma-

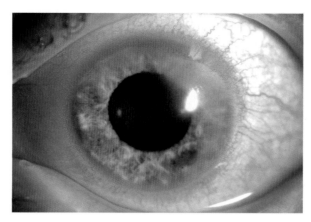

FIGURE 15.1 **Redness localised around the limbus (circumlimbal). This is ciliary injection caused in this case by a keratitis. The vessels running up to the cornea are all engorged while those further away appear relatively normal. Such a pattern of redness occurs with corneal and intraocular inflammation.**

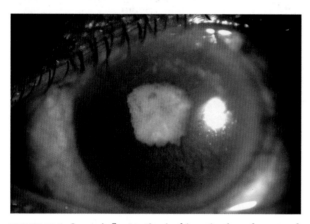

FIGURE 15.2 **Severe inflammation in this patient's eye has caused the iris to stick to the lens. This can be seen as the irregular pupil. The patient also has a dense white cataract because of the inflammation.**

tory cells into the anterior chamber. These cells float around the aqueous humour and are used to make the diagnosis at the slit lamp. Rarely, the patient may see them as tiny translucent objects floating around their field of vision (floaters).

Vision will be normal or mildly reduced.

Signs

The eye will be red, particularly around the limbus. This is called ciliary injection (figure 15.1).

The cells floating in the anterior chamber may be seen with the slit lamp.

These cells may stick to the inner surface of the cornea (the endothelium) in clumps, and are seen as white spots, called keratic precipitates.

The inflammation around the iris may cause it to stick to the anterior surface of the lens (posterior synechiae), which can result in an irregular-shaped pupil (figure 15.2).

The pressure inside the eye may go up if the drainage network becomes clogged by inflammatory debris. If the pupil becomes completely stuck, no aqueous will flow to the front of, and hence out of, the eye, and the pressure can rise dramatically, causing an inflammatory glaucoma.

Iritis can be idiopathic or acquired secondary to another medical condition. It is essentially the result of an autoimmune process, in which the immune system reacts against the iris tissue. Other systemic autoimmune diseases are often implicated, particularly HLA-B27 (human leukocyte antigen)-related disorders, and sarcoidosis.

Management

Address any underlying cause by treating any systemic disorder.

Give steroid drops topically to suppress inflammation.

Treat any pressure rise appropriately.

Dilate the pupil. This has a two-fold purpose: it gives symptomatic relief to the patient (i.e. stops their photophobia by paralysing the iris) and also prevents permanent adhesions developing between the iris and the lens.

Systemic steroids or steroid injections may be given around the eye if the inflammation is severe or fails to resolve.

Keratitis

Keratitis is inflammation of the cornea. There are

many causes, but the most serious, which requires identification and prompt treatment, is infective keratitis. Infective keratitis usually manifests as a corneal ulcer. An ulcer is defined as a break in a tissue's epithelium and, in this situation, is usually infective. Contact lenses are a major risk factor for corneal infections.

Symptoms

Because the cornea has many nerves, pain is usually marked. In some cases – e.g. when the ulcer is caused by the herpes simplex virus (a dendritic ulcer) – the nerves may be compromised, and the pain not so severe.

Vision will be anything from mildly to severely reduced, depending on the position of the ulcer. If the ulcer is directly over the visual axis (i.e. the part of the cornea that the patient actually looks through) vision will be dramatically reduced.

If the ulcer is small, the patient may simply experience a foreign-body sensation. Because of the generalised inflammation, the patient commonly experiences some degree of photophobia.

Signs

The cornea will be cloudy in the area of the ulcer.

Topical fluorescein will stain any corneal epithelial defect.

The pupil reactions will be normal in most cases.

If the inflammatory reaction is severe, as is common with an infective keratitis, the cellular reaction in the anterior chamber may be great. Large numbers of white blood cells are released and accumulate in the anterior chamber, possibly resulting in clinically visible settling and sedimentation. The white (pus) cells fall to the bottom of the anterior chamber and form a deposit called a hypopyon (figure 15.4). This is a sign of severe intraocular inflammation and requires urgent management of the aetiological cause.

Management

These patients usually require intensive (hourly) topical antibiotics.

It is important to try to identify the organism responsible before starting treatment because, if the ulcer does not respond, the treatment can be fine-tuned to target the particular pathogen responsible. A scrape is taken from the corneal surface in the area of the ulcer and samples sent for microscopy/gram staining and culture.

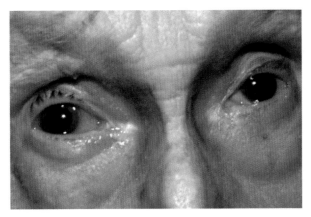

FIGURE 15.3 **This elderly lady has right angle-closure glaucoma. The eye is red, the pupil is fixed and mid-dilated, and the cornea is cloudy. Palpation will reveal an extremely firm globe.**

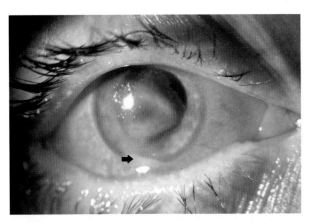

FIGURE 15.4 **A contact lens-related corneal ulcer. The arrow highlights the presence of a collection of pus cells (hypopyon) at the bottom of the anterior chamber.**

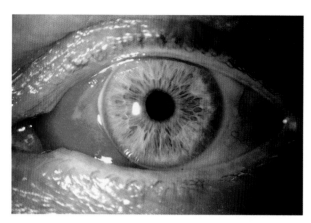

FIGURE 15.5　A subconjunctival haemorrhage. It is clearly seen that the blood is confluent and the redness is not due to engorged blood vessels as seen in inflammatory and infective causes of red eye.

If the ulcer is detected early, it will resolve with minimal scarring. However, an advanced ulcer will inevitably leave significant scarring, with concomitant loss of vision.

An untreated ulcer can erode right through the cornea and cause a perforation, thus putting the whole eye at risk. This is a major concern.

If the infection is severe and the cornea perforates, an operation is needed to replace the corneal tissue and maintain the integrity of the eye.

Other causes of red eye

Infective conjunctivitis

This is an extremely common disorder. The eye is red and sticky. The redness is confined mainly to the inferior fornix and pus may be visible. The patient does not usually experience pain, but slight discomfort is common. The eyelashes are frequently matted together in the morning. There may be a history of exposure to an individual with established conjunctivitis. Vision is unaffected, the pupil reactions are normal and the cornea is clear.

Conjunctivitis may be bacterial or viral. If bacterial, there is usually a significant amount of pus. Treatment with broad-spectrum antibiotic ointments or drops should lead to a speedy resolution.

Viral conjunctivitis is common and is sometimes associated with a flu-like illness or upper respiratory tract infection. The redness is usually more diffuse than in the bacterial variety, and pus is not a prominent feature. Patients tend to complain of an ache and discomfort with profuse watering, and they may have palpable pre-auricular lymph nodes. There is no treatment, but the condition is self-limiting and resolves in about two to three weeks. It is extremely contagious and easily spreads from one eye to the other. Commonly, the condition begins with redness in one eye and then, a few days later, the other eye becomes red. Sharing face towels or paper tissues can transmit the virus to other people. Babies and infants are potential sources of viral infections.

Subconjunctival haemorrhage

The clinical features of a subconjunctival haemorrhage are dramatic and can cause a surprisingly large amount of distress. Patients may feel a sudden, mild, foreign-body sensation or may be completely asymptomatic, and indeed a relative or a friend may be the first to notice the condition. The eye becomes rapidly blood-red, with the redness localised (figure 15.5) or involving the whole of the conjunctiva, obscuring all the white of the sclera. Close inspection will show that the redness is confluent and not caused by dilated blood vessels as in the inflammatory/infective conditions. It may be precipitated by coughing, sneezing or any form of straining, including constipation.

It resolves without treatment, yellowing initially and then disappearing over time, as any other bruise. Reassurance is the key intervention. If the patient is on warfarin or has a bleeding diathesis, it is worth checking coagulation status.

Episcleritis

Often of unknown aetiology, this condition causes localised inflammation/injection of the layer beneath the conjunctiva and adjacent to the sclera, hence the term 'episclera'. It results in an area of redness, which may be flat or have raised nodules. It is often associated with mild discomfort. It is self-limiting, but topical steroids are often given for symptomatic relief. It can be associated with systemic autoimmune disorders such as rheumatoid arthritis, and may be recurrent.

Scleritis

This is a more serious condition in which the sclera becomes very inflamed and injected. It is usually associated with advanced systemic autoimmune disorders. Severe pain is the key symptom that distinguishes it from episcleritis. Close inspection will show that the injected vessels are very deep and run through the sclera itself. A thorough search for an underlying cause should be undertaken. Active scleritis indicates that any systemic disorder is active. Immunosuppression, usually in the form of steroids initially (with adjuvant NSAIDs) at least, is required. Such scleritides may be necrotising or non-necrotising. In the necrotising variety, the redness has a white centre corresponding to an area of infarction/necrosis caused by the severe inflammation.

Allergic conjunctivitis

The conjunctiva has numerous areas of lymphoid tissue, responsible for policing the ocular surface by releasing immunoglobulins (usually IgA) into tears, with the subsequent identification and destruction of any invading organisms. In common with lymphoid tissue at other mucosal sites (e.g. the nasal mucosa) they may generate inappropriately severe reactions (hypersensitivity reactions) to certain antigens.

Pollen and the house dust mite are common antigens that can cause this reaction. The reaction is due to the presence of antigen (allergen) on the ocular surface. Resident cells cross-link and degranulate, releasing large amounts of histamine and inflammatory mediators. A florid allergic reaction may ensue, with redness of the conjunctiva associated with itching and serous discharge. Small nodules called papillae are often seen within the conjunctiva.

There is a spectrum within this disorder from mild self-limiting 'hayfever' to severe reactions resulting in corneal scarring.

Treatment is generally symptomatic with mild cases usually treated with antihistamine drops, such as sodium cromoglycate. Severe cases may require more aggressive treatment with steroids.

Topical steroids can make the condition worse. Only use them when the diagnosis is certain and adequate follow up arranged.

16 | Visual loss

When a patient presents with loss of vision, it is vital to be systematic and methodical. As with assessing all patients, begin by taking an accurate history.

History

- Time course and progression of the visual loss:
  - ☐ When did the visual loss occur?
  - ☐ Transient or permanent?
  - ☐ How long did it last?
  - ☐ How many episodes?
  - ☐ Is it getting better or worse?
  - ☐ Previous episodes?

- Description of the visual defect:
  - ☐ Central visual blur?
  - ☐ Central black patch in vision?
  - ☐ Visual field shadow?
  - ☐ Distortion?
  - ☐ Double vision?

- Other symptoms – ocular:
  - ☐ Pain? Redness? Photophobia? Flashes? Floaters? Haloes? Contact lens wear?

- Other symptoms – systemic:
  - ☐ Pain elsewhere?
  - ☐ Systems review.

The answers to the above questions should, in theory, reveal the most likely cause for the loss of vision.

It is important to understand which part of the visual pathway has been compromised.

Is it a problem of the front of the eye, blocking the light from reaching the back of the eye: cornea, anterior chamber and aqueous, lens or vitreous cavity?

Is it a problem within the retina itself: macular or peripheral or both?

Is it a problem with the transmission of impulses from the retina to the brain: optic nerve, optic chiasm, optic tract or optic radiation?

Is it a problem within the brain itself at the visual portion of the occipital cortex?

Lesions localised to each of the above areas will give very distinct symptoms and signs.

There are many possible causes for loss of vision and only a few are mentioned below. Other causes are discussed in the relevant chapters, and they include venous or arterial occlusions, age-related macular degeneration, and arteritic or non-arteritic ischaemic optic neuropathies.

Amaurosis fugax

This is a transient ischaemic attack ('mini-stroke') of the retinal circulation. Classically, patients develop sudden loss of vision that comes on over seconds and is often described as a curtain coming up or down over *one* eye.

It is important to note that this is not binocular, but occurs only in one eye. Binocular sudden loss of vision suggests pathology of the bilateral blood supply to the occipital cortex, namely both the vertebrobasilar arteries.

In amaurosis fugax, there is occlusion of the central retinal artery, resulting in transient ischaemia of the retina and thus retinal dysfunction and visual loss. The occlusion can have any one of several causes, but most commonly occurs when a fibrinoplatelet or cholesterol embolus passes from the heart or carotid arterial walls into the ophthalmic artery, and then into the central retinal vessels. There the embolus lodges, occluding the blood supply.

This blockage is by definition transient, and the interruption of the blood supply does not result in enough ischaemia to cause permanent problems. The embolus breaks up and passes through the central retinal circulation, thereby restoring the blood flow to the retina. The embolus might lodge within the visible retina and be seen lying within the lumen of peripheral retinal blood vessels or, more commonly, it will dissolve completely, leaving no sign.

Treatment is directed at the cause. Antiplatelet medication will help prevent further thrombo-embolic events and, it is to be hoped, minimise the risk of further ocular ischaemic events or formal cerebral stroke. If the patient is in atrial fibrillation, cardioversion or formal anticoagulation with warfarin may be required to prevent release of further emboli from the inner atrial wall.

If a carotid bruit is detected – although some clinicians question the value of listening for one – the patient should be sent for formal carotid Doppler study. The absence of a carotid bruit does not exclude the presence of significant carotid stenosis, and so patients with a convincing history of amaurosis fugax should be referred for investigation. If a significant stenosis is detected, the patient may benefit from carotid endarterectomy surgery from a vascular surgeon.

Vitreous haemorrhage

Vitreous haemorrhage is not a disease, but a manifestation of another pathology. Blood enters the vitreous cavity resulting in a variable degree of visual loss. If the amount of blood is small, the patient may only notice reddish/brown floaters in their vision, which are groups of red blood cells or clots. However, if the haemorrhage is severe, the patient's vision may be reduced to perception of light in the affected eye.

Intraocular blood vessels rarely rupture spontaneously and so any possible treatment depends on identifying a cause. Trauma can disrupt retinal vasculature, as can retinal detachment if there is a rip in the retina close to or over a blood vessel. The new blood vessels that develop in response to pathology (neovascularisation), particularly as a result of diabetic retinopathy, are abnormal and extremely susceptible to spontaneous bleeding, resulting in significant vitreous haemorrhages and loss of vision.

Some haemorrhages will settle without intervention, so conservative observation is indicated. Others, however, require surgery in the form of a vitrectomy (a procedure in which the vitreous is removed with intraocular instruments). Diabetic vitreous haemorrhages, in particular, may require early treatment if there has been no previous retinal laser treatment (see Chapter 20). In the absence of active intervention, the neovascular process will continue unabated, hidden behind the blood, thereby causing further, possibly irreversible, damage.

If the back of the eye is not visualised, it is important to assess the retina with an ultrasound scan in order to eliminate retinal detachment. This would require early surgery to reattach the retina and restore vision.

Optic neuritis

As the name suggests, in this condition the optic nerve becomes inflamed resulting in varying degrees of visual loss. Optic neuritis may be idiopathic or may be the result of a demyelinating process such as multiple sclerosis (MS). Local or systemic inflammatory conditions may involve the optic nerve directly or indirectly.

The primary complaint is loss of vision, classically in the form of a central positive scotoma where the patient notices a blur or black 'blob' in the centre of their vision. The vision may be severely affected, deteriorating to counting fingers or even hand motion. The patient may also experience some retro-ocular pain, particularly when they look rapidly from side to side. The patient's sight may become progressively worse over a week or two, before then gradually improving. Severe visual loss in young, otherwise well, patients can be extremely distressing, and it is important to reassure them that their vision is likely to recover.

Because the optic nerve is compromised, the impulses travelling along it are impeded and the brain does not 'see' images so brightly. The patient will see colours with their affected eye as 'washed out' and will manifest the clinical sign of 'red desaturation', a phenomenon whereby red objects viewed with the bad eye appear darker and less red than with the good eye. The patient will also have an RAPD (see Chapter 11, Pupil reactions).

The fundoscopic signs depend upon the exact site of the damage to the nerve. If the problem is anterior, as it is in one-third of cases, the optic nerve becomes swollen due to cessation of axoplasmic flow along the neurones that form the nerve. The disc margins become unclear, and the retinal vasculature may be visibly engorged. In contrast, in two-thirds of cases the optic nerve head remains normal, indicating that the nerve pathology lies more posteriorly. This latter condition is called retrobulbar neuritis.

The diagnosis is usually made clinically and initial management is conservative. The vision will improve progressively, with most patients recovering almost all their pre-morbid vision within six to 12 months. In some patients, the vision will improve but will not get quite back to normal. Patients often complain that colours remain less vivid, despite their recorded visual acuity indicating recovery. Repeated episodes of optic neuritis, as seen in patients with MS, will result in progressive stepwise deterioration in vision, as with each episode vision fails to return to baseline.

The major concern with patients with optic neuritis is that they are developing MS. If this is the patient's first episode and they have no other neurological history, then MS is usually not mentioned, as this can cause significant psychological morbidity. If the patient has other neurological symptoms or signs, then MS is more likely, and the patient should be referred to a neurologist to confirm the diagnosis and for counselling about the likely prognosis.

A magnetic resonance imaging (MRI) brain scan is the investigation of choice here, and this classically shows patches (plaques) of demyelination within the white matter of the brain or within the optic nerves themselves.

A large randomised, controlled study, the Optic Neuritis Treatment Trial (Beck RW, Cleary PA, Anderson MM, *et al*. A randomized, controlled trial of corticosteroids in the treatment of acute optic neuritis. *New Eng J Med* 1992; **326**: 581–8), found that, if the demyelinative changes described above are seen at an early-stage MRI, then treatment with high-dose intravenous steroids followed by oral steroids slightly reduced the likelihood of onset of MS within the first two years after the start of symptoms. The researchers also found, paradoxically, that oral steroids alone were detrimental. Because of the difficulty in obtaining MRI scans and the marginal benefit of the above treatment found by the study, a conservative approach is usually adopted.

17 | Age-related macular degeneration

The macula is the central part of the retina responsible for precise and detailed vision. It is the most important and physiologically active part of the retina. Here the retina consists almost solely of cones, the photoreceptors responsible for colour vision.

The photoreceptors lie on top of the retinal pigment epithelium (RPE). When we examine the fundus we are actually seeing the RPE layer, as a healthy neurosensory retina is clear and light passes through it without being reflected back. The RPE reflects and absorbs excess light. It should be a uniform red-orange colour throughout but may be slightly darker around the fovea. The fovea is the epicentre of the macula. It has no blood vessels, and, with the greatest concentration of cones, is responsible for very fine vision.

The photoreceptors are highly metabolically active, even in darkness and during sleep, and this continuous biochemical activity results in many by-products. These products are continually taken up by the adjacent RPE cells and recycled. In addition, the RPE layer supplies the photoreceptors with oxygen and other nutrients. RPE cells are effectively the caretaker cells of the neuroretina, responsible for the normal functioning of the photoreceptors and thus normal vision.

For an as yet unknown reason, the synergy between the RPE layer and the neuroretina breaks down in some people. The RPE cells fail to take up and recycle the metabolites, which then accumulate between the RPE and the photoreceptors. This accumulation eventually forms a pool of material, seen as a small yellowy/creamy area overlying the reddish RPE. This accumulation is called a drusen and is the result of a degenerative wear and tear process known as age-related macular degeneration (AMD) (figures 17.1 and 17.2). The photoreceptors in the area of the drusen are separated from the RPE layer and are therefore not in contact with their caretaker cells. As a consequence, they do not function correctly and eventually fail completely, resulting in blurring of vision. This is a manifestation of dry AMD.

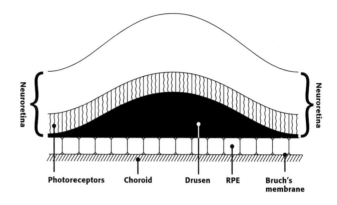

FIGURE 17.1 **Cross-section of the retina showing the abnormal collection of waste material that has collected between the retinal pigment epithelial cell layer and the photoreceptors forming a drusen.**

Apart from drusen, dry AMD may appear clinically as a pigmentary macular disturbance – small collections of black pigment in the RPE layer. This happens when the RPE cells lose control of their pigment production. When enough damage is done, atrophic lesions develop, appearing as very pale or white patches. These are seen because the sclera shows through the gap left by the degenerated neuroretina, RPE and choroid.

Vision in patients with dry AMD is usually only marginally reduced (around 6/12 Snellen) in the early stages. Indeed if the fovea is spared from the process, vision may be perfect (6/6), even with a large amount of drusen in the macula. Dry AMD is a chronic progressive disease, however, and the vision will usually slowly deteriorate. The loss is gradual and affects only the central vision. Navigational/peripheral vision is unaffected. Some degree of dry AMD is virtually universal in the elderly population.

Wet AMD

Some patients with dry AMD develop the more severe form, wet AMD. This occurs when blood vessels from the choroid layer (the vascular layer under the RPE) grow upwards and breach the RPE's basement membrane (called Bruch's membrane).

These pathological blood vessels suddenly break through the Bruch's membrane and penetrate the RPE layer to proliferate in the subretinal space (between the photoreceptors and the RPE), forming a subretinal choroidal neovascular membrane (CNVM). The pathological process is called choroidal neovascularisation (CNV). The exact cause is still unknown and is the subject of much research. These new blood vessels are abnormal, with no selective blood-retinal barrier to prevent the escape of fluid and unwanted molecules. They leak profusely, disrupting the retina's normal biochemical functions. The overlying photoreceptors are slowly and irreversibly damaged with concomitant severe visual loss (figure 17.3).

These blood vessels spread out in the subretinal space and affect a wide area. If the lesion is beneath the fovea, the vision is dramatically reduced. Because the fluid leaking out of these vessels lifts the retina, it often distorts central vision. The patient notices that straight lines appear bent. This is because the light is falling on a ballooned, irregular retina that sends images to the brain as if it were still flat and is called metamorphopsia.

This new blood vessel complex may haemorrhage and cause significant and sudden loss of vision, leaving the retina permanently scarred (figure 17.4). Haemorrhage is a poor prognostic sign. The end stage of all the damage is a disciform (disc-like/circular) scar involving a significant part of the macula with marked permanent loss of the central vision (figure 17.5).

Visual loss tends to begin with distortion and then rapidly progresses to the 6/36 level or worse. If the haemorrhage is significant, the vision immediately deteriorates to 6/60 or worse, with little chance of recovery.

There is no treatment for dry, 'gradual wear and tear' AMD. However, clinical trials show that multivitamins and antioxidants might slow progression of this disorder and minimise the patient's risk of developing the disastrous wet variety. Wet AMD is the main cause of severe visual loss in these patients, and the management of the neovascular membranes is a major challenge to ophthalmologists today.

If the CNVM develops in an area of retina away from the fovea, argon laser may be applied to burn the membrane. This leaves a scar and causes vision loss in the field corresponding to that part of the burnt retina, but it does prevent further leakage and proliferation of the blood vessels (CNV) and the risk of involvement of the fovea and loss of central vision. Unfortunately, however, the membrane often regrows after laser treatment.

Once the CNVM has grown under the fovea, any attempt at laser treatment kills the foveal photoreceptors, with associated iatrogenic severe visual loss. This was once the only option for a membrane under the fovea. It is not an elegant solution, and was, not surprisingly, unpopular with patients and ophthalmologists.

This dilemma spurred on a search for more targeted ways of attacking these membranes. Many methods have been tried, and many more are currently under investigation.

Lasers have been used on the lesions with limited success, and steroids have also been tried, particularly in younger patients, based on the theory that there is an inflammatory component to these new membranes, but again with variable results.

Recently, there has been much interest in a new technology called photodynamic therapy (PDT). A special dye is given intravenously, which attaches to the endothelial cells of the new blood vessels under the retina. A special laser is then applied to the area, which is taken up by the dye, causing the new blood vessels to thrombose and die. Patients often require treatment over several years, but studies indicate some success for this method in preventing further visual loss in a specific subset of patients with a particular form of CNV. This initial work appears promising. The dye is expensive, however, and there are economic implications for widespread treatment.

We are still unsure of the exact cause of AMD, but on-going research is looking at ways of targeting therapies to prevent onset and retard progression.

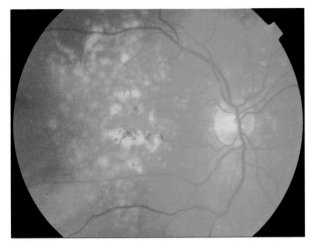

FIGURE 17.2 Dry AMD: colour fundus photograph of a patient with extensive changes of dry age-related macular degeneration. There are creamy drusen spread throughout the macula. There are also associated pigmentary changes around the fovea.

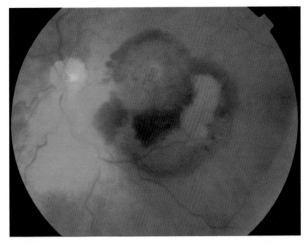

FIGURE 17.4 Wet AMD: colour fundus photograph of a patient with a left subretinal choroidal neovascular membrane. The yellow-green membrane is clearly seen with surrounding subretinal haemorrhage.

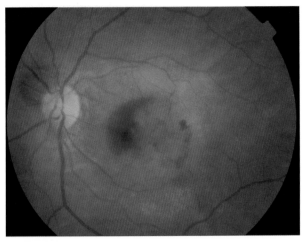

FIGURE 17.3 Wet AMD: colour fundus photograph of a patient with a left subretinal choroidal neovascular membrane. There is a subretinal haemorrhage and there are exudates in the inferior macula. The membrane can be seen as a greyish-yellow area approximately four disc areas in size in the middle of the macula.

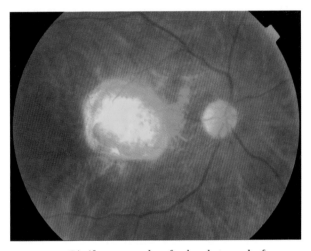

FIGURE 17.5 Disciform scar: colour fundus photograph of a patient's right eye showing the end stage after the damage caused with wet AMD. The subretinal choroidal neovascular membrane has disappeared but left behind a macular scar. There is a disc of scar tissue (hence the term disciform) in the middle of the macula.

18 | Cataract

Cataract means clouding of the lens in the eye. The cloudiness may be mild and visually insignificant or it may be complete and result in virtual blindness.

Causes

Lens opacities can be congenital or acquired.

Congenital cataracts can occur as a result of maternal infections (such as rubella), intrauterine infections, chromosomal or metabolic disorders. They may also be hereditary, following autosomal dominant or recessive inheritance patterns.

Trauma can cause a cataract to form without direct injury to the lens within a few days or many years later. Penetrating injury to the eye involving the lens capsule causes rapid development of a white cataract, as the lens fibres immediately soak up aqueous fluid. Intraocular surgery also slowly increases the process of cataract formation.

Inflammation in the eye, such as iritis or uveitis, can also cause a cataract by gradual damage to the metabolic processes of the lens.

Metabolic problems, particularly diabetes, will cause changes in the nutrient and metabolic milieu surrounding and bathing the lens, resulting in accelerated cataract formation.

Numerous drugs affect the lens. Particular culprits implicated in cataractogenesis are corticosteroids and antimetabolites.

Pathology of cataract formation

The lens is formed from specialised cells full of clear proteins called crystallins, together with large amounts of water. There is no blood supply and the lens relies on the surrounding aqueous fluid for nutrients and oxygen.

Over time and in response to trauma, the crystallin molecules change their structure and become more opaque. This is accompanied by changes in the

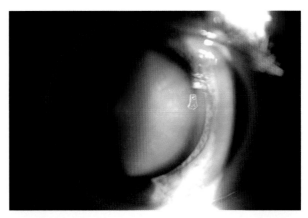

FIGURE 18.1 **Slit lamp view of a dense cataract. The slit view allows us to see deeper into the cataract and get a three-dimensional impression of it.**

hydration of the lens. With these changes, the refractive index of the lens may increase, thus giving the eye more focusing power and effectively making the patient short-sighted (*see* Chapter 7, The focusing mechanism of the eye [refraction]). Elderly patients who needed reading spectacles are occasionally surprised that they can suddenly see things close up clearly and read without their glasses (a hallmark of short-sightedness). This phenomenon has been described as 'second sight' and represents a myopic shift in refraction (*see* Chapter 7). Although the lens power increases for a short time, this benefit is short-lived, as the lens continues to change, leading to opacity and reduced vision.

Patients tend to complain of gradual onset of blurred vision and misting. Other symptoms include haloes or glare related to the disruption and scatter of the light passing through the lens. These symptoms are particularly noticeable in bright light and at night. Posterior subcapsular cataracts (lens opacities localised to the back of the lens) are especially troublesome because they cause haloes and glare. These symptoms alone may warrant cataract extraction, despite normal visual acuity.

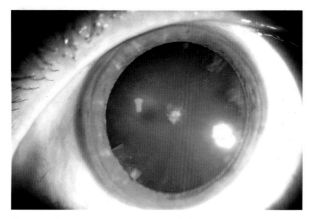

a)

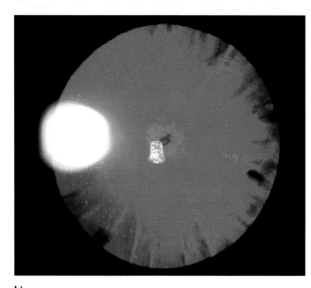

b)

FIGURES 18.2a and b **a) Anterior segment view showing the whitish appearance of the cataract. b) The cataract is seen much more clearly with the use of the ophthalmoscope. The red reflex is interrupted by black spoke-like opacities.**

Cataracts are best seen by examining the patient with a slit lamp (figure 18.1), but looking at the red reflex with the direct ophthalmoscope will allow you to make a reasonable assessment (figures 18.2a and b). The cataract is seen as black or grey opacities against the bright glow of the red reflex. If the cataract is extremely advanced it will appear white, giving the patient a leucocoria (white pupil).

Management

If the patient is experiencing symptoms and feels that a visual improvement would enhance their quality of life, they should be offered cataract extraction. Cataract surgery is not entirely without risk, but it is relatively safe. In common with any intervention, it is important to give the patient adequate information about risks and possible complications. The risks-versus-benefits ratio should always be considered, particularly when a cataract is not reducing vision excessively, or when there is concurrent ocular pathology.

When you see a patient with a cataract, take a thorough history and do a full ocular examination. It is not uncommon for patients with cataracts to have other concurrent pathology, particularly AMD. It is also important to ensure that the cataract is indeed responsible for the visual symptoms, as this will have implications for the decision to proceed with cataract extraction and will allow the ophthalmologist to give the patient realistic expectations about their vision after surgery.

In the past, the cataract was removed and the patient left without a lens (aphakia). This meant that the eye's focusing mechanism was grossly underpowered, and the patient had to wear very thick 'jam-jar bottom' glasses. With the advent of intraocular lens (IOL) technology, however, we are now able to replace the native lens with a synthetic one, allowing accurate focusing of incoming images on to the retina. This is called pseudophakia.

Intraocular lenses are made in many different powers. A series of complex calculations are done, based on many measurements including the length of the eye and the steepness (and thus power) of the cornea. The results are used to work out the power of lens needed to correct the focusing ability of the eye in question. It is thus possible to fit an IOL into the eye of a short- or long-sighted patient that cancels out their pre-existing refractive error, allowing them to see in the distance without spectacles.

The synthetic lenses do not change shape like natural lenses, and thus they keep a fixed power. Reading spectacles will be needed for near distance, however. This is not a major problem for older patients, who have probably been using reading spectacles for some time, but younger patients might be surprised that they cannot now see close up without glasses.

Surgical aspects

Historically, several techniques have been used for cataract extractions. Currently, two methods are used for surgical extraction: extracapsular cataract extraction (ECCE) and phacoemulsification. Phacoemulsification is the newer technique and is rapidly becoming the gold standard. As the technology advances, different techniques may develop, all aimed at removing the cataract with minimal trauma/disturbance to the eye and replacing the lens with a totally biocompatible material.

ECCE

This involves a large incision, involving almost one-third of the corneal circumference. A linear hole is made in the anterior lens capsule and the lens is expressed out through the corneal wound by pressure on the eye. The soft remnants of the cataract are then sucked out with a special instrument. A lens is then placed into the capsule – called the capsular bag. The corneal wound is sutured closed with non-absorbable material (figure 18.3). With such a large corneal wound, rehabilitation is quite lengthy and there are often problems with healing and with excessive irregularity of the cornea (astigmatism).

Phacoemulsification

With this new technology, a very small wound (about 3 mm) is made in the cornea to access the anterior chamber and thus the cataract. A round cut is made in the anterior capsule of the lens with a needle and forceps (called a continuous curvilinear capsullorhexis) and fluid is injected around the cataract to release it from its surrounding capsule. A phacoemulsification probe is then inserted in the anterior chamber.

Phacoemulsification involves using ultrasound energy to 'eat away' the cataract. Once the cataract is removed, an IOL of about 6 mm in diameter is inserted in the capsular bag. To allow this small-incision procedure, modern IOLs are pliable, allowing the surgeon to fold the lens in half or roll it into an 'injector' device and pass it through the 3 mm wound into the eye. The lens then unfolds in the capsular bag.

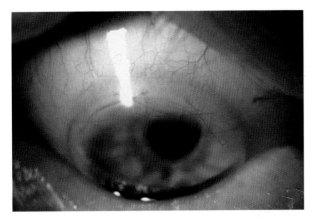

FIGURE 18.3 Colour photograph of the front of an eye that has undergone large-incision cataract surgery (extracapsular cataract extraction). The patient is looking down and the sutures for the corneal wound are clearly seen.

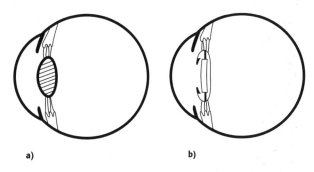

a)   b)

FIGURES 18.4 a and b a) Cross-section of the anterior segment of the eye. The cloudy lens (cataract) is clearly seen. b) The cataract has now been removed and has been replaced by a thin synthetic lens. The new lens rests within the capsule of the old lens.

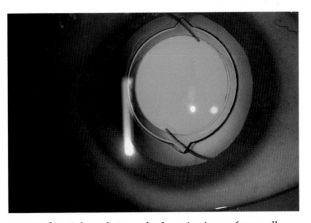

FIGURE 18.5 Colour photograph of a patient's eye after small-incision (phacoemulsification) cataract surgery and intraocular lens implantation. The new synthetic lens can clearly be seen against the red reflex. The clear portion is named the optic and is responsible for refracting the light. It is held in place within the capsular bag by blue arms (called haptics) seen superiorly and inferiorly.

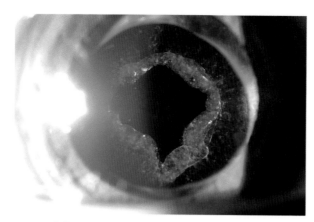

FIGURE 18.6 **The patient has undergone cataract surgery and lens implantation; however, lens epithelial cells have proliferated and caused posterior capsular opacification. A YAG laser has been used to cut a diamond-shaped hole in this thickened area of capsule.**

No sutures are usually required as the wound is self-sealing (figures 18.4a, 18.4b and 18.5).

Postoperative management

Patients are usually given an antibiotic drop and a steroid drop to use four times per day.

The main complication of concern is infection. Infection inside the eye, called postoperative endophthalmitis, is a disastrous problem that can be blinding. If it is caught early enough and appropriate treatment initiated, vision can be saved. Infection usually occurs between two and five days postoperatively. It presents as decreased vision, redness and pain. Any patient with these symptoms early in their postoperative course should be seen by an ophthalmologist as a matter of urgency.

Postoperative refraction

The eye usually takes approximately one month to settle after cataract surgery. At this stage, the patient may attend their optician for refraction and prescription of new spectacles. Usually when an IOL power is selected for implantation, the surgeon is aiming to give the patient unaided distance vision.

Occasionally, the patient's circumstances require a different approach. If the patient would rather have unaided near vision (thus needing spectacles for distance vision), the surgeon may choose an IOL power aiming for a refraction of –1 to –2 (*see* Chapter 7). If the patient has one eye with a significant cataract and the other with a clear lens, then a lens power that leaves the affected eye matching the unaffected eye may be needed, even if this means leaving that eye markedly short- or long-sighted. This is because a large discrepancy between the refractions of the eyes (e.g. more than two dioptres [dioptres are the measurement used to quantify spectacle power]) can lead to difficulty with cerebral integration of the two different-sized images from each eye.

Tight stitches from sutured wounds (e.g. after ECCE) may result in significant corneal irregularity and thus excessive astigmatism (*see* Chapter 7). Sutures may be removed allowing the cornea to regain its original sphericity once the wounds are adequately healed.

Posterior capsular opacification

When the hole is made into the front of the capsule surrounding the lens in order to remove the cataract and place the synthetic lens into the capsular 'bag', the posterior capsule is left intact to support the new lens. This is completely clear initially, but in about one-third of patients proliferating residual lens epithelial cells eventually cause this layer to become cloudy, usually years later. The vision deteriorates gradually, and the patient develops a 'second cataract' (not truly a cataract at all). This is easily detected on slit lamp examination and is treated by using a YAG laser to burn a hole in the cloudy layer, thus clearing the vision again (figure 18.6). Modern IOLs are designed to minimise this problem.

19 | Cornea

The cornea is the clear window of the eye and essential for vision. It also plays a vital role in the refractive mechanisms of sight (*see* Chapter 7). It is dome-shaped, measuring approximately 12mm in diameter with its horizontal meridian slightly wider than in its vertical dimension, and is only 0·5mm thick centrally and 1mm thick at its peripheries. The cornea is avascular, receiving nutrients and oxygen from the aqueous fluid circulating in the eye and the tear film/atmosphere.

The cornea retains its clarity through a relative state of dehydration. This dehydration is facilitated by the active pumping of water out of the corneal substance by the endothelial cells lining the inner surface of the cornea. These endothelial cells cannot replicate and thus over the years their numbers decrease irreversibly. This is only a problem if the density of endothelial cells falls below a certain critical value and the pump fails. The cornea then becomes too wet, thickens and loses clarity. This is called corneal oedema, and can occur in response to many different types of insult.

Infection

(*See also* Chapter 15, Red eye.)

The human cornea is relatively resistant to infection, but may be involved in bacterial, viral, amoebic and fungal processes. Very few bacteria are capable of infecting the native healthy cornea. Organisms that can produce infection in a healthy cornea include *Neisseria gonorrhoea*, diphtheroids and *Haemophilus* species. The greatest risk of infection occurs when the cornea's defences are weakened. Factors likely to lead to corneal compromise include excessive dryness, neuropathy, previous scarring, lid abnormalities, and most importantly contact lens wear.

Bacterial

Bacterial keratitis can occur after a corneal injury such as abrasion or laceration, particularly when there is retention of foreign material. It may also occur as a result of contact lens wear.

Once the epithelium is breached, the bacteria are able to invade the corneal stroma and form a localised abscess. This will manifest as a white, fluffy, localised opacity of the cornea with an overlying corneal epithelial defect. It may be associated with a collection of white pus cells settled at the bottom of the anterior chamber, called a hypopyon (figure 15.4).

Treatment involves intensive broad-spectrum topical antibiotics after a corneal scrape has been sent for microbiological culture. Unfortunately, even with speedy resolution, a corneal ulcer usually leaves a scar. If this scar is close to the visual axis (the central area of the cornea that the patient looks through) vision may be markedly reduced.

Viral

Herpes simplex keratitis (dendritic ulcer)

Herpes simplex virus infection can occur in childhood as a vesicular lid rash or may be entirely subclinical. The virus may then lie dormant in the trigeminal ganglia and reactivate at any time. When activated, the virus particles travel down one of the divisions of the trigeminal nerve and result in cutaneous involvement. If the virus attacks the mandibular division of the trigeminal nerve, the patient may develop a cold sore. If it travels down the ophthalmic division, it may cause vesicular lesions on the lid margin, or if it travels along the nasociliary division, it can reach the corneal nerves. Infection of the cornea results in mild pain, redness and blurring of vision. The epithelium overlying the infected corneal nerves breaks down and an ulcer forms. The ulcer is branch-shaped – the classical dendritic ulcer – and will clearly stain with fluorescein (figures 19.1a and b).

Treatment involves application of antiviral ointments such as aciclovir usually five times a day, which should lead to rapid resolution within about two

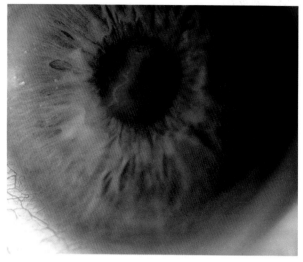

a)

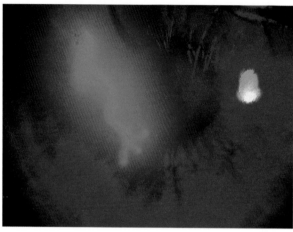

b)

FIGURES 19.1 a and b a) Colour photograph of a patient with a dendritic ulcer. The fine branching pattern is visible; however, it is much more evident when viewed with fluorescein staining and a blue light. b) Typical fine branching pattern of a dendritic ulcer seen with fluorescein staining and a blue light. (Courtesy of Mr R.M. Gregson.)

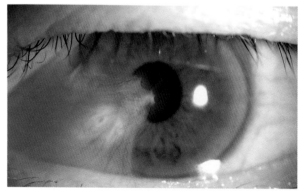

FIGURE 19.2 Colour photograph of a marked pterygium that is growing across to affect the centre of the cornea and thus vision.

weeks. Unfortunately, a visually significant scar can be left. We can never kill the virus but only inhibit its activity in the cornea. The virus will thus always lie dormant in the trigeminal ganglion and can reactivate with consequent recurrence of dendritic ulcers. Multiple episodes will result in progressive scarring, and if this compromises vision the patient may require a corneal graft. Steroids must *never* be given in isolation to patients with a dendritic ulcer, as this will cause a dramatic increase in the size of the ulcer.

Protozoal

Acanthamoeba

Acanthamoebae are free-growing protozoa. They live in brackish water, but can be found in any water, including tap water. They are usually implicated in corneal infections related to contact lens wear. Patients develop a markedly painful red eye. In contrast to bacterial infections, the pain usually outweighs the clinical signs. This condition is potentially sight threatening, and can be very hard to diagnose. It is usually related to contaminated contact lens fluids or contact lens cases. If suspected, it is important to culture the contact lens case to see whether any organisms can be isolated. The clinical appearance may resemble that of a bacterial infection, but certain features are visible on slit lamp examination that may help to secure the diagnosis. If a bacterial ulcer is not resolving despite a prolonged course of intensive antibiotic therapy, acanthamoeba keratitis should be suspected. Treatment is with an intensive course of specialised drops.

Fungal

Fungal keratitis is rare and usually associated with significant corneal compromise or trauma. Corneas suffering trauma involving organic matter (e.g. wood) are particularly prone to fungal keratitis, especially if foreign material, such as part of a thorn, is retained within the cornea. Clinically, the eye is red and inflamed. The cornea will show white, spreading, finger-like opacities within the stroma. Treatment is with intensive, topical antifungals.

Non-infective conditions

Pterygium

A pterygium is a benign degeneration of the conjunctiva that spreads to extend over the cornea (figure 19.2). The deeper conjunctival layers proliferate and begin to invade the superficial layers of the cornea. This condition is more common in tropical climates, and is associated with excessive exposure to ultraviolet (UV) radiation. It usually occurs at the 'three o'clock' and 'nine o'clock' positions of the cornea, as these areas are most exposed. The superior and inferior conjunctiva are protected by the lids. Pterygium is usually asymptomatic until the invading fleshy conjunctiva extends to the central cornea and affects vision.

The exact aetiology is unknown, but UV radiation and the human papilloma virus (HPV) have been implicated in pathogenesis. Patients may complain of the cosmetic appearance and request treatment. Surgical removal is required, but the patient must be warned that the lesion can recur.

Pinguecula

A pinguecula is similar to a pterygium in that it is a conjunctival degeneration. It manifests as single or multiple yellowy nodules lying on the conjunctiva adjacent to the cornea at the 'three o'clock' and 'nine o'clock' positions. In contrast to pterygia, pingueculae never encroach on to the cornea and are usually asymptomatic, requiring no treatment.

Band keratopathy

When the eye is exposed to chronic inflammation, the cornea reacts by losing its metabolic integrity, allowing salts, particularly calcium, to enter the anterior corneal stroma just beneath the epithelium. These white calcium crystals are deposited within the interpalpebral space (the area between the upper and lower eyelids), forming a white band that eventually extends right across the middle of the cornea. It begins at the three and nine o'clock positions, and then progresses across the visual axis, with concomitant visual loss.

If the vision is reduced enough to warrant an operation, the calcium is dissolved by applying chelating solutions to the anterior corneal stroma after the overlying epithelium has been removed in theatre. The chelating agents leave the corneal architecture unaffected. The corneal epithelium heals and corneal clarity should be restored, along with vision.

It is important to treat the underlying disorder in order to prevent onset or recurrence of the condition. Rarely, metabolic disorders such as hypercalcaemia cause band keratopathy because of the high levels of ambient calcium salts involved.

Corneal arcus

This is a common finding and not pathological. It is related to deposits of fat within the corneal periphery and manifests as a ring of white about 1mm in from the corneal limbus. It tends to occur in older patients, and is hence commonly referred to as arcus senilis. If found in patients under 40 years of age with no other ocular pathology, it may be a sign of familial hypercholesterolaemia and requires investigating.

Keratoconus

Keratoconus is a condition of unknown aetiology whereby the cornea progressively loses its gentle curvature. The central portion of the cornea thins and extrudes to form a cone shape (figure 19.3). This cone

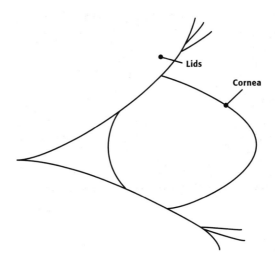

FIGURE 19.3 **Cross-section of the cornea showing the cone-shaped protuberance of the corneal surface resulting in abnormal refraction of light.**

cannot focus the light normally, and the patient develops a large degree of astigmatism (*see* Chapter 7) and, if uncorrected, progressive blurring of vision. The weakened central section of cornea is prone to sudden decompensation, which occurs when the endothelial cell layer develops a spontaneous rupture that allows fluid to enter the normally dehydrated cornea, resulting in sudden opacity with visual loss and pain.

Initially, the irregularity (and thus astigmatism) of the cornea may be corrected by spectacles but, over time, the irregularity becomes so marked that contact lenses are required to restore an acceptable refractive contour. Eventually even these will fail to correct vision, however, and a corneal graft (penetrating keratoplasty) will be needed. Patients who have this surgery tend to do well and have good visual results, but

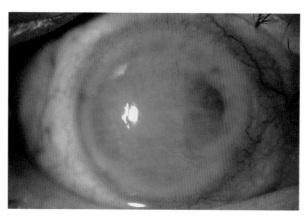

FIGURE 19.4 **The cornea is cloudy due to decompensation/failure of the endothelial cell pump. Water has entered the cornea resulting in oedema and a hazy appearance. The vision will be reduced due to the opacity.**

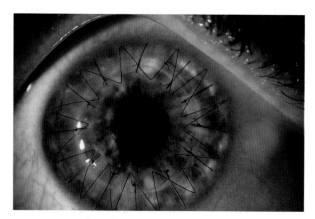

FIGURE 19.5 **Colour photograph of a corneal graft/penetrating keratoplasty. The sutures holding the new central graft tissue in place are clearly seen.**

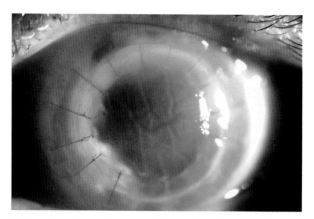

FIGURE 19.6 **Colour photograph of a patient who has undergone a previous corneal graft. The graft is failing and is thus opacified and hazy.**

the graft can still fail and significant visual morbidity is associated with complications. If at all possible, these patients are managed without resorting to surgery.

Pseudophakic bullous keratopathy

The endothelial cells are responsible for pumping water out of the cornea, thus maintaining corneal clarity. They are lost throughout life due to involutional/ageing changes. Ocular trauma, even in the form of a planned surgical procedure such as cataract extraction, results in attrition to the endothelial cells. Inevitably, there is some degree of cell loss. If the cornea has enough reserves, then the cell loss and consequent decrease in endothelial cell density will be subclinical. If, however, the cell count falls below a critical level, the cornea will become oedematous (excessively hydrated), with fluid-filled microcysts (called bullae) developing within the corneal stroma and epithelium (figure 19.4).

Postoperative corneal oedema is relatively common in the early stages, probably related to transient dysfunction of the endothelial cells. If this fails to clear, the patient has developed pseudophakic bullous keratopathy.

Sometimes hypertonic eye drops are used to help dehydrate the cornea and improve corneal clarity and thus vision, but this is a temporary measure with limited efficacy. Definitive management involves corneal grafting, but this is dependent upon the visual potential of the eye and the motivation of the patient.

Corneal grafts

If the cornea is irreversibly compromised in terms of clarity or contour, resulting in poor vision, the patient may be considered for corneal grafting (penetrating keratoplasty).

Corneal grafts are the most successful allotransplants in humans. Donated corneas are stored in central eye banks ready to be ordered when a graft is required.

Because of its avascularity and its immune-privileged site (not being in direct contact with the circulating white blood cells), the cornea does not need to be HLA-matched (human leukocyte antigen), unless there have been several previous graft rejections. A corneal 'button' is cut from the donor cornea (usually around 7·5 mm in diameter) and a slightly smaller area is cut (trephined) from the patient's cornea. The new cornea is then sutured in place (figure 19.5). Problems include early rejection, leakage from the wound and infection.

Patients do not require routine systemic immunosuppression, and are usually maintained on topical steroids for one to two years.

Rejection is the major concern and may occur early or late. It may affect the epithelial, stromal or endothelial component of the new graft. It manifests as decreased vision, redness and pain with oedema/haze of the graft tissue (figure 19.6). If untreated, the graft will fail and progressively vascularise and opacify. Treatment should be initiated early with high-dose, systemic and intensive topical corticosteroids guided by the severity of the problem. With appropriate treatment, the graft may be saved and vision preserved. Unfortunately, some patients have irreversible rejection and will require a second graft.

Loose stitches are a common problem and cause a foreign-body sensation (figure 19.7). Loose stitches can also stimulate graft rejection, and an ophthalmologist should remove them urgently.

Indications for grafting are mainly related to keratoconus, pseudophakic bullous keratopathy, corneal dystrophies and degenerations or infections.

If a cornea is about to perforate, or has already done so, because of uncontrolled infection, a graft may be required to remove the infective focus and restore the integrity of the globe. Penetrating keratoplasty in the presence of active infection is obviously risky, and should only be carried out by experienced hands.

Patients who have had a corneal graft because of scarring secondary to herpetic keratitis are at particular risk of graft rejection or recurrence of their herpetic disease.

Corneal dystrophies

These are a group of inherited corneal disorders that result in abnormality of the corneal endothelium, stroma or epithelium.

Endothelial dystrophies lead to endothelial cell loss and dysfunction. The commonest is Fuchs' endothelial dystrophy, which is seen clinically as a 'beaten bronze' appearance of the red reflex. In the early stages, the cornea maintains its clarity but over time the endothelial pump can fail and the cornea will become cloudy and oedematous, with visual loss. The condition is pain free unless the bullae (microcysts formed by the accumulation of fluid in the corneal substance) burst at the epithelial surface, resulting in a sharp pain. Patients with this condition already have a compromised cornea and are at risk of pseudophakic bullous keratopathy after cataract surgery. Treatment is with topical hyperosmotic solutions to dehydrate the cornea,

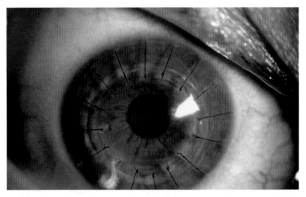

FIGURE 19.7 A loose corneal suture is seen to the bottom left of the picture. Mucus is adhering to it and it is probably causing a foreign-body sensation. Of more concern is that it may stimulate a graft rejection.

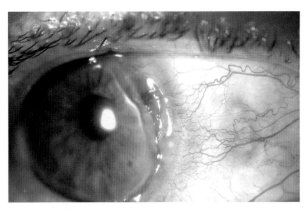

FIGURE 19.8 The cornea has begun to melt away and thin in a trough parallel to the corneal limbus due to rheumatoid arthritis. The eye need not be excessively inflamed or red.

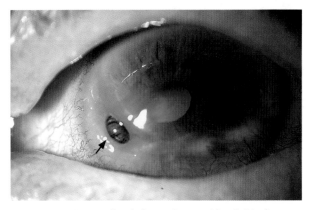

FIGURE 19.9 A corneal melt due to rheumatoid arthritis that has become full thickness resulting in a perforation. The aqueous has flooded out of the anterior chamber and the hole is plugged by iris tissue (arrow).

or corneal grafting.

A common dystrophy involving the epithelial layer is called Cogan's microcystic dystrophy. In this condition, the superficial epithelial cells are not correctly stuck down to the underlying stroma. Cogan's is related to abnormal junctions between the basal epithelial cells and the underlying basement membrane (the Bowman's membrane). Patients may experience sudden sharp stabbing pains caused by some of the superficial cells spontaneously detaching, effectively giving the patient a non-traumatic corneal abrasion. This can happen quite frequently, particularly if the cornea has been inadvertently damaged or scratched. The classical history is pain first thing in the mornings when the patient opens their eyes. The eye dries up over night and the inner surface of the upper lid sticks to the weakened epithelial cells. When the eye is opened, the lid rips off the cells, causing an abrasion. Treatment usually involves keeping the eyes well lubricated to prevent any tractional force on these fragile cells. Eye ointment at night may prevent morning dryness.

There are many other dystrophies that can lead to material being deposited in the cornea, with subsequent loss of corneal clarity. Some are related to systemic conditions, while others are localised to the cornea. Usually, treatment of any underlying cause and cornea grafting restores vision.

Corneal involvement in systemic disease

Corneal melt

The cornea is composed of collagen and is thus susceptible to damage associated with systemic connective tissue disorders such as rheumatoid arthritis. Patients with active disease may develop sterile corneal ulcers or loss of corneal stromal collagen, leading to progressive thinning (figure 19.8) and even perforation (figure 19.9). Treatment is related to control of the systemic inflammatory process and ensuring adequate wetting of the cornea with preservative-free lubricant drops. Any perforation can be treated with a special corneal glue to prevent the aqueous fluid leaking out of the eye.

Kayser-Fleischer ring

This is a symptom of Wilson's disease, a disorder that causes the body to retain copper. The Kayser-Fleischer ring is the result of deposits of copper at the periphery of the cornea, and appears as a thin, copper-coloured ring within the cornea. It is best seen with a slit lamp.

20 | Diabetic eye disease

Complications of diabetes are the commonest cause of blindness in the Western world. Patients with insulin-dependent diabetes (IDD) are usually diagnosed early in life and tend to be spared diabetic eye problems in the first years of their disease. Later on, however, more and more of these patients develop eye problems, with as many as 90% having diabetic eye disease by the fifteenth year of diabetes. Patients with non-insulin-dependent diabetes (NIDD) on the other hand may have significant ocular pathology at diagnosis. As a general rule, they tend to get a maculopathy, whereas those with IDD are more prone to neovascularisation (new blood vessel formation) and complications of the peripheral retina.

A large study (the Diabetic Control and Complications Trial) (The effect of intensive diabetes treatment on the progression of diabetic retinopathy in insulin-dependent diabetes mellitus. The Diabetes Control and Complications Trial. *Arch Ophthalmol* 1995; **113**: 36–51) has shown that the progression and severity of diabetic eye disease is related to the patient's degree of diabetic control. The tighter the control, the smaller the risk of developing ocular complications of diabetes and of progression of any existing diabetic eye disease.

There are several risk factors for the development and progression of diabetic eye disease:

- Duration of disease. The longer the patient has diabetes, the more likely they are to develop diabetic eye disease.
- Poor control. The worse the control, the more likely the patient is to develop problems and lose vision. Individual control may be objectively assessed by measuring the serum levels of glycosylated haemoglobin (HbA$_{1c}$). In the normal population this should be less than 6·5%, but in patients with poorly controlled diabetes it may reach 10%.
- Hypertension. Even a small degree of hypertension

increases the risk of diabetes-related eye and systemic disease.
- Smoking.

Attention to the above factors can help to reduce the risks of diabetic eye disease. Unfortunately despite this, patients can still develop significant problems, even progressing to bilateral blindness.

The effects of diabetes on the eye

Pathology of background diabetic retinopathy

Diabetic retinopathy is the result of changes in the microvasculature of the eye. The capillary walls become weakened. Their basement membranes thicken and the capillaries lose their supporting pericyte cells (these cells surround the retinal capillaries and are responsible for the tight blood-retinal barrier). These pathological changes have two effects. As the basement membrane thickens, the passage of red blood cells through the narrowed inflexible lumen of the capillaries is restricted.

The loss of pericytes and the changes in the basement membrane also cause breakdown of the physiologically vital blood-retinal barrier (analogous to the blood–brain barrier). Tight control of the nature and volume of fluid passing out of the capillaries into the retinal milieu is essential for the retina to work properly. When this selective filter system fails, excessive fluid leaks out and causes retinal oedema (swelling) with retinal dysfunction. The excessive extravascular flow of fluid contains fat and other unwanted materials, which are taken up by groups of macrophages in the retina. The lipid deposits remain while the continued extravasation of fluid persists, but can be cleared once the leakage is stopped.

Diabetic retinopathy has a wide spectrum of severity. It begins with the subtle changes of mild background diabetic retinopathy and then moves through moderate to severe background diabetic retinopathy. Of greatest concern to the ophthalmologist is the subsequent development of proliferative diabetic retinopathy and maculopathy. Proliferative retinopathy may result in bleeding and scarring that can seriously affect vision, while maculopathy may result in marked dysfunction of the macula with reduction or even loss of central vision. There are several clinical signs of diabetic retinopathy that are discussed below.

Microaneurysms

These are usually the first sign of diabetic retinopathy and used to be called dot haemorrhages. As the walls of the capillaries weaken, they are susceptible to the effects of the blood pressure and may 'blow out' and form a small, localised aneurismal dilatation. They expand abnormally and dilate focally within the retina, seen as a small red dot on fundoscopy (figure 20.1).

Haemorrhage

If these microaneurysms 'pop', they leave a haemorrhage within the retina. This is called a blot haemorrhage, and is seen as a large red blob against the orange background of the retinal pigment epithelium layer reflection (figure 20.1). Over time, this haemorrhage may disappear. If the blood vessel bursts in the superficial layer of the retina, it will spread along the nerve fibre layer (see Chapter 5, Basic anatomy), forming a feathered-edge flame shape, unsurprisingly called a flame-shaped haemorrhage.

Exudates

Lipids released by the leaking retinal vasculature are deposited as localised lakes within the retinal substance. This lipid-filled retina is seen as a glossy yellow area, and is called a hard exudate. Such deposits begin as isolated areas, but may coalesce to form much larger exudates. Occasionally, they are seen surrounding a leaking microaneurysm in a circular pattern, called a circinate exudate (figure 20.2).

Cotton-wool spots

These used to be called soft exudates, but actually represent localised retinal infarction, leading to secondary damage to the overlying nerve fibre layer (NFL). As the blood supply to the nerve fibres is interrupted, the fibres become ischaemic, and their axoplasmic flow is compromised. The collection of axoplasm in the ischaemic portions results in localised opacification of the NFL (figure 20.3). This is visualised as a white 'fluffy' appearance to the superficial retina and tends to have feathery edges – hence the term cotton-wool spot. They are not true exudates.

Changes in venous vasculature

As the retinal circulation is progressively compromised, the blood flow becomes more and more sluggish. The veins dilate, and may become beaded with sections of dilatation interspersed with sections of constriction (venous beading). Such veins can even form loops that project up off the retina (venous looping).

Intraretinal microvascular abnormalities (IRMA)

These are clusters of weakened dilated capillaries within the retinal substance, and may be thought of as areas of arteriovenous shunting between the arterioles and venules. These lesions indicate significant diabetic retinal ischaemia. They are flat and lie within the retinal substance, thus differentiating them from new vessels/neovascularisation.

Proliferative diabetic retinopathy

Pathology of neovascularisation

The progressive damage to the microvasculature of the retina results in hypoperfusion and ischaemia of the many highly metabolically active retinal cells. The ischaemic retina becomes starved of oxygen and reacts by releasing cytokines and other chemical messengers in an attempt to stimulate the growth of new blood vessels (neovascularisation). Although the retina is trying to survive, this is a pathological process and is responsible for the significant visual morbidity associated with proliferative diabetic retinopathy.

The local retinal blood vessels react to the stimulus of the cytokines by producing new blood vessels (neovascularisation) composed initially of proliferating vascular endothelial cells. These new blood vessels are deformed, and do not have the appropriate blood-retinal barrier (figure 20.4). They usually project up above the retina into the vitreous cavity and leak profusely. They are immature and fragile, and are thus prone to rupturing. If they do burst, they can be the source of significant sight-threatening haemorrhage, usually into the vitreous cavity.

In addition to the vascular effects, the released cytokines also stimulate fibrous proliferation. The growing fibrous tissue may result in tugging/tractional forces on the retina, with subsequent distortion of the usually smooth retinal surface or even frank retinal detachment (figure 20.5).

The new blood vessels usually develop at the optic disc, but they can form anywhere in the retina or even in the iris.

Maculopathy

Maculopathy indicates diabetic changes within the macula. Changes in the macular blood vessels, resulting in fragility and leakage, may lead to macular oedema, haemorrhages and exudates. These will eventually result in reduction of vision, particularly if these changes spread to the fovea (figure 20.6). Any diabetic changes in the macula warrant the need for close follow up as the disease may rapidly progress to affect vision. Before these pathological changes reach the fovea and affect vision, laser therapy may be given to arrest progression (see below).

Background versus proliferative diabetic retinopathy

The distinction between proliferative and background, otherwise known as non-proliferative diabetic retinopathy, is important, as the management of these two levels of diabetic change is different.

Clinical findings of background (non-proliferative) diabetic retinopathy

- Microaneurysms (dot haemorrhages).
- Exudates.
- Cotton-wool spots.
- Blot haemorrhages.

Clinical findings of proliferative diabetic retinopathy

- Neovascularisation at the disc or elsewhere in the retina.

With a greater understanding of the pathology and progression of diabetic retinopathy, a new category has come into common use. Pre-proliferative diabetic retinopathy, also called severe non-proliferative diabetic retinopathy, is a degree of diabetic retinal disease now recognised as the precursor of neovascular/proliferative diabetic retinopathy. Changes such as IRMA, venous beading and severe haemorrhages in all four quadrants of the retina are classified as pre-proliferative diabetic retinopathy. Such changes require close follow up by an ophthalmologist for signs of progression or may even warrant early laser treatment (see below).

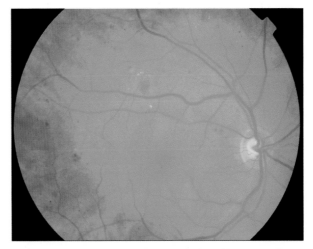

FIGURE 20.1 Colour fundus photograph of mild background diabetic retinopathy. There are microaneurysms (dot haemorrhages) and blot haemorrhages scattered around the posterior pole. The macula is relatively spared.

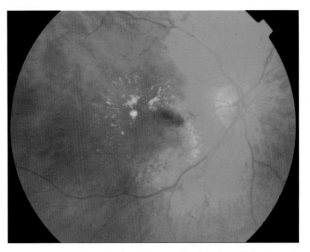

FIGURE 20.2 Colour fundus photograph of marked diabetic maculopathy. There is a large ring of exudates surrounding a leaking point in the macula. The exudates are also affecting the fovea and thus vision is probably reduced and certainly threatened.

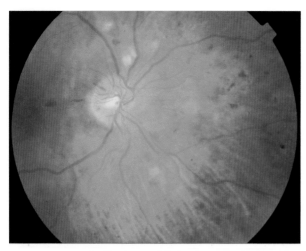

FIGURE 20.3 **Marked background diabetic retinopathy with dot and blot haemorrhages, and extensive cotton-wool spots.**

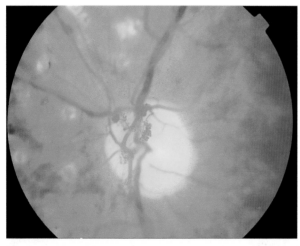

FIGURE 20.4 **Proliferative diabetic retinopathy. New blood vessels have developed at the optic disc. These vessels are abnormally friable and may rupture, causing a vitreous haemorrhage and marked reduction in vision.**

Treatment

Maculopathy

The aim of treating diabetic maculopathy is to decrease the amount of macular oedema and prevent the spread of exudates and haemorrhages to the fovea, thus preventing permanent loss of vision. The only proven treatment shown to be of benefit in macular oedema is laser photocoagulation. Steroids injected around or into the eye are proving effective in some situations where the maculopathy is resistant to standard laser treatments.

Laser energy is applied to the retina to make controlled burns. These burns seal the leaking blood vessels and result in resolution of the intraretinal oedema and resorption of the exudates. This laser energy obviously cannot be applied to the fovea, as a burn there will result in immediate dramatic loss of vision. It is important to treat the abnormal areas of retina before oedema becomes established at the fovea and particularly before exudates develop there. Lasering the retina within the macula can cause a small visual field defect (scotoma). However, the brain rapidly adapts to this and, as with the blind spot, it is hardly noticeable (it becomes a negative scotoma). By selectively treating non-essential areas of the macula, the ophthalmologist attempts to preserve the fovea and thus the most sensitive part of the retina.

Management of diabetic maculopathy is based upon a large study called the Early Treatment Diabetic Retinopathy Study (ETDRS) (Photocoagulation therapy for diabetic eye disease. Early Treatment Diabetic Retinopathy Study Research Group. *JAMA* 1985; **254**: 3086). The ETDRS defined certain clinical characteristics of macular oedema that were indicative of the potential for progression to visual loss. The presence of these features, called clinically significant macular oedema (CSMO), warrant laser treatment to the affected area of retina to preserve sight.

In order to visualise the affected area better, an intravenous fluorescein angiogram (IVFA) may be undertaken. A dye, sodium fluorescein, is injected intravenously into the arm, and photographs are taken of the back of the eye. The passage of the fluorescent dye through the arteries, capillaries and veins of the eye is easily seen with a light, and photographed. The abnormal leaky parts of the retina are easily spotted and laser treatment can be directed to these areas to 'dry' the macular oedema.

Proliferative diabetic retinopathy

The stimulus for the proliferation of blood vessels is hypoxia of the retina. In an inelegant solution to this problem, ophthalmologists kill off this starving retina, rather than try to help it. By destroying large amounts of the peripheral retina (pan-retinal photocoagulation – PRP) with laser, the hypoxia is alleviated and the stimulus for neovascularisation is removed. Moreover, the cells that were secreting the cytokine stimulus to cause the proliferation are destroyed. The balance between oxygen supply and demand in the retina is restored, and the new vessels, deprived of their stimulus to grow, disappear. The burnt areas of retina form scars, seen as variably pigmented pale patches, scattered throughout the peripheral retina and coming up to, but not usually crossing, the vascular arcades around the macula (figure 20.7). Because the scars consist of dead tissue, the patient has no vision in this area. Patients will lose some peripheral visual field and, if a large amount of laser is required, they will suffer markedly constricted fields, and might no longer be allowed to drive.

There is some evidence that patients with severe non-proliferative or pre-proliferative diabetic retinopathy may benefit from PRP laser, but this is controversial and most ophthalmologists wait for new blood vessel changes before treating.

Vitrectomy

If the new blood vessels haemorrhage into the vitreous, then the vision will be suddenly reduced. If a large amount of blood enters the vitreous cavity, the loss may be severe, possibly even reduced to perception of light (PL) visual acuity. The haemorrhage may clear over time but, if it is dense, this may take years, if it happens at all.

Not only will the vision be reduced, but also the ophthalmologist will be unable to give the much-needed PRP laser treatment. In order to apply the laser, the ophthalmologist needs an adequate view of the retina. If blood obscures that view, then laser treatment has to be delayed, and this delay allows the proliferative process to progress unchecked under the cover of the vitreous haemorrhage.

In these cases, an operation may be required to clear the blood, restore vision and allow laser treatment. This operation is called a vitrectomy and involves cutting/chopping up the vitreous jelly and sucking it out, along with the blood. Aggressive laser therapy is then given.

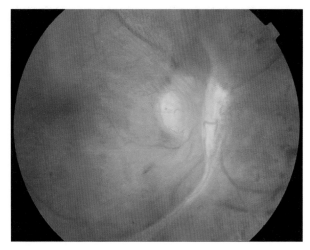

FIGURE 20.5 Proliferative diabetic retinopathy. Here the new blood vessels have grown along with fibrous tissue. This fibrous tissue is causing traction and folding of the retina.

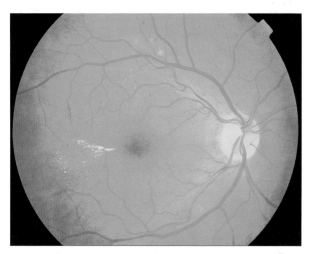

FIGURE 20.6 Background diabetic retinopathy with significant maculopathy. The exudates from a leaking patch of retina in the temporal macula are 'pointing' and progressing towards the fovea.

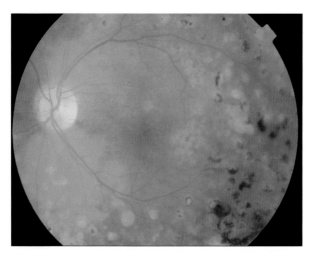

FIGURE 20.7 **Pan-retinal photocoagulation scars are seen in the peripheral retina. These are seen as regular, round, pale patches with or without surrounding pigment changes.**

Other diabetic problems

People with diabetes have an increased incidence of vascular problems, such as central retinal vein or artery occlusions.

They also have an increased incidence of cataracts at a younger age, possibly caused by the glycaemia affecting the hydration and metabolism of the lens. Not only do diabetics get cataracts earlier, but also surgical removal may stimulate progression of their diabetic retinopathy. These patients require adequate stabilisation of their pre-operative diabetic retinopathy and careful follow up to detect progression.

New vessels may also develop in the anterior segment (on the iris or in the drainage angle), as a result of diffusion of the vascular proliferative factors from the hypoxic retina through the vitreous to the front of the eye. These new blood vessels may result in fibrovascular blockage of the aqueous drainage system, resulting in rubeotic glaucoma (*see* Chapter 21, Glaucoma).

Diabetic screening

Patients with diabetes should be screened regularly for diabetic retinopathy. This may be done by an optometrist or diabetes physician. Patients with maculopathy, severe non-proliferative diabetic retinopathy or proliferative diabetic retinopathy should be immediately referred to the ophthalmology services for follow up.

21 | Glaucoma

In order to keep the spherical shape necessary for sight, the eye must maintain a certain level of internal pressure. Most of the globe is filled with vitreous jelly that is static in volume. The pressure is created, maintained and changed by the amount of aqueous fluid in the anterior chamber. Aqueous fluid is produced by the ciliary body and drains into the trabecular meshwork that lies within the internal angle where cornea meets iris.

A simple comparison is with water in a bath. The ciliary body can be seen as a continuously running tap and the trabecular meshwork as the plug hole, which constantly empties the bath. The intraocular pressure depends upon the amount of aqueous (i.e. the amount of water in the bath), which, in turn, depends on the inflow-versus-outflow ratio.

In normal eyes, the production of aqueous corresponds to the drainage, and is maintained at a relatively constant level (tap flow = plug flow). Normal intraocular pressure (IOP) is between 14 mm and 22 mm of mercury (mmHg). Normally, there is a diurnal fluctuation in IOP, with the pressure highest in the morning, which then reduces throughout the day.

In some people, the balance between production and drainage is disturbed: either the aqueous production is excessive or the drainage is deficient.

Any imbalance will result in raised IOP, with a variety of consequences depending on the degree of pressure rise, its rapidity of onset, and the individual susceptibility of the patient's eye to that raised pressure.

Measuring intraocular pressure

There are two main methods used in clinical practice: applanation tonometry and 'air-puff' tonometry.

Applanation tonometry

When you indent a balloon with your finger, the rigidity/firmness of that balloon is proportional to the pressure inside. Low pressure makes a soft balloon; high pressure, a hard balloon. The Goldmann applanation tonometer is used to measure IOP in the hospital setting. This consists of a tonometer head attached to a spring-loaded lever. After application of anaesthetic and fluorescein dye, the tonometer head is brought into contact with the cornea. The force exerted by the spring mechanism may be altered until the head indents the cornea by a certain pre-set amount. At this point, the force required to indent the cornea (read off a dial) is equal to the IOP (opposing equal forces).

Air-puff tonometry

Here a pulse of air is used to indent the cornea, and the degree of indentation is measured by reflection of light. A calculation is made about how 'stiff' the eye is, and thus the IOP measurement. Optometrists commonly use this method to measure IOP in the community, but unfortunately it tends to give false high readings, resulting in inappropriate referrals to hospital eye services.

Recently, evidence has emerged indicating that corneal thickness is an important factor in IOP measurement. The thinner the cornea, the more likely we are to underestimate the true pressure inside the eye. Thus, if a patient has a central corneal thickness of 0.45 mm (the normal being 0.55 mm) and a measured pressure of 20 mmHg, their pressure is actually likely to be higher. This is because the calculations used for Goldmann applanation tonometry are based on the standard corneal thickness.

Clinical tip: in the absence of equipment, you can arrive at a gross estimation of IOP by a digital method. An eye with pathologically high pressure will feel extremely firm, like a cricket ball, when compared with a normal eye. Close your eyes and palpate your own globe. It should 'give' slightly, indicating normal IOP. This is a clumsy method and will not detect the moderately raised pressure of chronic glaucoma but should help in detecting acute, particularly angle-closure, glaucoma.

Glaucomatous damage

Glaucoma is an optic neuropathy that we do not yet fully understand. For some reason, the optic nerve starts to malfunction and the patient begins to lose nerve fibres. This manifests as optic disc changes and a specific pattern of visual field loss.

There is much research into the exact reasons for these changes and the consequent visual loss. We do know that raised IOP is a risk factor for glaucomatous damage, and this is the only factor that we can currently modify in order to prevent progression of the disease. In simple terms, the high pressure inside the eye occludes the fine capillaries supplying blood to the optic nerve head, resulting in death of nerve fibres and consequent patches of visual field loss.

The optic nerve head reacts to the raised pressure by 'bowing out', resulting in a cup at the optic disc. This cup represents loss of retinal nerve fibres as they dip down and enter the optic nerve (figure 21.1). Changes in the cup-to-disc ratio of the optic nerve head are often the first sign of glaucoma damage. The vertical dimension of the cup is compared with overall vertical top-to-bottom distance of the disc to give the cup–disc ratio (figure 21.2).

Visual field changes represent the other main feature of glaucoma, and one that results in the ocular morbidity. The lost nerve fibres all project from the retina and are responsible for carrying the impulses from those photoreceptors to the optic nerve, and hence to the brain for analysis. When these nerve fibres degenerate and die, the area they serve becomes 'blind' and a visual field defect, or scotoma, develops.

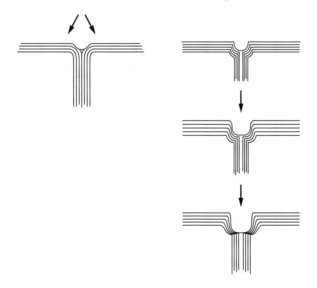

FIGURE 21.1 **Cross-section of the optic disc showing that continued pressure on the optic nerve head causes progressive damage and loss of nerve fibres. This is seen clinically as increased cupping.**

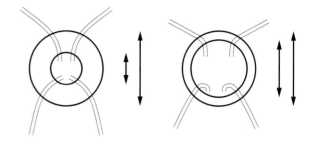

FIGURE 21.2 **The cup–disc ratio is described according to the vertical dimensions of the cup itself compared with the overall vertical size of the disc. The cup–disc ratios here are 0·5 and 0·8.**

Measuring visual fields

Visual fields may be assessed by clinical examination (*see* Chapter 10) or with automated equipment. There are many types of equipment that measure the visual field. The mainstays are the Goldmann and the Humphrey automated perimeters.

The Goldmann visual field test involves the patient looking into an illuminated bowl. The patient keeps looking straight ahead while light targets are moved from the peripheries to the central field of vision. The patient presses a button when they see the light coming into their field of vision, and the areas where the targets are seen are plotted on paper. The light targets can be changed in size and intensity to assess the sensitivity of the visual field.

The Humphrey automated perimeter is the current gold standard of visual field testing. Again, the patient stares into a diffusely light bowl. Lights then flash up automatically in various parts of the bowl corresponding to areas of the patient's visual field. If the patient sees the light, they press a button and this is recorded by computer (figure 21.3). The light at each point may be varied in intensity and the minimum illumination seen is recorded, and thus the light sensitivity of that part of the retina is determined. A reliability indicator also gives the examiner an objective assessment of the patient's degree of co-operation, and thus the reliability of the result. Each plot may also be compared with standardised population data to give statistical information as to 'normality' or the likelihood of a statistically significant visual field defect being present.

The classical visual field defect caused by glaucoma is called an arcuate scotoma (figure 21.4a). It is a negative scotoma (*see* Chapter 10) lying at about 15° above or below the fovea. It occasionally extends from the blind spot and is described as an arcuate scotoma because it arcs around the central vision. As with the blind spot,

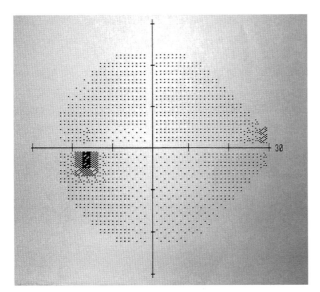

FIGURE 21.3 A printout from an automated visual field machine showing a normal visual field. The black areas are the areas the patient cannot see while the white areas are areas seen by the patient. The localised black area on the left is the patient's blind spot and represents an absolute scotoma (hence it is black). The test goes out to approximately 25° in each direction away from the fovea (represented by the centre of the cross-lines).

the patient does not realise that they have a patch of missing sight as the brain fills in the gap for them. In addition to the loss of this 'arcuate' area, the peripheral visual field also begins to deteriorate. If the process is unchecked, the patient may progress to develop true tunnel vision, where they have only a central small island of vision left (figure 21.4b). Eventually even this can be lost, and the patient goes blind.

Classification of glaucoma

Acute versus chronic

Glaucoma is acute or chronic, depending on the rapidity of onset and progression of the pressure rise.

Rapid rise in pressure causes:

- Pain
- Redness
- Nausea and sometimes vomiting
- Decreased visual acuity due to corneal oedema
- Fixed mid-dilated pupil due to iris ischaemia (the high pressure compromising iris blood supply).

If untreated for a long time this leads to irretrievable visual loss.

With a gradual rise in pressure:

- Patient usually asymptomatic
- Commonly found at a routine optician check-up

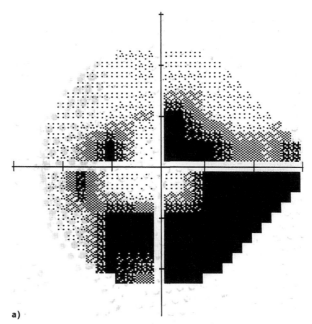
a)

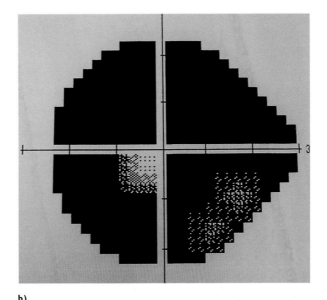
b)

FIGURES 21.4 a and b a) A typical arcuate scotoma seen in glaucoma. b) Severe glaucomatous damage resulting in preservation of only a small central area of vision.

- The major pathology associated with a long-standing rise in IOP is irreversible, gradual and progressive loss of the visual field.

Chronic glaucoma is of gradual onset and slowly progressive, with an IOP usually in the region of 24–34 mmHg.

Acute glaucoma is due to a rapid rise in IOP associated with significant symptoms and visual deterioration. This condition is an ophthalmological emergency and requires rapid lowering of IOP to avoid permanent blindness through infarction of the optic nerve head.

Open-angle versus closed-angle

These terms refer to the pathology underlying the pressure rise, centring on the drainage angle of the anterior chamber. As mentioned above, the trabecular meshwork lies in the angle and is responsible for draining aqueous fluid from the eye. Any process that causes the angle to be physically blocked (e.g. peripheral iris in patients with a narrow angle or by a fibrovascular membrane, as seen in some inflammatory glaucomas) will lead to angle-closure glaucoma. If the angle is open, the pathology must lie within the trabecular meshwork itself at a more microscopic level, and the patient has open-angle glaucoma.

Primary versus secondary

In common with many other medical conditions, glaucoma can be caused by a primary problem inherent to the individual's eye or secondary to another pathological process.

Gonioscopy

Ophthalmologists can visualise the angle and decide whether it is open or closed by means of a gonioscope. Total internal reflection of light in the peripheral cornea does not allow direct visualisation of the angle structures. A contact lens containing a mirror is therefore placed on the eye, allowing a reflected view of the trabecular meshwork.

Ocular hypertension

As mentioned above, an individual eye responds very variably to pressure. In some patients, the IOP is high according to our measurements, but the patient has none of the pathological problems associated with glaucoma. Here we cannot give the patient a diagnosis

of glaucoma because their optic discs are normal and their visual fields are intact. The pressure is high, but this is 'normal for the patient' and well tolerated. The patient has ocular hypertension and is at risk of developing glaucoma, but is by no means certain to get it. They may warrant treatment to lower the pressure, thus reducing the risk of developing glaucomatous damage, but such decisions are based upon the whole clinical picture and not just the high pressure.

Chronic open-angle glaucoma (COAG)

This is also called primary open-angle glaucoma or chronic simple glaucoma. The pressure is above normal (usually in the region of 24–34 mmHg) despite the patient having open angles on gonioscopy, and there is no underlying pathology to be found. The patient's eye is typically not red or painful. Such patients are usually completely asymptomatic and it is picked up at a routine optician check-up.

If untreated, the patient will progressively and painlessly lose visual field, with concomitant changes (cupping) of the optic disc. Eventually, these patients lose vision completely in the affected eye. As the pathology occurs in the form of negative scotoma, the patient does not notice any problem until the central vision is affected, by which time they have lost all of their peripheral vision, as well as some central vision irreversibly. As this is commonly a bilateral disorder, the potential for bilateral blindness is high when the condition is not diagnosed and treated early enough.

COAG is quite a common condition, affecting about one in 200 people over 40 years of age. It is hereditary in that if there is a family history of glaucoma, the patient is at increased risk of developing glaucoma. No specific gene has been isolated and no specific inheritance patterns have been identified globally. Certain paediatric/congenital glaucomas have, however, been linked to specific genes.

The precise cause of open-angle glaucoma is unknown, but we do know that there is some blockage to the normal functioning of the trabecular meshwork. As the meshwork acts as a sieve, filtering the aqueous fluid as it drains it, the sieve can become blocked over time, thus resisting the outflow of aqueous with a subsequent pressure rise.

Primary angle-closure glaucoma

Some people have shallow anterior chambers (a short distance between the back of the cornea and the lens surface), leading to a shallow drainage angle.

When the pupil dilates (e.g. in the dark) the iris can 'ruffle up' in the peripheries of the anterior chamber and cause a physical blockage to aqueous outflow and an acute rise in pressure – this is acute angle-closure glaucoma, a form of primary glaucoma (figures 21.5a and b).

The condition presents with a red, painful eye. The pupil is mid-dilated and the patient may be vomiting. Medical treatment is given to lower the pressure inside the eye. Topical miotics (to constrict the pupil) are applied, but can only take effect once the pressure is reduced and the sphincter pupillae muscle is re-perfused and functional. With miosis, the iris is pulled out of the angle and the blockage temporarily relieved. Definitive treatment is required in the form of a laser or surgical peripheral iridotomy (a hole in the iris). Laser energy is applied to burn a hole in the peripheral iris, creating a short cut for the drainage of the aqueous, thereby restoring flow and drainage (figure 21.6). The peripheral iridotomy stops the iris from blocking the angle even if the pupil is dilated.

If the above measures fail, a drainage operation or lens extraction may be required. By removing the lens and replacing it with a thin, synthetic intraocular lens, the iris is made to fall back and the angle opens.

As the cornea tends to be flatter in patients with narrow angles, it has less refractive power and so these patients tend to be long-sighted. This is more common in patients of Far Eastern origin, as they tend to have flatter corneas and consequently shallower anterior chambers with narrower angles.

Normal-tension glaucoma (NTG)

This condition (also called low-tension glaucoma) may be thought of as the opposite of ocular hypertension. Pressures are high in patients with ocular hypertension, but they tolerate this well, with no evidence of glaucoma damage. In NTG, the pressure measurements are repeatedly within the normal range, but the patient develops optic disc changes and visual field loss consistent with glaucomatous optic neuropathy. These patients are difficult to diagnose and may present late, as the pressures are repeatedly reassuringly normal when measured by the optometrist. For some unknown reason, even these normal pressures cause damage, and the patient needs pressure reduction. Lowering the IOP by at least 30% slows down the progression of glaucomatous damage. These patients can be very hard to treat as their pressures may already be low.

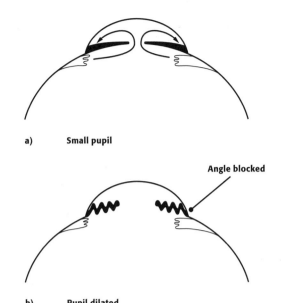

a)   **Small pupil**

b)   **Pupil dilated**

FIGURES 21.5 a and b a) The normal flow of aqueous is from the ciliary body through the pupil and out of the drainage and trabecular meshwork. When the pupil is small in eyes with shallow anterior chambers there is usually still enough space for aqueous drainage. b) When the pupil dilates the iris may ruffle up in the angle and block the aqueous outflow. The pressure goes up dramatically and the patient develops angle-closure glaucoma.

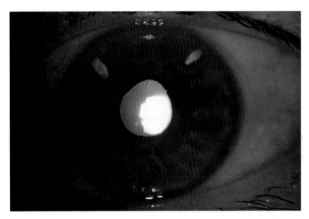

FIGURE 21.6 Laser holes have been burnt in the iris by YAG laser to cause peripheral iridotomies. The red reflex is seen clearly shining through the gaps. This has been done prophylactically to prevent (or treat) angle-closure glaucoma.

Secondary glaucoma

Certain conditions affecting the eye can lead to blockage of the trabecular meshwork and consequently increased IOP.

Inflammatory glaucoma

Intraocular inflammatory disorders can lead to exudation of plasma and inflammatory blood cells into the anterior chamber. Normal aqueous flow will result in the accumulation of this inflammatory material over and within the trabecular meshwork. This can result in a physical blockage of the drainage apparatus, thereby causing a pressure rise. Aqueous outflow may be restored when the inflammation has resolved, but sometimes the angle is permanently blocked by the inflammatory matter (e.g. fibrin) or by the formation of a fibrovascular membrane. In these cases, the pressure remains high, and an operation is often required to reduce the pressure and preserve sight.

Rubeotic/neovascular glaucoma

This is a form of glaucoma in which new blood vessels form within the drainage angle. These vessels do not form in isolation, but are accompanied by fibrous tissue. This fibrovascular proliferation may grow over the angle structures and increase the pressure inside the eye by means of two mechanisms. It may block the drainage of the aqueous by covering and infiltrating the trabecular meshwork or it may cause the tissues to contract, resulting in closure of the angle (see above).

The commonest cause of rubeotic glaucoma is a central retinal vein occlusion (CRVO). The retina becomes ischaemic, prompting the release of numerous vasoactive compounds that stimulate angiogenesis. These substances, e.g. vascular endothelial growth factor F (VEGF), diffuse from the retina through the vitreous cavity and into the anterior chamber, stimulating pathological fibrovascular proliferation. This process can occur very rapidly (often within three months of the CRVO, hence the old name of '90-day glaucoma'). It is usually associated with a large pressure rise (*see also* Central retinal vein occlusion, Chapter 26).

Rubeotic glaucoma can also be related to diabetic retinopathy or any other ischaemic retinal process.

Pigmentary and pseudo-exfoliative glaucoma

These two conditions involve pathological liberation of material from the iris into the anterior chamber. In the former, the underlying condition is called pigment dispersion syndrome. The pigment arises from the posterior surface of the iris by trauma related to the approximation of the iris to the zonular fibres that suspend the lens, with subsequent persistent rubbing.

The pigment is deposited on the inner surface of the cornea and in the trabecular meshwork, causing a physical blockage to aqueous drainage and, therefore, glaucoma.

In pseudo-exfoliation syndrome, an amyloid-type material is liberated from the iris and again deposited throughout the anterior chamber. This material also occludes the trabecular drainage mechanism and can result in glaucoma.

These patients are usually treated medically, but surgery may become necessary if the pressures cannot be controlled.

General management of glaucoma

The goal of management is to reduce the intraocular pressure to a level at which there will be no further damage. The precise level of IOP required in each patient varies. Ophthalmologists tend to aim for a pressure reduction of around 30%, but in some patients this may not be enough. If after the IOP has been reduced by this amount, the glaucoma continues to worsen, the pressure needs to be lowered further. This is why glaucoma patients should be followed up for life; despite apparently successful treatment (as measured purely by IOP readings) glaucoma may still progress, with the risk of eventual onset of blindness.

IOP reduction is first tried by medical means (usually drops) but if this fails by surgery.

Therapy aims to decrease the production (turn off the tap) or increase the drainage (open the plughole) of aqueous flow.

There are several eye drops that aim to decrease IOP in different ways. Below, the most common are discussed.

Beta blockers

Topical beta blockers work by decreasing the amount of aqueous produced at the ciliary body. These drugs are usually effective and relatively cheap. The dose is usually twice daily, and the drops are well tolerated in most patients. Timolol, which is available in 0·25% or 0·5% strengths, is most commonly used.

The main problems with beta blockers are that they can lose their effectiveness with long-term use, and they can have systemic side effects. While it seems unlikely that such a small amount of drug administered in liquid form to the eye could have significant systemic effects, some patients experience a worsening of their bronchospasm or congestive cardiac failure. Significant asthma, chronic obstructive airways disease or cardiac failure are relative contraindications to the use of topical beta blockers.

Alpha agonists

These drugs act on the alpha-adrenergic receptors to decrease ciliary body production of aqueous. Brimonidine is an example of alpha agonist drops.

Pilocarpine

Although this drop is becoming less popular, many patients are still using it. The dose is usually four times a day. It causes miosis of the pupil, and is thought to work by mechanical traction on the trabecular meshwork, opening the spaces and facilitating aqueous outflow.

Topical carbonic anhydrase inhibitors

Carbonic anhydrase inhibitors block the production of aqueous at the ciliary body. They work well, but cause an allergic reaction in some patients. Dorzolamide is an example.

Prostaglandin analogues

These drugs are relatively new, and appear to be a potent addition to the arsenal of weapons against glaucoma. There are several preparations available, all of which act to increase aqueous outflow of the eye. Interestingly, they do not act on the conventional trabecular drainage mechanisms but facilitate aqueous egress from the eye through the uveoscleral route (via diffusion through the iris). Latanoprost, travoprost and bimatoprost are all examples.

Oral preparations

There is only one commonly used drug that is given orally to bring down IOP. Acetazolamide is a carbonic anhydrase inhibitor that suppresses biochemically the ciliary body production of aqueous. This drug affects several other organ systems, however, and must be used with caution. It can stimulate a significant diuresis and also cause hypokalaemia and other unpleasant side effects. For these reasons, it is usually only prescribed as a short-term measure.

Sometimes in an acute situation, an osmotic agent such as mannitol is given intravenously to bring the pressure down.

Laser

Recently, it has been seen that laser applied directly to the trabecular meshwork using a gonioscopy lens reduces the pressure in the eye (argon laser trabeculoplasty). The exact mechanism of this pressure reduction is unknown, but the treatment probably stimulates changes in the trabecular sieve, reducing its resistance to aqueous outflow.

Laser may also be applied to the ocular surface in the region of the ciliary body to cause direct thermal damage, reducing its ability to produce aqueous (a process called cyclodiode laser). The laser involved is called a diode, and it is able to penetrate the sclera to cause a direct burn to the ciliary body. It can cause a lot of inflammation and even some visual loss, so it tends to be used only when the pressure is out of control in eyes that are already blind. In this situation, treatment is aimed at relieving the pain of markedly raised IOP.

Surgery

If the patient is intolerant of drops or if there is progression of glaucomatous damage despite maximal medical therapy, the patient requires surgery to bring the IOP down to acceptable levels and thus preserve sight.

Several operations are possible, but the commonest is the trabeculectomy. Here the small flap of sclera is dissected and a puncture hole made in the eye. The sclera is then sutured back in place to form a flap valve. This valve allows aqueous fluid to pass from the inside of the eye to the subconjunctival space. The area of the subconjunctival fluid becomes raised, forming a dome or 'bleb' (figures 21.7 and 21.8), and the aqueous in this bleb gradually diffuses away via the blood vessels of the sclera and episclera.

One potential problem with this type of surgery arises because the body tries to heal this abnormal communication between the inside of the eye and the subconjunctival space. This would, of course, cause the procedure to fail. To overcome this, antifibrotic or antimetabolite agents can be given to stop the scarring process by inhibiting fibroblast activity, either intra-operatively or postoperatively. The most common such drugs are mitomycin-C or 5-fluorouracil.

These procedures are extremely dangerous, how-

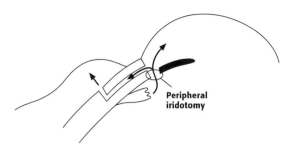

FIGURE 21.7 **Cross-section of the superior sclera and cornea. A trapdoor has been formed in the sclera allowing egress of aqueous fluid from the anterior chamber into the subconjunctival space forming an elevated bleb. A hole has also been created in the iris (a peripheral iridotomy) to facilitate flow of aqueous.**

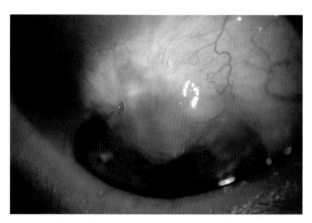

FIGURE 21.8 **A trabeculectomy bleb has been formed. The bleb seen is a ballooning of the conjunctiva where the aqueous is draining from the anterior chamber thereby lowering the intraocular pressure. This bleb is quite cystic in nature.**

ever, and not to be undertaken lightly. The potentially sight-threatening complications include overdrainage, infection and haemorrhage.

If a standard trabeculectomy fails, it can be tried again. If the second attempt fails, a drainage tube can be sutured to the eye within the anterior chamber. The Molteno tube and the Ahmed valve are among those used. This tube allows fluid to flow out of the eye, thus controlling IOP. Because the implant is a foreign body, the eye often tries to expel it over time. A tube can also become blocked months or years after implantation.

Glaucoma drop problems

Glaucoma drops can cause local and systemic complications despite the small volume of drugs administered. Topical beta blockers may lead to exacerbation of airways disease or cardiac problems, and other glaucoma formulations may have numerous adverse effects. In order to minimise the risk of systemic complications patients may be advised to apply pressure over the side of their nose immediately after drop administration. This closes the lacrimal sac and prevents the passage of the drug into the nose, and, hopefully, absorption into the blood stream.

It is not uncommon for allergy to occur after prolonged drop use. Despite no early problems, patients may develop their first episode of allergy several years after commencing a drop. If a patient develops a red, itchy eye with lid swelling they may have developed a drop allergy. Sometimes the allergenic element is the preservative used in the drop formulation. Some drops are available without preservatives.

In the great majority of patients there is no problem with temporary cessation of treatment to allow the allergy to settle. Glaucoma damage in the majority of individuals takes many years to worsen and the effect of a higher pressure for a short period of time will be minimal. Thus if the patient has the symptoms and signs of allergy it is reasonable to stop their drops and await their next review appointment at the hospital. If their next follow up is several months away then it is advisable to contact the hospital to try to expedite a follow up appointment. In patients with end-stage or severe glaucoma it is more prudent to contact the hospital for advice rather than stop the drops.

22 | Lids and lacrimal apparatus

The lids protect the front of the eye and ensure the ocular surface stays hydrated and clean. The lids are covered with normal skin that is susceptible to the same conditions as the skin on the rest of the face. Tears are produced by the lacrimal gland in the superotemporal part of the orbit and bathe the eye continuously to keep it healthy. The tears drain via the nasolacrimal duct down into the nose. Insufficient tears will lead to dryness, while excessive production or poor drainage will lead to a watering eye.

Neoplasms

The skin surrounding the eye, like that covering the rest of the body, can be affected by neoplastic processes, including malignant melanomas and squamous cell carcinomas. Specific neoplasms related to the lids and periocular skin include basal cell and sebaceous cell carcinomas. The above conditions are discussed in Chapter 24.

Malposition of the eyelid

The lids have a vital function in protecting the ocular surface by acting as a physical barrier and also by sweeping across the cornea to remove any foreign bodies or debris. Their other important role is to distribute tears and maintain the correct level of hydration required by the conjunctiva and the cornea. If the lids are not in the correct position, they may fail in the above tasks with deleterious consequences.

Ectropion

In this condition, the lower lid becomes droopy and sags down (figure 22.1).

This usually occurs as an involution change due to ageing of the tendons that hold the lid in place. It may also occur as a result of a sixth nerve palsy or of the contracture of a scar below the eye or because of a large heavy lesion on the lower lid, resulting in a mass gravitational effect.

Apart from the cosmetic appearance, an ectropion has two major sequelae:

1) Tears are not propelled towards the puncti and nasolacrimal system but pool in the inferior fornix and overflow, causing excessive watering.

2) The lids protect the cornea and the position of the lower lid ensures that the cornea is bathed in tears and kept moist. If the lower lid sags, it cannot bathe and protect the ocular surface, and excessive exposure may occur. Drying of the cornea leads to damage to the corneal epithelial cells, causing redness and 'grittiness', and eventually possibly corneal ulcers or even perforation.

Treatment

Keeping the eye wet with topical lubricants will protect the cornea and may alleviate some of the symptoms. Surgical correction is usually required. The lower lid has to be repositioned either by shortening with a wedge resection of lid tissue or tightening the lateral lower lid tendon.

Entropion

Here the lower lid turns in (figure 22.2). This is usually as a result of involutional/ageing processes, but it can also occur through persistent conjunctival infection or inflammation that results in scarring and inward traction of the lid margin.

When the lid margin is turned in, the eyelashes now point backwards, rubbing up and down the cornea with each blink. This causes progressive damage. Initially, the result is irritation and superficial drying of the corneal epithelium. Over time, however, the cornea is permanently damaged and a scar develops. Even worse, a significant corneal infective keratitis may ensue with a real risk of permanent visual loss.

Treatment

Topical lubricants are used to keep the cornea moist and protect it from the abrasive effect of the lashes. Taping the lower lid to the cheek is often a good temporary measure as it pulls the lashes away from the eye. Surgery is required to correct the abnormality and provide long-term protection from the lashes, however.

There are many ways in which this can be done. The simplest involves sutures to pull the lower lid out (everting sutures), but this procedure often has to be repeated after about a year. Other more permanent procedures involve shortening the lower lid or making full-thickness horizontal cuts along the lid and placing sutures in order to redirect the muscles to pull the lid out into a normal position.

Trichiasis

Trichiasis describes a condition in which the eyelashes point in the wrong direction (i.e. backwards). This sometimes occurs even when the lower lid is in the correct position. The lashes scrape up and down the cornea with each blink, and can cause significant damage and scarring as described above.

Patients will experience redness and a foreign-body sensation or 'grittiness'.

Treatment

Treatment is directed at protecting the cornea with topical lubricants. The lashes have to be removed either by temporary epilation (plucking) or by more permanent electrolysis of each hair follicle. In severe cases, surgery may be required to split the lid margin and redirect the lashes outwards.

Trachoma

Trachoma is the commonest cause of blindness in the developing world. It is a form of chronic conjunctivitis but warrants mention here because its blinding effect is caused by the resulting entropion and trichiasis. Trachoma results from chronic infection with *Chlamydia trachomatis*, which leads to scarring of the conjunctiva and fibrosis of the accessory tear glands. The lower lid turns in as a result of the fibrosis and the lashes begin to rub on the cornea. The eye is already dry because of the damage to the tear glands and so the cornea is rapidly damaged. It becomes vascularised and opacifies, resulting in blindness.

The disease is propagated by poor hygiene, and the major intervention required is prevention by cleanliness and better public health facilities. In the acute stages, tetracycline ointment helps in eliminating the organism. Surgery may be required later to correct the lid abnormality. Trachoma is endemic in many developing countries, and is a major cause of preventable blindness, making it a prominent worldwide health issue.

Blepharitis

This is a condition of the lid margins, whereby they become mildly inflamed and develop dandruff-like flaking of the skin (figure 22.3a). Numerous meibomian (fat) glands line the upper and lower lids, and secrete fat for the outer layer of the tear film. When these do not function correctly, they can become partially blocked. This is called meibomian gland dysfunction, and it contributes to the pathology of blepharitis (figure 22.3b).

The inflammation causes attrition to the ocular surface and the cornea, and the patient complains of irritation, a burning feeling or a foreign-body sensation.

Treatment

Lubricants can minimise the irritation.

Most of the debris on the lid margin is composed of fatty material and skin flakes. Thus, warm bathing of the eyelids can be very beneficial. The warmth melts the fat and the gentle washing of the lid margins removes the dandruff, allowing the margin to return to normal. Occasionally, an antibiotic ointment may be required to settle any infection.

Dry eyes

Dry eyes is a very common complaint. The cornea needs a certain level of moisture to keep it healthy. This is provided by tear secretion from the lacrimal gland and numerous other accessory glands throughout the conjunctiva. If this tear production is inadequate, the cornea becomes dry and the superficial epithelial cells suffer.

Patients experience symptoms of grittiness, burning, foreign-body sensation and occasionally sharp stabbing pains. The eyes may be slightly red or they may be completely white. When fluorescein dye (with topical anaesthetic) is placed on to the cornea, it may stain small pinpoint patches of the surface, indicating that the epithelium has been worn away in those areas. These are called superficial punctate erosions (figure 22.4). The patient does not need to have this evidence of corneal damage to be plagued with marked symptoms of dry eye disease.

There are many lubricant drops available, each with their own characteristics. There are also many artificial teardrops available over the counter.

A Schirmer's test is used to measure tear production. This involves placing a thin strip of blotting paper over the lower lid margin and leaving it in place for several minutes to soak up tears. The amount of liquid taken up by the blotting paper is measured, and this gives some indication of the amount of tears being produced.

If simple topical drops are ineffective, the puncti (nasolacrimal drainage holes) can be occluded, either temporarily with absorbable gelatin rods or more permanently with silicone plugs or even surgery.

Chalazion

The meibomian glands lie within the tarsal plates of the upper and lower lids, and secrete fat on to the ocular surface via ducts that open on to the lid margin. If these ducts become blocked, the meibomian gland swells and forms a cystic mass called a chalazion, meibomian cyst or tarsal cyst (figure 22.5). The patient usually notices this mass or is conscious of a mild irritation. The condition may resolve spontaneously if the duct unblocks by itself or it may require intervention.

Warm bathing of the eye can increase the temperature of the fatty matter within the chalazion and allow drainage via the meibomian duct with resolution. If the cyst remains, however, or increases in size, it may require incision and curettage. Local anaesthetic is injected around the cyst and the lid everted. A stab incision is then made through the internal conjunctiva and the cyst curetted from within.

If the chalazion bursts within the lid, fatty material leaks into the surrounding tissue and causes an inflammatory reaction. The cyst becomes red and painful, and may get bigger. Infection can then set in, as well as frank cellulitis, requiring oral antibiotics. Even an inflamed chalazion may settle with conservative measures such as warm bathing, however. A topical antibiotic is usually given as an adjunct.

Stye

A stye is an infected eyelash root and is sometimes mistaken for a chalazion. Treatment is with topical antibiotics. A stye usually resolves with no sequelae, but if it causes a cellulitis, systemic antibiotics may be needed.

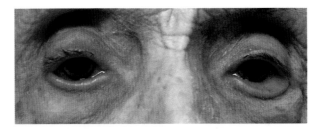

FIGURE 22.1 **This elderly lady has bilateral ectropions of her lower lids related to lid laxity.**

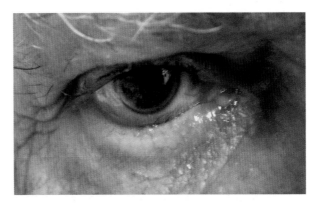

FIGURE 22.2 **A right entropion. The lower lid is turning in causing the lashes to abrade the ocular surface. There is a mucous discharge but the eye has been protected (hence it is not red) by the use of lubricant gels and drops.**

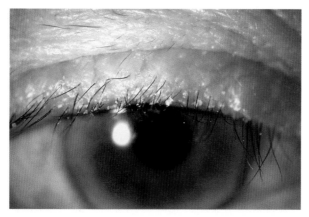

a)

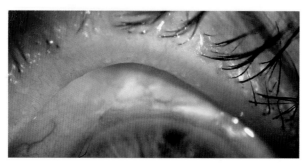

b)

FIGURES 22.3 a and b a) Blepharitis with crusting of the lid margin. b) Blepharitis with blockage/capping of the meibomian fat glands.

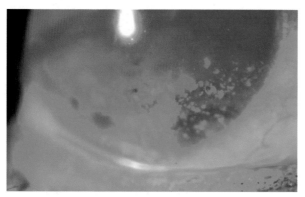

FIGURE 22.4 Severe drying of the inferior cornea has resulted in areas of epithelial cell loss, clearly seen with a blue light as patches of fluorescein staining.

Ptosis

A ptosis is a droopy upper eyelid (figure 22.6). It may be congenital or acquired.

Congenital ptosis can occur as a result of malformation of the levator muscle of the upper lid.

Acquired ptosis can be involutional (as a result of ageing), myogenic (as a result of a muscle problem) or neurogenic (as a result of denervation).

Involutional ptosis

The levator muscle inserts into the top of the tarsal plate of the upper lid. Ageing and attrition result in gradual stretching and disinsertion of the levator tendon. This results in the upper lid drooping. Patients complain of the cosmetic appearance and also of poor vision if the lid drops over the visual axis. Surgery may correct the lid position by reinserting the tendon into the tarsal plate and lifting the lid up. It is hard to achieve a perfect lid level and, if it is overdone, the lid will be too high, resulting in difficulty in closing the eyes, with subsequent corneal exposure problems.

Myogenic ptosis

Patients with myotonic dystrophy may have a myogenic ptosis due to an abnormality of the levator muscle. One type of myogenic ptosis is related to myasthenia gravis (MG). MG can affect the whole body or be local to the eye (ocular myasthenia). In the eye, it can cause a ptosis or diplopia due to ocular muscle imbalance. The classic feature of this type of ptosis is fatigability. The degree of droopiness is variable and tends to get worse with prolonged eye opening and when the patient is tired (e.g. towards the end of the day). When examining a patient with MG and a ptosis, if you ask the patient to look up for an extended period, you will notice the upper lid gradually drooping even further. This is called fatigability and is the hallmark of this disorder. The diagnosis may be confirmed by a positive serum anti-acetylcholine receptor antibody titre.

Neurogenic ptosis

There are two sources of innervation to the muscles of the upper lid. The levator muscle (the most important muscle for upper lid position and movement) is supplied by the third (oculomotor) cranial nerve. There is also a minor muscle that helps lid elevation, called the Muller's muscle. This muscle receives its innervation from the sympathetic plexus, and is part of the 'fight or flight' stress response.

In stressful situations, where the sympathetic system is foremost, the individual needs their eyes wide open to see the predator or prey, so the Muller's muscle contracts, opening the eyes wide. If the sympathetic supply to the eye is interrupted, this muscle relaxes and the lid droops by about 2mm. This is called Horner's syndrome and is usually accompanied by a constricted (miosed) pupil. It occurs as a result of interruption of the sympathetic nerves that emerge from the thoracic spine and rise up through the neck to the eye. A rare cause of Horner's syndrome is a malignant tumour of the lung apex (Pancoast tumour).

A third nerve palsy will result in a complete ptosis, an oculomotor palsy (where the eye is in the down and out position) and may result in a dilated pupil (*see* Third nerve palsy, Chapter 12).

Watering eye (epiphora)

There are two levels of tear production. Basal tear production continues throughout the day and night, and keeps the ocular surface moist. When extra tears are required, however (e.g. to wash away a foreign body), then reflex tear secretion occurs. If basal secretion is compromised, the eye becomes dry and the patient may complain of a gritty feeling.

Tears drain into the lacrimal puncti – two small holes placed medially on the lid margins, one on the upper lid and one on the lower. These puncti drain into ducts (canaliculi) that run medially to enter the lacrimal sac. From there, tears drain down via the nasolacrimal duct into the nasal cavity (figure 5.4).

Epiphora describes the symptom of tears that overflow out of the eye. This may be because tear production exceeds the draining capacity of the nasolacrimal system or because nasolacrimal drainage is obstructed.

In children

A membrane lies at the bottom of the developing nasolacrimal duct, at the point where it enters the nasal cavity. This membrane breaks down with interuterine growth, and is usually gone at birth. A small proportion of babies are born with this membrane still intact, however. This causes a blockage, and the tears cannot drain into the nose. The baby has a watery and frequently sticky eye. This membrane usually disappears, typically by the age of one year. If it has not disappeared by then, or if infection develops in the nasolacrimal sac due to stagnation of tears, a

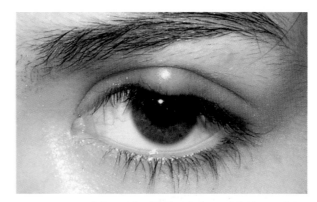

FIGURE 22.5 A chalazion localised to the upper lid. The overlying redness is not infective but is inflammatory.

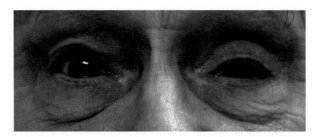

FIGURE 22.6 This patient has a left-sided ptosis. The lid is droopy and obscuring the corneal reflection on the left-hand side.

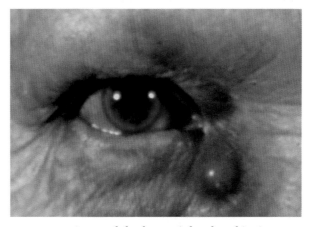

FIGURE 22.7 A mucocele has become infected resulting in dacrocystitis. (Courtesy of Mrs L.C. Abercrombie.)

probe is passed down the nasolacrimal duct under general anaesthesia to perforate the membrane. This procedure can cause substantial trauma, however, and is best deferred to allow nature to take its course.

In adults

Ageing can cause scarring and blockage of the fine tubes of the nasolacrimal apparatus. This is compounded by the frequent upper respiratory tract infections encountered in temperate climates. If the duct is completely blocked, the eye will water continually. The amount of epiphora, and thus the concern that it causes the patient, is dictated by the amount of basal and reflex tear production.

Patients may be offered surgery if they are motivated and sufficiently bothered by their symptoms. The procedure is called a dacrocystorhinostomy (dacrocysto = lacrimal sac, rhino = nose, ostomy = make hole between), and involves creating a new channel between the puncti, canaliculi, lacrimal sac and the nose. This can be done externally, but recently laser and endoscopic technology has progressed to allow a new drainage tract to be created from inside the nose. However it is done, this is a fairly large operation, and often requires prosthetic tubes to be in place for up to six months to prevent re-stenosis of the new drainage tracts.

Mucocele and dacrocystitis

Because the tear drainage system is blocked, excess tears can collect in the lacrimal sac, which can produce a swelling in the medial canthus between the eye and the bridge of the nose. This is called a mucocele, and is usually asymptomatic except for the cosmetic appearance. Pressure applied on the swelling can cause the mucus and tears in the sac to pass through the puncti on the lid margins back on to the eye. Stagnation of tears and mucus in the sac may encourage bacterial colonisation and infection (figure 22.7). It is therefore important to advise parents to keep the sac as empty as possible. Indeed, in paediatric patients massage of the nasolacrimal system in a superior-to-inferior direction may force tears into the nasolacrimal duct and stimulate opening of the membrane that is obstructing the tear flow.

If the nasolacrimal sac is frankly infected, it becomes a red and painful swelling. Pressure on this will be painful but may result in pus passing through the upper and lower puncti on to the eye. Treatment is with systemic antibiotics, but if the swelling is extremely large it may require incision and drainage under local anaesthetic. In such cases, the nasolacrimal system is inevitably blocked due to secondary scarring and the eye will water once the infection has settled. The patient may require a dacrocystorhinostomy to prevent tearing and reduce the risk of further infective complications.

23 | Orbit

The orbit is the area surrounding the globe within the orbital fossa/eye socket. It can be directly affected by local or systemic disease, or indirectly by spread from adjacent structures, particularly the sinuses and the nasopharynx.

Proptosis

The globe is held within the orbit by numerous fine ligaments but mainly by the action of the extraocular muscles. As the globe must be mobile to allow the eye to move, the attachments are lax and the optic nerve emerging from the back of the eye is extra long, giving it some slack. The globe thus has some scope for anterior movement. Orbital problems that cause increased pressure behind the eye will push the globe forwards. This is called proptosis, and it can be unilateral or bilateral.

Several problems can result from this forward movement of the eye. The major concern is visual loss secondary to stretching or direct compression of the optic nerve. Once the slack in the optic nerve is taken up and the nerve is pulled taut, any further forward pressure on the eye will stretch and damage the nerve (figure 23.1). If the eye is held firmly by the extraocular muscles, then this anterior movement may be resisted, causing excessive pressure in the orbit and direct pressure on the nerve. Thus optic nerve damage may occur, even if the degree of proptosis is not great.

Proptosis may have other consequences apart from damage to the optic nerve. The front of the eye may become compromised because the cornea is too far forward to allow the lids to fulfil their protective and lubricative function. The blink reflex then becomes ineffective as the lids cannot physically cover the whole ocular surface. The resulting corneal exposure can lead to drying and ulceration.

If the optic nerve is compromised or if there is significant corneal exposure, emergency treatment is required to move the eye back under cover or to decompress the nerve and release the stretch or pressure, thus preventing permanent visual loss.

Lastly, significant chronic proptosis may result in major cosmetic concerns, particularly in young women.

Exophthalmos is the term for proptosis caused by thyroid eye disease (see below).

Thyroid eye disease

Thyroid eye disease is an autoimmune disorder characterised by circulating autoantibodies to thyroid antigens. This results in stimulation of thyroxine production and hyperthyroidism. Cross-reactivity between the autoantigens targeting the thyroid also results in attack upon the orbital tissue. The pathological thyroid antibodies appear to attack the fibroblasts within the orbit. This results in inflammation and swelling within the retro-ocular and orbital tissues, with vast amounts of oedema and deposition of mucopolysaccharides.

Systemic thyroid disease may precede, occur simultaneously with, or follow the development of thyroid eye disease. Strangely, patients sometimes display the ocular features of thyroid eye disease without the thyroid features.

The disease is characterised by an active and a chronic phase, the hallmark of which is inflammation. The eye is painful and red, the globe is pushed forward (exophthalmos) by the retro-ocular inflammation and swelling, and eye movements may be painful because of involvement of the ocular muscles. In addition, the excessive sympathetic stimulation to the eye results in lid retraction, where the upper and lower lids are pulled back allowing the sclera to show above and below the limbus (scleral show). Forward movement of the globe will further compound the problem of the lid position, as the lids are pushed further from the cornea.

In the active phase, the patient is at risk of optic

nerve compromise by either stretching or compression of the nerve. It is important, therefore, to treat this condition aggressively with systemic steroids to suppress the inflammation. If vision is reduced due to the effect on the optic nerve, the patient needs decompression of the orbit to release the pressure on the nerve. This is tried medically first by systemic immunosuppression but, if this fails and vision is not improved or it deteriorates, the patient may need surgery.

Surgery aims to remove the bony walls of the orbit to create more space and thus reduce the retro-orbital pressure. The orbit has four bony walls and it is possible to decompress them all. The number of walls tackled will depend on the severity of the inflammation and the degree of exophthalmos.

Although the optic nerve is important, it is vital to remember that the cornea may become exposed and damaged, requiring lubricant drops to protect it.

Once the active inflammation settles, it is possible to assess the permanent chronic damage. The active inflammation may have resolved, but may have left the patient with significant residual exophthalmos, due to a permanent increase in retro-ocular tissue volume (figure 23.2). In addition, the extraocular muscles may respond to the inflammation with scarring and fibrosis. This in turn may cause severe oculomotility problems, including significant squints and troublesome continuous double vision. Surgery to attempt to correct the squint is possible.

Cosmesis is a major concern, as this disorder typically affects young women and may result in significant abnormalities in the position of the lid and eye. Lid reconstruction should be left until the globe position and ocular alignment have been stabilised satisfactorily.

When examining these patients, it is vital to check the health of the cornea; ensure the health of the optic nerve by checking visual acuity, visual fields, colour vision and pupil reactions; and assess eye movements.

Imaging of the orbits is usually by CT scan, showing the anatomy of the nerve, orbital walls and orbital apex.

Idiopathic orbital inflammation

This condition used to be called orbital pseudotumour. The precise cause is unknown, but it manifests in otherwise healthy people with sudden onset of a red, painful, swollen, restricted and proptosed eye. The optic nerve can rapidly become compromised, and the condition needs emergency treatment. It is a diagnosis of exclusion once other causes of orbital inflammation have been ruled out.

It is virtually impossible to differentiate this condition clinically from infective orbital cellulitis. These patients tend to be less systemically unwell compared to those with infective orbital cellulitis, but the first line of treatment is still usually with antibiotics. Imaging can often highlight significant localised infection, but diffuse orbital cellulitis may mimic idiopathic orbital inflammation.

This is an inflammatory disorder and so treated with systemic steroids. If the inflammation, redness and proptosis do not rapidly resolve, the diagnosis must be questioned.

Carotid-cavernous fistula

The carotid arteries pass through the cavernous venous sinus within the cranium. Rarely, an abnormal connection develops between the carotids and the cavernous sinus. This can happen suddenly or gradually, and be of a high flow (free, direct communication) or lower flow (connection via other fine vessels, thus limiting flow). In either case, the cavernous system and the veins that drain into it are not prepared for the high pressure of the arterial circulation. Rapid venous dilatation occurs, resulting in back pressure to all the veins that drain into the cavernous sinus.

The orbital veins become engorged and fail to drain. The eye becomes red, the intraocular pressure goes up as aqueous cannot pass out of the eye due to the high orbital venous pressure, the globe becomes proptosed and, finally, vision is threatened due to optic nerve compression and stretch, and corneal exposure. A bruit may be auscultated over the eye due to the high abnormal flow of blood into the orbit. Also, the oculomotor nerves run within or in the walls of the cavernous sinus and abnormal dilatation may result in oculomotor nerve palsies affecting nerves three, four and six. If severe, this will cause an immobile 'frozen' eye.

The condition can occur spontaneously in elderly patients or be related to head trauma. Treatment should be instituted as a matter of urgency if the vision is threatened, and usually involves neuroradiologically guided embolisation.

Orbital cellulitis

Orbital cellulitis is infection of the orbital tissues surrounding the eye (figure 23.3). True orbital cellulitis is a sight-threatening ocular emergency, requiring rapid antibiotic treatment to prevent permanent visual loss. Bacteria somehow gain access to the orbit and spread throughout the loose connective and fatty tissue surrounding the globe. The result is optic nerve compression, ophthalmoplegia (reduced ocular movements) and proptosis. Patients are usually systemically unwell.

The nasal sinuses are the usual source of the bacterial inoculum responsible for orbital infection. Infection within the sinuses (sinusitis) may occur subclinically, only causing problems when it breaches the orbital walls to enter the orbit and spread rapidly, causing orbital cellulitis. Computerised tomography may reveal a localised infection or subperiostial abscess requiring surgical drainage.

Patients should receive high-dose systemic antibiotics and be monitored closely for signs of optic nerve compromise.

Preseptal cellulitis

Preseptal cellulitis is often confused with orbital cellulitis, but is an infection of the lid tissue and not the orbit itself. It is of much less clinical severity and in isolation is not sight threatening. Preseptal cellulitis easily progresses to orbital cellulitis and loss of vision, however, so it should be treated carefully and followed up.

The lid tissue is separated from orbital tissue by a fibrous septum that acts as a block to the spread of the infection posteriorly into the tissue around the eye. This septum may be breached spontaneously and the bacteria responsible for the preseptal cellulitis may invade the orbit, causing orbital cellulitis, with risk to sight.

In preseptal cellulitis, the upper or lower lid usually becomes erythematous, hot and oedematous. If the upper lid is involved, it may result in a partial or total ptosis (figure 23.4). The key differentiating features from the more vision-threatening orbital cellulitis are that underlying eye/globe/sclera are white, the ocular movements are full, vision is normal when the lids are opened, and the pupils react normally. If the eye itself is red, the vision reduced or the ocular movements limited, the patient has orbital cellulitis and requires emergency imaging, along with high-dose parenteral antibiotics and surgical drainage of any collection, if appropriate.

In children over five years of age and in adults, the condition may settle with oral antibiotics. If the eye becomes red, the patient may have developed orbital cellulitis, which requires admission, imaging and intravenous antibiotics or surgical drainage of any collection.

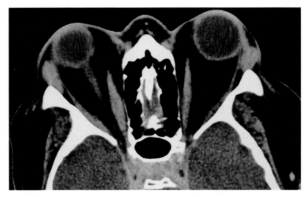

FIGURE 23.1 CT scan of a patient with severe bilateral thyroid eye disease. The exophthalmos is stretching the optic nerve and threatening vision. (Courtesy of Mrs L. C. Abercrombie.)

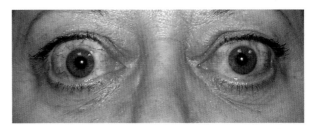

FIGURE 23.2 This lady is in the inactive phase of thyroid eye disease. She has significant bilateral exophthalmos and lid retraction. She is at risk of corneal drying and exposure, and may seek surgical intervention for cosmetic rehabilitation. (Courtesy of Mr G. Ainsworth.)

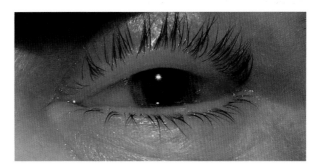

FIGURE 23.3 The lids are swollen and red. When the eye is opened it is seen that the eye itself is also red. This is early orbital cellulitis.

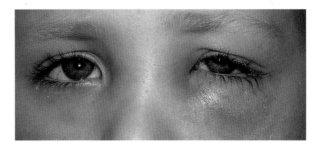

FIGURE 23.4 Preseptal cellulitis of the left eye. The lower lid is markedly erythematous and swollen. Close inspection shows that the globe itself is completely white and the eye movements are intact. Vision is also normal and the patient is well in himself.

Cavernous sinus thrombosis

The cavernous sinus is a venous lake lying within dural folds into which several of the cerebral veins drain. Running within the walls of the cavernous sinus are several key cranial nerves, most importantly the third and fourth, and branches of the ophthalmic division of the fifth. The sixth nerve runs free within the sinus and is therefore at particular risk of damage from cavernous sinus pathology.

A cavernous sinus thrombosis will result in venous congestion of the brain with headache, will compromise the sixth cranial nerve and can damage the other cranial nerves. Imaging, usually by magnetic resonance angiography (MRA), is required to confirm the diagnosis, and liaison with a physician about anticoagulation is necessary. The prognosis for recovery of the function of the oculomotor nerves is variable.

Management of orbital problems

In general, the management of orbital pathology involves treating the underlying cause. If the pathology is infective, then antibiotics and removal of any foci or source of infection is required. If the aetiology is inflammatory, then suppression of this process is needed before the nerve and vision are threatened. While this is being done, it is vital to prevent permanent visual loss by keeping a high index of suspicion for optic nerve or corneal compromise. The globe itself is well protected by the scleral envelope from the orbital tissue. The ocular muscles and optic nerve are not so privileged, and may become involved, either directly or secondarily.

Protect the eye by treating any exposure of the ocular surface (particularly the cornea) and decompress any pressure or stretch upon the optic nerve, either medically or surgically. Once the active pathology is controlled, any scarring or residual cosmetic defect can be dealt with.

24 | Ocular oncology

The eye is not spared the risk of cancer and other neoplastic conditions, either as a primary site or by direct spread from adjacent structures (particularly the nasopharynx) or metastasis.

Lids and periocular skin

The periocular skin, like that of the rest of the body, can develop a variety of neoplasms, including malignant melanomas and squamous cell carcinomas. The face's potential for excessive exposure to UV radiation may be a risk factor for periocular dermatological malignancy.

Malignant melanomas may develop *de novo* or from a pre-existing naevus. Treatment is with wide local excision to ensure clear resection margins.

Squamous cell carcinomas present as red blistering skin around the eye and may be mistaken for blepharitis (*see* Chapter 22).

Basal cell carcinoma

Basal cell carcinoma (BCC) is the commonest tumour of the eyelids. These usually occur on the lower lids and manifest as a raised mass with a pearly rolled edge (figure 24.1). They grow slowly and are locally invasive, hence their other name, rodent ulcers. They are malignant in that they continue to grow and may invade and destroy adjacent tissue, but they do not metastasise, and so local clearance is usually curative as long as the histological margins are clear.

The treatment is local excision. If the resection margin is clear, the patient should be cured. A large lesion may require extensive surgery to reconstruct the lid and/or face. Radiotherapy can be used for recurrent disease or in the rare cases where the patient is unsuitable for surgery. Radiotherapy is, however, a suboptimal treatment and should be considered palliative rather than curative.

The need for clear resection margins, but also for good cosmesis and the preservation of healthy tissue, has led to the use of surgical techniques such as Mohs micrographic surgery and frozen section. The first stage is to remove the tumour along with a small amount of healthy surrounding tissue. The tissue is then sent for rapid histological analysis. If the resection margin is clear, closure, with or without reconstruction, is carried out. If not, more tissue is removed in the area of the lesion (i.e. the involved resection margin). This technique should result in better clearance and decreased risk of recurrent disease.

Recurrent disease is always a concern, and these patients may require long-term follow up. Recurrence may occur within the previous scar tissue, making early identification difficult. Surgery for recurrent disease is often fraught with difficulty, and so it is paramount to ensure that the tumour is completely removed during the first procedure.

Sebaceous cell carcinoma

This form of carcinoma develops in the sebaceous and meibomian glands surrounding the eye. It usually occurs within the lid and may be mistaken for a chalazion. Any rapidly recurrent chalazion that occurs after surgical treatment must raise the suspicion of a sebaceous cell carcinoma, particularly in elderly patients, and warrants a full-thickness lid biopsy. Pagetoid spread of carcinoma cells on to the skin can result in a red, scaly appearance that may be mistaken for a blepharitis.

Intraocular malignant melanoma

Malignant melanoma can affect any of the melanocyte-containing tissues within the eye. The iris and the choroid are most at risk, but the choroid is much more likely to be affected.

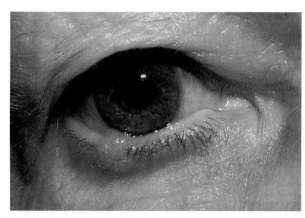

FIGURE 24.1 **Typical appearance of a lower-lid basal cell carcinoma. Loss of lashes (madarosis) in the area is an important sign that this is not a benign process.**

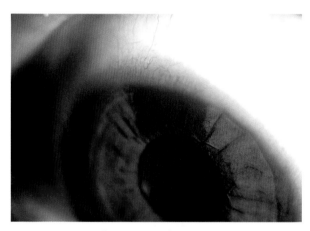

FIGURE 24.2 **Typical appearance of an iris naevus in the upper portion of the patient's iris. The pupil margin is not distorted indicating that this is probably benign.**

Iris and choroidal naevi consist of groups of melanocytes, and manifest as flat or slightly raised brown areas on the iris surface (figure 24.2) or within the choroid under the retinal pigment epithelium (RPE) (figure 24.3).

Iris naevi may be numerous and very hard to identify on brown irides. Growth is the key feature of concern. If they become larger and particularly if they begin to distort the normal anatomy of the iris and pupil, they are likely to be malignant and require definitive diagnosis and excision.

Choroidal naevi are not uncommon and appear as well circumscribed, flat, variably pigmented areas under the retina and RPE layer. They often have overlying yellow plaques (drusen). Growth or excessive size and elevation are indicators that this melanocytic lesion is likely to be malignant and requires treatment (figure 24.4).

As with moles elsewhere on the body, the diagnosis of malignancy is sometimes difficult. While a patient may observe a mole on the back of their hand themselves and elect to have it removed because this is easily done, a suspicious choroidal naevus will require follow up by an ophthalmologist, while removing it 'just in case' is clearly not an option.

Treatment of malignant melanomas depends on their size and position. Resection or plaque radiotherapy are options. The latter involves the surgical placement of a small radioactive plaque on the outside of the eye overlying the tumour to deliver a high dose of radiotherapy directly to the mass. If the tumour is very large, removal of the eye may be the only course possible.

Metastases

The choroid is the most vascular tissue in the body, so it is not surprising that this is a common site for haematogenous spread from distant primary neoplasms. Common sources of metastases include breast, bowel, lung, liver and prostate. These metastases appear as raised, dome-shaped yellow lesions beneath the retina. They are often surrounded by a retinal detachment and are indicative of widespread systemic metastases, particularly if multiple. The presence of ocular metastases is a poor prognostic indicator.

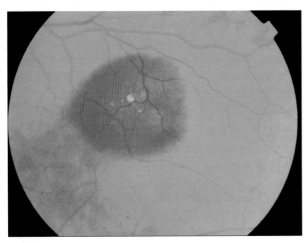

FIGURE 24.3 Colour photograph of a choroidal naevus. The pigmented area is flat and there are typical drusen overlying it. These are both reassuring features that this is indeed a benign naevus.

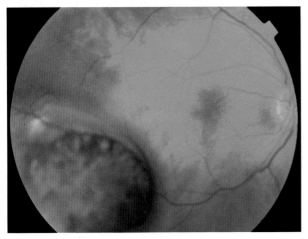

FIGURE 24.4 Colour fundus photograph of a choroidal malignant melanoma. The abnormal area is pigmented and markedly raised. There are also folds in the surrounding retina.

25 | Neuro-ophthalmology

The eye is closely related to the central nervous system (CNS). Four of the cranial nerves supply the eye, and the retina is a part of the CNS. More importantly, the retina is the only part of the CNS we may observe directly and examine morphologically. If any evidence of a neurological problem is found when the eye is assessed, the patient should have a complete examination of the CNS and peripheral nervous system (PNS).

Optic neuritis

(*See also* Chapter 16, Visual loss.)

This is inflammation of the optic nerve. It may be idiopathic or related to a demyelinating disorder such as multiple sclerosis.

The optic nerve becomes compromised and fails to conduct visual impulses from the retina to the brain. The exact pattern of visual loss varies and depends upon which part of the nerve is involved. Usually, the patient develops a central visual field defect (scotoma) with significant visual loss. The vision can be reduced to counting fingers, which is very distressing, particularly for the young adults who are commonly affected by this condition.

The clinical findings are minimal. In about one-third of patients the optic disc is swollen (true optic neuritis), and in the other two-thirds the disc is normal (retrobulbar neuritis), indicating a more posterior site for the inflammation. *See* Chapter 16 for diagnosis and management.

Papilloedema

This term is applied to swelling of the optic nerve head as a result of raised intracranial pressure (ICP). It is a diagnosis, and the term should not be used to describe a swollen optic disc unless it is definitely secondary to raised ICP. It is assumed that the rise in ICP is transmitted along and around the optic nerve

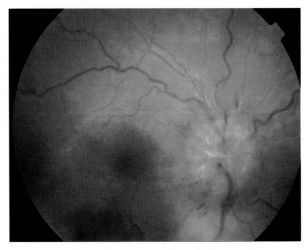

FIGURE 25.1 **Classical appearance of papilloedema with marked disc swelling and some flame-shaped haemorrhages around the disc.**

sheaths, resulting in compression of the nerve and compromised axoplasmic flow. This blocked axoplasmic flow manifests clinically as swelling of the optic nerve head/optic disc, with or without localised retinal haemorrhages around the disc (figure 25.1).

Vision may be completely unaffected, but some patients experience transient visual 'fluctuations' with transient blurring, occasionally associated with rapid standing. Long-standing raised ICP with consequent prolonged pressure on the optic nerve can result in damage to the patient's visual field, with progressive potentially irreversible peripheral field loss.

The raised ICP may be related to numerous pathologies, but cerebral tumours, intracranial haemorrhage or benign intracranial hypertension (BIH) should be considered.

Benign intracranial hypertension

Here, the intracranial pressure is raised but there is no structural abnormality in the brain detected on imaging, and the composition of the cerebrospinal fluid

(CSF) is normal. Some type of functional blockage to CSF drainage within the CSF drainage network (the arachnoid villi) is presumed. The diagnosis is made by normal cerebral imaging in association with a raised opening pressure on lumbar puncture (LP) and normal CSF biochemistry.

This condition may be related to the use of some oral contraceptives, NSAIDs or steroids.

The optic discs are swollen (papilloedema), but initially the vision remains normal. If the increased ICP persists, the patient will progressively lose visual field. Patients often have a headache, which is worse in the mornings.

Treatment consists of reducing the ICP. Repeated therapeutic LP with removal of a volume of CSF will reduce the ICP, but this is a temporary measure and unpleasant for the patient. More definitive treatments consist of surgical decompression via cerebroperitoneal shunts (insertion of a tube to drain CSF from around the brain into the peritoneum for absorption) or optic nerve sheath fenestration (surgical opening of the optic nerve's dural sheath to release excessive pressure and decompress the nerve).

Pseudopapilloedema

This is not a disease entity but a normal variant. Here the optic nerve appears swollen but is not. The posterior segments of small eyes, such as those that are markedly long-sighted, are crowded with nerve fibres and neurones squeezing into a small optic nerve head, making the optic disc appear raised and swollen.

Occasionally, there are calcific deposits within the substance of the nerve at the optic nerve head (called optic nerve head drusen). These are seen as yellow-white 'glistenings' within the optic disc, and may elevate disc contour to give the appearance of disc swelling. The distinction can be hard to make clinically, particularly in young eyes. A fluorescein angiogram will give the definitive answer, as the truly swollen disc will leak fluorescein, unlike the normal (and psuedopapilloedematous) disc.

Headache

Patients often present to their ophthalmologist or optometrist complaining of headaches or pain localised to, or around, the eye. In the great majority of cases there is no identifiable ocular pathology, but some conditions can cause this type of pain and thus require exclusion. Most are associated with a red eye and are discussed in Chapter 15.

The ophthalmic division of the trigeminal nerve is responsible for sensation and thus pain from the eye. Its relatively broad territory makes referred pain localised to the ocular region a common phenomena, necessitating assessment of teeth, sinuses and ears if no ocular pathology is found.

Uncorrected refractive errors may lead to eye 'strain' and dry eyes may result in significant ocular pain and discomfort.

Migraine

Migraine usually begins in adolescence, often with a positive family history. Certain triggers may bring about an attack. These triggers vary from individual to individual but alcohol, chocolate and cheese are common culprits. Patients may experience visual auras consisting of flashing lights, hazy vision or other curious visual or auditory phenomena.

Photosensitivity and flashes of light are common symptoms. The aura is thought to be due to cerebral vasoconstriction followed by vasodilatation, and the headache is thought to be secondary to stretching of the nerves within the vessel walls.

Patients often have an intense headache associated with photophobia that is frequently localised behind one eye. Nausea and vomiting are common.

Cluster headaches

Cluster headaches are severe headaches occurring on several successive occasions usually over a period of weeks and concentrated around one eye of middle-aged, usually male, patients.

Assessment

Optic nerve assessment involves assessing the patient's visual acuity, colour vision, visual fields and pupil reactions.

Assessment of the pupil reactions is described in detail in Chapter 11. Thorough assessment of the other cranial and peripheral nerves is vital.

Some of the pathologies associated with the pupil reaction are outlined below.

Argyll Robertson pupil

This is associated with neurosyphilis. The patient has a small pupil with no reaction to light but preserved reaction to accommodation.

Holmes-Adie pupil

This myotonic pupil is large and reacts sluggishly to light and accommodation. Poor focus (accommodative power) and loss of tendon reflexes are common.

Horner's syndrome

Horner's syndrome is characterised by a small pupil (miosis), ptosis (droopy lid), anhidrosis (loss of sweating on one side of the face) and apparent enophthalmos. It results from the interruption of the sympathetic nervous supply to the eye, and causes include neoplasia, infection and inflammation. A Pancoast tumour of the lung apex must be excluded by imaging. A painful Horner's syndrome should raise the suspicion of a carotid artery dissection.

Third nerve palsy with pupil involvement

The presence of a third nerve palsy with a poorly reactive dilated pupil is an ominous sign, and should be considered an aneurysm of the posterior communicating artery until proven otherwise. These patients need urgent imaging as a ruptured aneurysm is potentially life threatening. This is discussed further in the examinations section in Chapter 12.

The motor nerves to the eye and their oculomotor supplies are also discussed in Chapter 12, as are the common oculomotor palsies seen in clinical practice.

Nystagmus

Nystagmus is the involuntary repetitive oscillation of one or both eyes. It is clinically described in terms of its direction, speed and frequency. It occurs when a lesion causes dysfunction of the mechanisms that initiate or modify eye movement.

Eye position and stability are controlled by several inter-related neurological factors. Vision is a key component and is responsible for fixation on a target and the pursuit of targets in motion. Saccades are movements that bring objects lying in the peripheral visual field to the fovea, i.e. moving the eyes to look at an object. All the above rely on good vision in order to function properly.

The ear also plays a vital part in ocular stability. Otoliths are ear organs that monitor the position of the head in space and work in conjunction with the semicircular canals to assess the movement and position of the head, and thus the relative positions of the eyes.

The cerebellum is the final dictator of ocular position and stability, and exerts its influence via the vestibular nuclei. It fine-tunes eye movements and ensures ocular stability.

Nystagmus may be pathological or physiological.

There are several forms of physiological nystagmus, but the most important are end-point nystagmus – which occurs when the 'normal' individual gazes to the extreme right or left – and optokinetic nystagmus (OKN), which occurs when the individual repeatedly fixates and follows a moving target.

Ocular nystagmus

Ocular nystagmus is related to very poor vision. In this condition, the eye movements are roving and searching, oscillating back and forth. This sign in infancy is particularly worrying, and indicative of severe visual impairment. The eyes are starved of visual stimulus and move constantly, attempting to find something to view.

Pathological nystagmus

Pathological nystagmus usually consists of a fast and slow phase, but its direction is always described and documented in that of the fast phase.

Cerebellar nystagmus

Cerebellar nystagmus is the commonest form of pathological nystagmus seen in clinical practice. Its precise nature depends upon which lobe of the cerebellum is damaged. The eyes lose the fine control required to keep them stable while gazing to one side or the other, resulting in a coarse nystagmus. The patient should be scanned to exclude a space-occupying lesion or cerebrovascular accident.

Optic atrophy

Optic atrophy is a clinical finding related to damage or death of the optic nerve. Loss of neurones leads to progressive uncovering of the underlying sclera at the optic nerve head (optic disc). The optic disc becomes paler and paler until it appears white. The patient often has a relative afferent pupillary defect (RAPD), confirming significant optic nerve damage. Many conditions assault the optic nerve and result in neuronal loss and nerve death. Investigations should be directed according to history and associated clinical signs.

Conditions that can cause optic atrophy include neoplastic compressive lesions (e.g. cerebral tumours), vascular events (e.g. anterior ischaemic optic neuropathies), inflammatory conditions (e.g. optic neuritis), metabolic disorders (e.g. certain vitamin/nutritional deficiencies) and glaucoma.

Neurological visual field loss

The assessment and interpretation of common visual field defects are discussed in the examination section in Chapter 10.

Retinal field defect

This defect is localised to the area of retina that is damaged.

Optic nerve lesions

Optic nerve lesions can result in a broad spectrum of visual field defects, depending upon exactly which neurones are affected. Patients may develop a central scotoma, or lose a vertical half of their visual field (called an altitudinal visual field defect) or their temporal or nasal visual field. These hemianopic lesions are distinguished from optic radiation, optic tract or occipital cortex lesions by the fact that they are unilateral and do not obey the vertical midline (i.e. they cross the vertical line down the centre of the vision of either eye).

Optic chiasm lesions

Compressive lesions of the optic chiasm compromise the decussating (crossing) nerve fibres, resulting in bitemporal hemianopias.

Optic tract and radiation lesions

Such lesions result in homonymous hemianopic defects. These can be virtually identical and symmetrical in each eye (congruous) if the lesion is quite posterior, or can be quite different in shape (incongruous) if the lesion is anterior, before matching visual fibres from each eye have organised to run together.

Occipital lobe lesion

Occipital lobe lesions involving the visual cortex result in a contralateral congruous symmetrical homonymous hemianopia. The macular fibres, and thus central vision, are often preserved, even if an entire vertical half of vision is lost.

26 | Vascular diseases

Hypertensive retinopathy

The way that the eye responds to hypertension is related to its effects on the retinal vasculature, particularly on the arterial vessels.

The responses of the young eye are different from those of the older eye. Young patients tend to develop the classical changes of hypertensive retinopathy, whereas in older patients involutional sclerosis and fibrotic changes of the arterioles limit the ability to react in the 'classic' way.

In common with blood vessels throughout the body, the retinal arterioles attempt to regulate the blood flow by vasoconstricting in response to raised blood pressure. This narrowing of the retinal arteries and arterioles may occur in segments or be diffuse. In the normal population, the retinal veins are 50% larger than the arteries, therefore the arteriovenous ratio is 2:3. In hypertension, this ratio can change and the arteries can become much narrower than the veins – this is arteriolar attenuation.

Over time, the vessel walls hypertrophy and increase in thickness and muscular content. The thickened walls glisten metallically when viewed through the ophthalmoscope, and are often said to resemble silver or copper wiring.

Changes begin to develop where the retinal arteries cross the retinal veins and where they share a common adventitial sheath. The thickened arteries are carrying blood at high pressure and they compress the adjacent vein at the arteriovenous (AV) crossings. This compression is seen as localised nipping or squeezing of the vein wall (AV nipping).

As the blood pressure goes up, the artery and arteriole walls lose their integrity and begin to leak fluids, leading to retinal oedema and causing lipids to be deposited in the retinal tissue. These lipids are seen as yellow exudates similar to those seen in diabetic retinopathy. In severe cases, these lipids collect in the macula where, because of the orientation of the macula's retinal layers, they may take on the shape of a star pointing towards the fovea (macular star).

Haemorrhages may occur and their clinical appearance will vary, depending on in which retinal level they lie. If they occur deep within the retina, they will form a red blob (blot haemorrhage), but if they occur in the superficial nerve fibre layer, they will appear flame-like (flame-shaped haemorrhage) (figure 25.1).

Localised infarction of the retina – caused by localised occlusion of critically attenuated arterial vasculature – will result in cotton-wool spots, white feathery lesions of the nerve fibre layer (figure 26.1).

In its end stage, hypertensive retinopathy produces swelling of the optic disc.

As explained above, the changes will manifest to a much greater degree in the young eye and will be blunted with ageing.

Grading

Of the many different systems for grading retinal findings in hypertensive patients, the commonest is Keith and Wagener, below.

Stage 1

Focal narrowing of retinal arterioles.

Stage 2

Generalised arteriolar attenuation.

Stage 3

Haemorrhages, exudates, cotton-wool spots, retinal oedema.

Stage 4

As above, plus optic disc swelling.

Stage 4 is classified as malignant or accelerated hypertension and is indicative of severe hypertension with marked end organ damage (renal and cardiac).

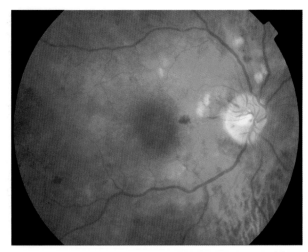

FIGURE 26.1 **Grade III hypertensive retinopathy. There are retinal haemorrhages, exudates, and cotton-wool spots. The retinal arteries are thinned and attenuated. Arteriovenous crossing changes are seen with thinning of the vein where it crosses the artery (best seen in the upper vessels).**

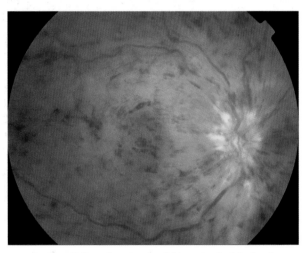

FIGURE 26.2 **Colour photograph of this patient's right fundus showing extensive haemorrhages spread throughout the retina and macula, typical of a central retinal vein occlusion. The disc is also swollen.**

Severe hypertension may result in a central retinal vein or artery occlusion, with potentially catastrophic consequences for vision.

Management

Patients should be referred to a physician for management of their hypertension. Retinal features will resolve with time once the blood pressure is brought down to normal. There may, however, be significant permanent damage if the hypertensive changes were marked or were present for prolonged periods of time.

Retinal venous occlusions

Central retinal vein occlusion (CRVO)

CRVO occurs when the venous outflow from the retinal vasculature becomes completely blocked. Back pressure results in rupture of venules with resulting extensive haemorrhages throughout the retina (figure 26.2).

The vein is thought to be compressed and blocked where it leaves the eye with the artery at the lamina cribrosa (the area of sclera that is thinned and perforated to allow the vessels and optic nerve to enter and exit). Excessive pressure on the vein at this point may predispose to CRVO. Thus hypertension (resulting in a high pressure in the adjacent central retinal artery) or raised IOP (pressure within the eye exerting a compressive effect) are risk factors for venous occlusion.

The patient's vision is usually poor and the optic disc is often swollen with an RAPD. Haemorrhages are scattered throughout the retina and vary greatly in degree, depending upon the severity of the occlusion.

The amount of retinal damage resulting from a CRVO depends upon the severity of the blockage. If venous outflow was completely occluded, then no arterial blood is able to enter the eye and perfuse the retina. Consequently, parts of the retina die and the long-term visual prognosis is very poor. This variant is called an ischaemic CRVO. If there is still some flow, allowing oxygenated blood to enter the retina, the damage may not be so severe. The latter situation is called non-ischaemic CRVO and has a better prognosis.

In an ischaemic CRVO, the retina is deprived of oxygen and thus releases chemical signals to encourage new blood supply. These vasoactive compounds diffuse to the front of the eye and cause new blood vessels to grow on the iris and within the drainage angle. This fibrovascular proliferation can block the drainage of aqueous fluid, causing rubeotic glaucoma, classically as early as 90 days after the onset of the CRVO (*see* Chapter 21).

Branch retinal vein occlusion (BRVO)

If the blocked vein lies away from the optic disc in the retina, the back pressure, retinal haemorrhages and potential ischaemia will affect only part of the retina (figure 26.3).

The symptoms and signs will depend on the site of the venous occlusion and, more importantly, how close it is to the optic disc and central retina. If the blockage is in the retinal periphery, it may be clinically completely silent. If one of the major retinal veins is involved close to the optic disc, a large section of retina will be affected together with part of the macula, resulting in significant visual loss.

The ruptured blood vessels never fully regain their correct blood-retinal barrier function. They may leak fluid and exudates that can result in macular oedema and prolonged visual deficit. Laser treatment to the site of the leaks and ischaemia sometimes improves vision.

In BRVO, the ischaemic retina can also release enough vasoactive chemical messengers to cause new blood vessels to form in the retina, at the optic disc or on the iris.

Retinal arterial occlusions

Central retinal artery occlusion (CRAO)

In this condition, the central retinal artery becomes blocked by an embolic phenomenon, compression or inflammation. The retina is deprived of its oxygen supply and rapidly dies. Irreversible catastrophic damage usually occurs within 90 minutes of arterial compromise.

This condition comes on very suddenly and the patient loses sight rapidly until the eye is virtually blind. The patient classically describes a curtain descending or ascending across their vision, identical to that experienced during an amaurosis fugax attack. However, unlike the TIA of amaurosis fugax, in this case the vision does not return.

The blockage is usually related to a large embolus that travels through the internal carotid and ophthalmic arteries to occlude the central retinal artery. These emboli can be calcific, atheromatous or fibrinoplatelet, and may have a cardiac or carotid source. Atrial fibrillation or valvular pathology can result in an embolus

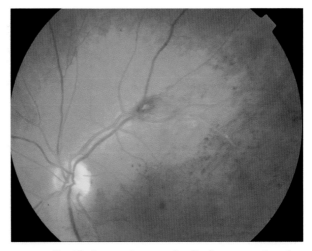

FIGURE 26.3 The haemorrhages are localised to one portion of the retina. The area of venous blockage is probably at the point the artery crosses the vein just proximal to the large retinal haemorrhage.

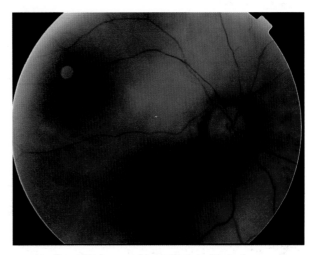

FIGURE 26.4 The cherry-red spot of a central retinal artery occlusion. The retinal arterioles are closed down and the retina is cloudy and creamy in appearance. The normal darker colour of the fovea clearly shows through as a 'cherry-red spot'.

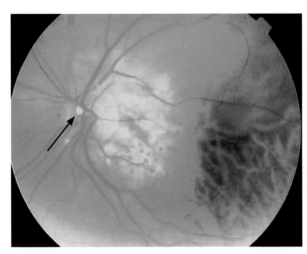

FIGURE 26.5 **A central retinal artery occlusion with a cholesterol embolus clearly visible impacted in the central retinal artery at the optic disc (arrow).**

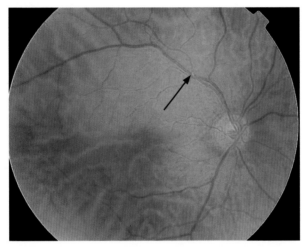

FIGURE 26.6 **A small embolus has lodged in the superotemporal retinal artery (arrow) and caused a branch retinal artery occlusion. The distal retina is cloudy and ischaemic. Part of the macula (and thus central vision) has been affected.**

passing out of the heart towards the eye. Significant carotid stenosis can also result in emboli that can put the eye at risk.

The retina fails to pass any light impulses to the brain, thus there is no effective pupillary light reflex. There is usually a dense relative afferent pupillary defect or even a total afferent pupillary defect.

The dead retina swells and fills with axoplasm, giving it a white, creamy appearance. At the fovea, the retina is extremely thin, composed of a thin layer of bare photoreceptors. Within this central area, the creamy oedematous retina is absent and thus does not block the normal underlying colour. The clinical appearance is of a creamy white retina with a red disc or spot at the fovea, called a 'cherry-red spot' (figure 26.4). Sometimes the embolus itself is visible within the retinal circulation (figure 26.5). A cherry-red spot is seen in other conditions where the retina becomes white and cloudy, such as certain metabolic storage disorders (e.g. the mucopolysaccharidoses).

Treatment is, unfortunately, usually fruitless, and the prognosis tends to be very poor indeed. If the patient is seen soon after onset of symptoms, attempts should be made to re-establish the retinal circulation. Vigorous ocular massage may help dislodge an embolus, or measures can be taken to decrease the intraocular pressure in the hope of 'flushing' an embolus through. Medical IOP-lowering agents are usually administered, and a needle paracentesis (needle aspiration of aqueous fluid from the anterior chamber to lower the pressure immediately virtually to zero) is often tried.

It is important to follow up these patients and watch for the onset of ocular complications, such as neovascularisation. The mainstay of management is to treat any underlying cardiac or carotid aetiology, and minimise the risk of further vaso-occlusive events with antiplatelet medication, formal anticoagulation treatment or even surgical carotid endarterectomy, if significant carotid stenosis is discovered.

Branch retinal artery occlusion (BRAO)

If an embolus is small enough, it can enter the retinal circulation and will only impact and cause occlusion when it lodges in a vessel of sufficiently narrow calibre. When this happens, the embolus impacts and blocks off the blood supply to the distal retina (figure 26.6). The symptoms and signs depend on where the blockage occurs and, more importantly, how proximal it is to the origin of the central retinal artery. If the blockage is in the retinal periphery, it may be clinically completely silent. If one of the major retinal blood vessels is involved close to the optic disc, a large amount of retina will be affected as well as part of the macula, resulting in significant visual loss.

If the patient is seen early, attempts can be made to dislodge this blockage, as in the management of CRAO. The mainstay of management is to treat any underlying cardiac or carotid aetiology and minimise the risk of further vaso-occlusive events as described above.

Ischaemic optic neuropathy

In this condition, as the name suggests, the blood supply to the optic nerve itself becomes compromised. This may be due to a microvascular event, such as a diabetic mononeuropathy or microembolic infarction, or secondary to involvement of the blood supply of the nerve by an inflammatory process.

Visual loss tends to be rapid, and patients may lose parts of their visual field, while other parts are spared. For example, patients commonly lose the upper half of their visual field, with sparing of the lower half of their vision, or vice versa – an altitudinal visual field defect.

As the optic nerve is compromised, the axoplasmic flow ceases and the optic disc usually becomes swollen.

There are two forms of ischaemic optic neuropathy: arteritic and non-arteritic.

Arteritic ischaemic optic neuropathy is an ophthalmic emergency and requires urgent treatment to avoid bilateral blindness. It is related to infarction of the optic nerve, secondary to a vasculitic process affecting the posterior ciliary arteries that deliver most of its blood supply. This vasculitic process is part of giant cell or temporal arteritis (GCA/TA) and requires immediate treatment with high-dose steroids (see below).

The non-arteritic (non-GCA-related) version of this disorder tends to have a better prognosis for final vision. For an unknown reason, the blood supply to the optic nerve is compromised, presumably related to a microembolic event.

Patients should be started on antiplatelet medication if there is no contraindication, as this should decrease the risk of further ischaemic pathology affecting the optic nerve. All cardiovascular and cerebrovascular risk factors should be addressed.

Giant cell arteritis

GCA is a systemic disorder characterised by generalised inflammation of large and medium-sized arteries. Patients tend to be over 55 years of age, with a female preponderance ratio of 2:1. The inflammatory process attacks the elastic lamina of blood vessels throughout the body, but intracranial vessels, which do not have elastic lamina, tend to be spared.

Systemic features include malaise, fever, weight loss, scalp pain, headache, polymyalgia rheumatica, tender temporal arteries and jaw claudication. A definite history of jaw claudication (a phenomenon related to masseter ischaemia, where talking or eating causes pain that disappears when jaw movement stops) is a relatively specific symptom of GCA.

Ocular involvement is usually secondary to inflammation of posterior ciliary arteries, causing an arteritic anterior ischaemic optic neuropathy. Diplopia may be a feature because of the involvement of small vessels supplying extraocular muscles or arteritis of the vasa nervorum of ocular motor nerves. Rarer sequelae include CRAO.

The classical presentation is sudden visual loss in one eye with a preceding history of systemic features. Typical clinical findings are a swollen optic disc with an RAPD and a tender non-pulsatile temporal artery. When one eye is affected, the other eye is at high risk, often within days and nearly always within six weeks of onset of symptoms.

This is an ophthalmic emergency and requires immediate investigation and appropriate management. Westergreen erythrocyte sedimentation rate (ESR) is high (usually more than 80 mm hour^{-1}) but 10% of patients will have normal levels. The C-reactive protein (CRP) is usually universally raised. Patients may have an anaemia of chronic disease.

When the condition is suspected, temporal artery biopsy is indicated. A 3 cm length should be excised and sent for histopathological analysis within two weeks of initiating corticosteroid treatment. If the biopsy is done when the patient has been on a long course of steroids, the histopathological features may be masked by the action of the drugs.

Histopathology shows granulomatous inflammation of the vessel wall with abundant epithelioid cells, lymphocytes and giant cells.

Treatment should start as soon as the diagnosis is suspected, with systemic corticosteroids being the mainstay. Treatment will probably be intravenous for the first 48 hours, and then oral corticosteroids at a starting dose of 1 mg/kg/day will be given, with the dose adjusted according to serial measurements of inflammatory indices and to clinical condition.

The prognosis for the affected eye is usually poor but early and long-term treatment is usually effective in preventing involvement of the other eye.

27 | Miscellaneous conditions

Myopia

Myopia (short-sightedness) is not strictly a disease. A small degree of myopia is not uncommon and may be regarded as physiological. In pathological myopia, the eye is excessively long and the sclera abnormally weakened and stretched. Because the eye is too long, the image is focused too far in front of the retina (*see* Chapter 7, The focusing mechanism of the eye [refraction]).

The weakness of the sclera predisposes the patient to many problems. The retina may begin to degenerate (myopic degeneration), resulting in extensive atrophic patches, leaving the underlying white sclera showing through (figure 27.1). This occurs mainly around the optic disc, but can also occur in the macula with concomitant visual loss. Patients can also develop retinal detachments or even choroidal neovascular membranes that are not due to age-related macular degeneration (*see* Chapter 17). Such eyes are also prone to damage because of their abnormally thinned sclera.

There is no treatment except refractive correction, observation and rapid appropriate management of any complications.

Retinitis pigmentosa

This is a hereditary condition that can be inherited in an autosomal dominant, autosomal recessive or even x-linked fashion. It can also be sporadic. It causes degeneration of the rod photoreceptors with gradual loss of the peripheral field of vision. As already described, the rods are responsible for night vision and so patients with this condition experience great difficulty seeing dim light and may complain of night blindness (nyctalopia). Eventually all peripheral vision is lost, and only the cones in the macular remain. These patients see with only 10° or 15° of central vision, which is true tunnel vision.

The typical findings of retinitis pigmentosa are bone spicule pigmentation, disc pallor described as 'waxy' and arteriolar attenuation (figure 27.2). The bone spicule appearance is due to degeneration of the retinal pigment epithelial cells that release their pigment into retina as linear clumps when they die. This is said to resemble the spicules seen on light microscopy of bone.

Unfortunately there is no treatment, and the condition tends to be progressive. Age of onset and disease progression varies considerably. As a general rule, the later in life the disease presents, the better the prognosis. Patients need counselling about the condition and the likely course of the disease. A specialised electrodiagnostic test of retinal function can be used to confirm the diagnosis and assess severity. Patients who have, or are planning to have, children should receive genetic counselling.

Albinism

As with cutaneous albinism, the ocular form manifests as a relative or absolute lack of melanin in the pigmented tissues of the eye. In ocular albinism, the retinal pigment epithelial layer is extremely pale and does not perform its proper functions of absorbing excess light and supporting the retina metabolically. The patient does not see well, due to excessive light absorption and scatter. The iris is also very pale (usually blue), and allows light through because its rear surface, which is normally pigmented and blocks the light, is absent. It is thus possible to see the red reflex shining back through the iris tissue.

Ocular albinism affects only the eye, while patients with oculocutaneous disorder have fair hair and their skin has the classic bleached-white appearance.

There is no treatment, and vision usually remains subnormal but static.

Choroidal melanocytic lesions

The choroid, like the skin, may harbour many different types of pigmented lesions. A choroidal naevus is sim-

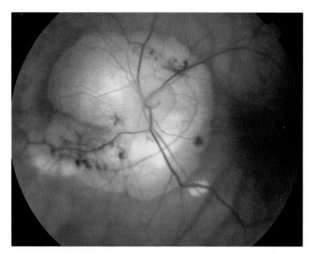

FIGURE 27.1 **A pathologically myopic fundus. There is extensive atrophy around the disc allowing the white sclera to show through. This atrophy may spread to involve the macula and thus reduce vision.**

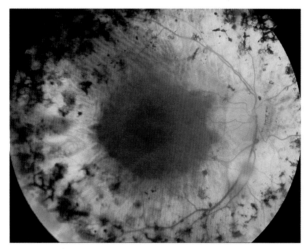

FIGURE 27.2 **Severe retinitis pigmentosa. The whole peripheral retina has degenerated resulting in only a central island of functioning retina within the macula.**

ilar to a benign mole on the skin. It may be flat or elevated and is seen as a dark red-brown lesion beneath the RPE layer (figure 24.3). It is usually asymptomatic, and picked up as an incidental finding on routine ophthalmoscopy. The key concern with such lesions is the presence of growth. If a lesion is seen to be growing, and particularly if it becomes more and more elevated, there is a risk that it may be a growing choroidal malignant melanoma.

A choroidal melanoma is the most common intraocular malignancy that occurs in one eye of patients over 50 years of age. If neglected, this lesion can grow to fill the entire eye and may metastasise haematogenously, usually to the liver. It can cause a retinal detachment or other complications such as secondary glaucoma.

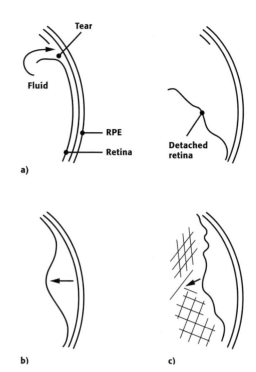

FIGURES 27.3 a–c **a) A hole or tear is made in the retina and fluid from the vitreous cavity is allowed to enter the space under the retina causing it to peel away. b) Fluid from the retinal pigment epithelial layer causes lifting off of the retina without a retinal break. c) Fibrous bands create traction and pull the retina gradually from the retinal pigment epithelial layer causing a firm detachment but no retinal break.**

Diagnosis can be extremely difficult, particularly if the melanoma is slow growing.

Treatment used to be radical surgery, but more conservative although equally effective treatment is now used. Limited resection together with radiotherapy, usually in the form of a radioactive plaque implant, means that the eye can be spared to some degree and some residual vision maintained.

Always remember that a mass in the eye might be a metastasis from a distant site.

Retinal detachment

The neurosensory retina is a clear layer, lining the whole inside of the eye. It is in direct contact with the RPE, but can become detached and pull away. This leads to retinal dysfunction, as the photoreceptors are no longer receiving their nutrients and oxygen from the RPE.

There are several ways in which the retina can come away from the RPE (figures 27.3a–c):

- A hole or tear forms in the retina, which allows fluid from the vitreous cavity to seep under and peel it away

- Fluid is secreted from the RPE as part of an exudative or inflammatory process into the space between the RPE and the retina, thereby lifting the retina and detaching it
- Tractional forces physically pull the retina away.

All three of these phenomena cause the retina to separate from the RPE with visual loss. If the process begins at the peripheries, the patient may notice a visual field defect at the edge of vision, often described as a curtain or black shadow that gets gradually larger. As detachment progresses, the macula will eventually come off, with concomitant severe reduction in central vision. Patients with retinal detachment can experience symptoms of flashing lights (photopsia) or floaters (little semi-translucent or solid objects floating in their vision).

The commonest cause of a retinal detachment is a tear or hole in the retina. This occurs because of abnormal attachments between the retina and the vitreous jelly. In youth, the vitreous is a semi-solid, gel-like structure, formed of numerous collagen fibres with high-molecular-weight substances and liquid suspended in between. Over time, the vitreous becomes more liquid as the gel and collagen structure breaks down. This process is called syneresis and is a natural ageing phenomenon.

As the collagen structure degenerates and the gel is replaced with water, the vitreous shrinks and collapses (figure 27.4a). This is called a posterior vitreous detachment (PVD) and occurs naturally. It usually happens suddenly and patients may or may not experience transient symptoms such as flashing lights or floaters. These symptoms are the same as those for retinal detachment. In isolated PVD, these symptoms tend to be short lived, and the floaters fewer, but dis-

tinguishing between the two conditions is difficult without a thorough examination of the retina.

If there are no abnormal attachments between the retina and the vitreous (vitreoretinal adhesions), then the PVD occurs without any pathological sequelae. If there are abnormal vitreoretinal adhesions, when the vitreous collapses, the PVD can cause tugging on a focal point of retina, causing a hole or tear (figure 27.4b). This allows the liquid from the watery vitreous to enter the subretinal space and peel off the surrounding retina, causing a retinal detachment.

A retinal detachment requires surgery to flatten the retina and seal the hole. This may be done externally, where the sclera is indented by an external piece of rubber sutured on to the eye and the hole is frozen or lasered (and thus sealed) into place.

Alternatively, the vitreous can be removed surgically to stop gel tugging on the retina.

If the hole is spotted before a detachment occurs, laser can be applied around the break to form scar tissue that holds the retina down and prevents the entry of subretinal fluid, and thus retinal/RPE separation and detachment.

The longer the retina remains detached, the less likely it is to survive, and it should be restored to its normal position as soon as possible. If the macula has been detached, then the visual prognosis is uncertain as, even when the macula is flattened, it may have sustained permanent damage.

There are many risk factors for retinal detachment, the most important of which is myopia or short-sightedness. Myopic eyes are too big and the ocular tissues tend to be imperfectly formed, with an excessively thin retina in places. Such areas of weakness are prone to holes and tears. As well as this inherent weakness, there are often areas of abnormal vitreoretinal adhesions, which means that a PVD can cause retinal breaks with subsequent detachment. The greater the degree of short-sightedness, the greater the risk of retinal detachment.

There are several congenital conditions that predispose to retinal detachment, such as Marfans and Stickler syndromes. Blunt trauma can cause a shock wave strong enough to tear the retina, and penetrating injuries can result in direct disruption. Patients who have had cataracts removed, particularly when an intraocular lens implant has not been placed into the eye (aphakia), are also at increased risk of retinal detachment.

Fundoscopy reveals corrugation and whitening of the retina in the detached area (figure 27.5). Usually

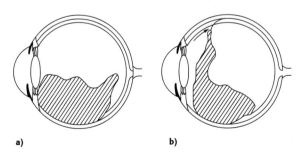

a)   b)

FIGURES 27.4a and b a) The clear vitreous has collapsed down in its own transparent bag. The remaining space in the vitreous cavity is immediately replaced by clear fluid that was originally in the vitreous bag. b) Once more the vitreous has collapsed and detached from the back of the eye. In this case an area of abnormal adhesion has caused the retina to come away forming a tear. This tear can allow fluid (arrow) to peel the retina off and cause a retinal detachment.

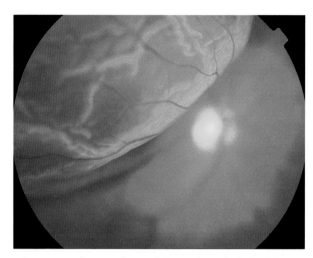

FIGURE 27.5 **The retina has peeled away from the back of the eye and has become raised, creamy and corrugated in appearance. The macula has already been detached and thus vision is markedly reduced. The optic disc can be seen out of focus in the background.**

the tear or hole is peripheral, so it may be quite hard to see with the direct ophthalmoscope.

Tractional retinal detachments occur through fibrosis of the retina or fibrous processes within the vitreous cavity physically pulling the retina off. The commonest causes are inflammation and proliferative diabetic retinopathy.

Exudative retinal detachments occur, as the name suggests, because of exudation of fluid into the subretinal space, usually through the body of the retinal pigment epithelium. This is secondary to underlying choroidal tumours, as a result of choroidal vascular defects or choroidal inflammatory processes.

Herpes zoster ophthalmicus (HZO)

After the viraemia associated with chickenpox, the herpes zoster virus can lie dormant in many nerves throughout the body. Reactivation of the virus in the ophthalmic division of the trigeminal nerve leads to shingles, with a vesicular rash in the cutaneous distribution of that nerve, i.e. over the forehead and upper eyelids. Vesicles form, followed by pustules with thick crusts. The patient usually experiences marked pain and a burning sensation.

The virus can involve any of the anterior structures of the eye, and conjunctivitis, keratitis or even iritis can occur. The eye is not always involved, however. If the eye becomes red while the patient is suffering from HZO, direct involvement of the eye must be suspected. A risk factor for ocular involvement is cutaneous disease involving the tip of the nose. This area is supplied by the nasociliary nerve (a branch of the nerve supplying the eye itself), so its involvement raises the suspicion that the eye is also involved. This is called Hutchinson's sign.

Even after HZO has resolved, the patient may experience neuralgic pain, which, although usually self-limiting, can be very distressing.

Myasthenia gravis

Myasthenia gravis (MG) is an autoimmune disorder characterised by the presence of anti-acetylcholine receptor antibodies. These antibodies compete with the acetylcholine (ACh) molecules released at the neuromuscular junction for the ACh receptor sites on muscles. The effect of the ACh is blocked and so the muscles are not stimulated effectively and tire rapidly. Muscular weakness can affect any part of the body. It is typically worse in the evenings and increases with prolonged exertion.

MG can occur as a systemic condition or may solely affect the eye. Ocular features are a variable fatigable ptosis or intermittent oculomotor muscle imbalance, resulting in a changeable squint and double vision.

This condition classically affects older people, and can be associated with thyroid autoimmune disease or, in younger patients, with the presence of a thymoma.

The diagnosis is based on clinical features and the presence of serum anti-ACh antibodies. A Tensilon test used to be common. This involves injecting an anti-acetylcholinesterase (edrophonium chloride) intravenously, resulting in a dramatic increase in ACh at the neuromuscular junctions as normal breakdown is blocked. If the muscle weakness is reversed, the diagnosis is confirmed. This is a dangerous procedure, however, as the increase in ACh activity may have adverse cardiac effects (a small dose of atropine is often administered to try to minimise this risk). Adequate resuscitation equipment should always be available.

28 | Paediatric ophthalmology

Paediatric ophthalmology is a highly specialised subject and a speciality in its own right. Many of the problems that affect the adult eye can affect the paediatric patient but with different manifestations. Children are different in that their eyes are growing continually and thus at risk of developmental problems. Naturally congenital disorders are also most likely to manifest in this age group. The child's developing nervous system and cerebral pathways are continually evolving in the early years, and any pathology may have significant deleterious effects on normal development.

Examining adult eyes can sometimes be difficult due to lack of co-operation, but these challenges are much greater with children. Generally, as children get older, they become more co-operative and tests of visual function can be more complex, and thus usually, but not always, more informative.

Assessing visual acuity in pre-verbal children is difficult. First, it is important to ask witnesses about the child's visual behaviour. Parents are the natural first source of information and are usually able to make accurate judgements about whether their baby or small child can see, and the likely level of vision.

- Does the baby respond to smiles?
- Can they recognise the mother's face?
- Does the baby fix on (stare at) and follow an object?
- Do the eyes wobble? (Nystagmus?)
- Are the eyes always straight? (Squint?)
- Does the child reach for and pick up objects? How big are these objects?

These questions are likely to yield a wealth of information because parents observe their offspring throughout their waking time, while the examining doctor may only have a few minutes in which to make an assessment.

There are several tests to determine vision in children who are too young to co-operate with normal testing, such as the Snellen chart. Examples include preferential looking tests, where a baby is presented with a card, half of which is blank while the other half has a visual stimulus on it. If the baby looks at the side with the stimulus they must be able to see it, while the size of the stimulus gives an indication of their degree of vision. Older children may be able to use cards placed at a distance showing pictures of animals or common objects. If they can see the image, they can match it to those on a card held close to them.

Remember that children are individuals and will co-operate and perform tests to different degrees. As the child gets older, the test results become more reliable and truer evaluations of visual acuity are possible.

As with any paediatric speciality, examining a child requires a certain degree of playmanship and a good level of rapport with youngsters. Time is limited and so toys and games should be used to keep a child's attention and co-operation during the examination. If a child refuses to be examined, trying to force them is unlikely to result in valuable information and such measures will certainly not endear you to the parents.

Cataract

A clinically significant cataract is an opacity of the lens that results in visual reduction. There are several opacities that do not involve the visually important portions of the native lens, and thus do not reduce vision. Such lens opacities are usually of no immediate concern or clinical significance. The growing lens is prone to develop cloudiness in reaction to local factors or systemic disorders.

In one-third of cases, a cataract in a baby is inherited, while in about another third of cases, the condition is related to a systemic disorder. In the remaining third it is sporadic, with no underlying aetiology or systemic disorder.

Disorders that can result in cataracts include chromosomal abnormalities, intrauterine or maternal infections, diabetes, galactosaemia, glucokinase deficiency and neonatal hypocalcaemia.

Neonates are highly dependent upon visual stimuli being presented to the eye and transmitted to the brain in order to lay down the appropriate visual pathways for vision. If in early life these visual stimuli are blocked (e.g. by the presence of an opacity, such as a cataract, interrupting light transmission to the retina), the visual pathways cannot form and the vision will remain poor even if the opacity is removed. The most sensitive time is the neonatal period, and a cataract can rapidly result in irreversibly poor vision if not removed quickly. If untreated, the baby will develop nystagmus as the eyes 'search' for stimulus. This is a poor prognostic sign, indicating that the visual potential has already been markedly impaired.

Checking for the presence of cataracts is part of the standard neonatal examination. Cataracts can be detected by a reduction in the red reflex seen within the pupil. This red reflex is formed by light reflecting back from the retina and is the reason why 'red eye' develops in flash photography. Shining a light (preferably the ophthalmoscope light, while looking through it) will elicit a red reflex that should be symmetrical between each eye. Sometimes in Afro-Caribbean babies, the red reflex is hard to see because of the large amount of dark pigmentation within the fundi.

If in any doubt, refer to a paediatric ophthalmologist for further assessment. A cataract should be surgically removed as soon as possible to allow light into the eye and facilitate development of the normal visual pathways. It is sometimes inadvisable to place an intraocular lens into the eye of a very young child, as severe inflammation and consequent complications may ensue. Instead, some young cataract patients are left without a lens (aphakia) and their vision corrected with contact lenses. Later in life, it is possible to place a lens into the eye surgically (pseudophakia).

Children with prolonged intraocular inflammation (such as uveitis) are also at significant risk of developing cataracts and, if these are visually significant and if the inflammation is adequately controlled, a cataract extraction should be undertaken.

Infantile glaucoma (buphthalmos)

In glaucoma, the pressure within the eye is raised and damages the optic nerve, resulting in visual field loss. In adults, the eye is fully grown and thus high intraocular pressure does not result in a change in globe size. In contrast, the neonatal eye is continually growing, and any significant period of raised intraocular pressure will have a direct effect on the size of the developing eye. As the scleral coat is not completely formed, the eye stretches and enlarges. Such eyes become abnormally big and have been compared with a bull's eye, hence the term buphthalmos. If untreated, this condition can result in bilateral blindness. The high pressure in the eye can rupture the inner layer of the cornea, allowing fluid to enter, causing swelling and cloudiness.

The aetiology of this condition is thought to be related to remnants of a membrane over the drainage angles preventing egress of aqueous from the anterior chamber (*see* Chapter 21, Glaucoma).

The corneal swelling and subsequent corneal surface irregularities related to the high pressure cause the baby to develop lacrimation (excessive watering), blepharospasm (excessive forceful blinking) and photophobia (sensitivity to light). These three signs raise the clinical suspicion of congenital glaucoma.

Treatment

The pressure must be reduced, but it is important to confirm that the pressure is indeed high. Naturally, the baby will not co-operate with standard methods of measuring intraocular pressure. These babies have to be examined under general anaesthesia to allow accurate measurement of the globe (particularly corneal diameter), and intraocular pressure. Surgery is then required to open up the drainage angle.

Retinoblastoma

Retinoblastoma is a malignant tumour of the eye and affects approximately one in 20,000 births. It usually presents in babies under three years of age with leukocoria (white pupil) or a squint. The leukocoria is usually noticed by the parents, and occurs because the white retinoblastoma mass is visible through the pupil. Squints occur because vision in the affected eye is significantly reduced, and thus fails to be kept straight by cerebral control.

There is a one-in-three chance of bilateral retinoblastoma, and so the other eye must be thoroughly examined. This is an inherited condition caused by a mutation in a tumour suppressor gene. Thus offspring of survivors of retinoblastoma are at increased risk of the condition, as are their siblings.

Prognosis and management depends upon the presence or absence of bilateral disease, the localisation of the tumour and the extent of local and systemic spread.

Juvenile idiopathic arthritis (JIA)

Juvenile idiopathic arthritis (also called juvenile chronic arthritis) is, as its name suggests, an arthritis affecting children. It appears to be an autoimmune disorder, and many of the children affected have anti-nuclear antibodies (ANA) in their blood. The disease can affect many joints (polyarticular) or only four or fewer joints (pauciarticular). There is also a systemic group of patients who are spared the risk of ocular problems.

Children with the pauciarticular or polyarticular disorder require long-term follow up by an ophthalmologist because they are at risk of developing a severe anterior uveitis (iritis), which can lead to glaucoma, corneal scarring or cataract. Such patients are unusual in that their severe intraocular inflammation can be completely silent. Adults who develop iritis will have a red eye and significant other symptoms. In JIA patients, the eye may be severely inflamed but totally white and the child will be completely asymptomatic. Only examination at a slit lamp will detect the inflammation.

Patients with pauciarticular JIA and a positive ANA are at greatest risk of severe ocular inflammation and require ophthalmic examination every two to three months, usually for more than seven years after onset of their disease. Any inflammation should be treated aggressively both locally and systemically, in consultation with a paediatric rheumatologist.

Coloboma

A coloboma is a congenital abnormality related to failure of the normal development of the eye. The eye forms by embryonic tissue wrapping round to form a closed tube and then a sphere. In some cases, this process fails and the tube/sphere fails to form because the edges do not fully come together. The rest of the eye develops normally, but the structures in the area of incomplete closure do not form and are replaced by plain connective tissue.

This problem may result in an abnormal optic disc, retina, choroid, iris or lens. If the coloboma does not directly involve the macula, the vision may be relatively normal. This is a non-progressive disorder.

Retinitis of prematurity

Retinitis of prematurity (ROP) is a disorder affecting premature neonates who tend to have low birth weight, low gestational age and a history of oxygen supplementation in early life.

In utero, the retina develops initially at the optic disc and then grows outwards in a wave, to spread and eventually cover the whole back of the eye. It is thought that hypoxia of the uncovered patches drives the migration of the developing retina towards the peripheries. This process is almost complete by term, but in premature babies the retina has not yet spread to cover the whole back of the eye.

High concentrations of inhaled oxygen (which is often given to these babies in the special care units) inhibit the normal spread of retina by negating the normal hypoxic drive to retinal growth. When this extra oxygen is discontinued, the area not covered by retina becomes suddenly markedly ischaemic and releases vasoactive chemical messengers that stimulate neovascular proliferation. These new blood vessels can bleed and cause excessive scarring. If this is untreated, blindness is a significant risk.

If the condition is detected and is deemed to meet special clinical criteria, laser may be applied to kill off the ischaemic areas in the periphery of the retina. This has been shown to reduce the risk of blindness dramatically. Babies weighing less than 1500 g (1250 g in some centres) or of less than 32 weeks gestation are deemed to be at greatest risk and warrant examination/screening by a specialist ophthalmologist.

Strabismus

A strabismus is the clinical term for a squint and occurs when the eyes do not point in the same direction. In order for the brain to receive virtually identical overlapping images for processing together, the eyes must be orientated so that the same objects are projecting their images within the same parts of the macula and peripheral retina. If this does not happen, the brain will get conflicting images from each eye.

The adult brain reacts to this by 'seeing' both images and trying to force them into one coherent picture. Usually this is impossible, and the patient ends up seeing double (diplopia). In the growing child, the brain is able to switch off one of the images and ignore it. Thus, a child may not get double vision, even though their eyes are pointing in completely different directions.

In a normal child, both eyes point in the same direction when they are looking at a distant object. As an object gets closer, the eyes are required to swivel in slightly or converge (move in towards the nose) in order to stay targeting on the object. This is one of the features of accommodation where the lens power of the eye increases to focus on the closer object and the eyes converge (move in).

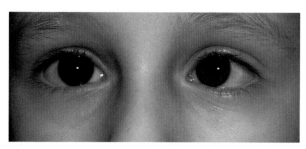

FIGURE 28.1 **A child with a convergent squint (esotropia). The corneal reflexes are clearly asymmetrical with the right corneal light reflex resting centrally on the pupil whereas the left lies at the pupil margin. The left eye is thus the deviating eye. (Courtesy of Mr T.K. Butler.)**

In a child with a squint, one eye is usually looking at the object of regard and this is called the fixing eye, as it has fixed on the target. The eye that is not looking straight is called the deviating or squinting eye.

A squint may be present all the time, i.e. the eyes are never straight, or it may be intermittent.

As already described, the brain is able to ignore the image received by the deviating eye in order to prevent the child experiencing diplopia. This has the unfortunate effect of preventing the normal visual pathways developing for the deviating/squinting eye. Without a visual stimulus to promote the formation of normal neural connections, the eye becomes lazy and may be left with a permanently poor visual acuity, even if the squint is later corrected.

Amblyopia, or lazy eye, usually only develops if the squint is constant, and if the child continually favours one eye and ignores the other. Sometimes the child may 'swap' between the eyes subconsciously. They may fix with the right eye and ignore the left eye, and then change to fix with their left eye and ignore the right. This is called cross-fixation. In this case, both eyes are receiving adequate visual stimulus (albeit for half the usual time) and the neural pathways are able to develop normally for each eye. Neither eye will develop amblyopia.

The deviating eye may be turned in (a convergent squint or esotropia) (figure 28.1) or turned out (a divergent squint or exotropia).

Squints are measured by assessing how far the deviating eye is turned in or out, using prisms placed in front of the eyes. These prisms bend incoming light by a fixed amount until the light is entering the eye through the centre of the cornea. The units of measurement are called prism dioptres. More than 45 prism dioptres of squint is a large squint. Orthoptists are allied health professionals with particular expertise in assessing strabismus patients, as well as evaluating all aspects of the child's visual system.

When a child looks at a close object, the eyes accommodate and some convergence takes place. It is therefore important to measure the degree of squint when the child is looking at an object close by (thus while they are accommodating) and while they are looking at an object in the distance (no accommodation active). The degree of squint can vary significantly, and indeed sometimes the eyes are straight for distance but squint markedly when the patient looks at an object close up.

Treatment

The major concern with a squint in childhood is the development of a lazy eye. If the child cross-fixates and thus maintains good vision in each eye, there is no immediate concern. If, however, the child favours one eye, and the other eye is becoming lazy, the child needs treatment to prevent irreversible amblyopia and thus long-term poor vision.

Correction of the squint by surgery (explained below) will result in both eyes receiving the same images, thus allowing both to develop normally. It may be better to treat the amblyopia first and 'kick-start' the lazy eye's development before embarking on surgery. This 'kick-starting' usually involves patching the good eye. By covering the normal eye (the one the child uses to fixate), the child is forced to use the deviating eye for sight. The brain now forces this eye to become straight and uses it to fix, thus giving it the correct visual input and allowing normal neural development with reversal of amblyopia. Care must be taken not to cover the good eye for too long, because if it is too deprived of visual stimuli then it too will become lazy. Once the amblyopia is reversed, surgery should be considered.

It is generally best to wait as long as possible before undertaking squint surgery, as the more developed the child's eyes and brain, the more predictable and reliable surgery will be. As explained above, if amblyopia is occurring despite attempted treatment then surgery should be done sooner. Another indication for surgery is cosmesis, thus it is usually best to undertake surgical correction of a squint before the child reaches school age to avoid social stigma and bullying.

Surgery

The horizontal alignment of the eyes is maintained by the four horizontal recti muscles: right medial rectus, right lateral rectus, left medial rectus and left lateral rectus. Squint surgery aims to tighten or loosen these muscles in order to alter the horizontal position of the eyes.

In order to strengthen a muscle, the muscle is identified and dissected clear of the surrounding tissue. It is detached from the sclera and a segment cut out of it. The muscle is then sutured back on to the sclera. Shortening the muscle in this way increases its strength. This operation is called a resection procedure.

Weakening a muscle is done by dissecting it clear and detaching it from the sclera as above. Rather than cutting a segment out, however, the muscle is left whole and sutured back on to the sclera but further back than its original position. The muscle has been effectively lengthened and thus weakened. This procedure is called a recession, as the muscle has been recessed further back.

If the patient has a convergent squint then one eye or both eyes are pointing too far in. To rectify this, the eyes must be made to point further out and thus straighter. This involves either weakening the muscles that pull the eyes in (the right and left medial recti) or strengthening the muscles pulling the eyes out (the lateral recti). Two operations are commonly used for a convergent squint in childhood. The medial recti muscles of both eyes can be weakened (bimedial recession) or, alternatively, the medial rectus of one eye (usually the deviating eye) can be weakened with concurrent strengthening of the lateral rectus of that same eye (called a medial-rectus-recess, lateral-rectus-resect procedure).

If the patient has a divergent squint, then one eye or both eyes are pointing too far out. To rectify this, both lateral recti can be weakened or both medial recti strengthened. More commonly, a recess–resect procedure is carried out on the diverging eye, where the lateral rectus is recessed (weakened) and the medial rectus resected (strengthened), thereby pulling the eye in.

Role of hypermetropia – accommodative squint

Accommodation is the process used to focus on near objects. When an object is close, the eyes must turn in slightly (converge) so that both are able to look at it. The pupils constrict (miose) and the lens changes shape to increase its focusing power, thus allowing the light from the object to be accurately focused on to the macula. There is a relationship between the quantitative increase in focusing power on the lens (more plus power) and the amount of convergence: the closer the object, the more the eyes need to converge and the more plus power the lens must exert.

Occasionally this system causes problems. If the child is long-sighted (hypermetropic), then in the rested state (fully relaxed lens) the light from objects in the distance is focused too far back behind the retina. The child must, therefore, exert some of the focusing power of the lens simply to be able to see clearly in the distance. When the child looks at something close up, the magnitude of lens power needed increases even further to very high levels. The link between the lens power and convergence (the process of accommodation) means that the eyes may be forced to converge too much by this large change in lens power. The eyes are thus forced into a convergent squint (esotropia) for near sight.

This squint may be fully or partially corrected by spectacles. The spectacles correct all of the child's long-sightedness and cancel out the need for accommodation. This also negates the need for their pathological excessive accommodative convergence. The child may no longer squint at all, or the magnitude of the squint may be markedly reduced by spectacles – a fully accommodative convergent squint or partially accommodative convergent squint, respectively.

Children with a convergent squint (esotropia) should be assessed by an optometrist to see if they are long-sighted (hypermetropic). If this is the case, then full spectacle correction should be given to see whether this straightens the eyes. If the squint disappears completely, the child should be regularly followed up with frequent assessment. As the child grows, the eyes may become progressively less long-sighted and eventually spectacles may no longer be needed.

Children with a partially accommodative squint may still require surgery to correct this residual ocular misalignment.

Pseudosquint

A pseudosquint is present when the child appears to have a squint or deviating eye, but the eyes are in fact straight (figure 13.1). There can be many reasons for this, usually related to the individual's facial architecture, the commonest being prominent epicanthal folds in babies (folds of skin at the medial aspect of the eye adjacent to the nose). These folds obscure the medial part of the sclera and make the eyes appear to be pointing in (cross-eyed/convergent squint). As the baby grows, the folds become less prominent and the pseudosquint disappears.

It is important to examine these patients correctly. Gross examination may be misleading, and the best way to assess true eye position is to assess corneal reflections (see below).

Examining a strabismus case

It is important to take an accurate history from the parents, including a birth history and history of any congenital or acquired diseases.

All these cases require a dilated fundoscopy by an ophthalmologist to ensure that there is no underlying cause for the squint. A pathology that is causing reduced vision in an eye (e.g. a cataract or a retinal tumour) will prevent the brain from maintaining normal 'straightness' and cause the eye to deviate. This needs to be excluded completely as a first stage.

The patient should be examined by means of a cover test, with particular attention to the corneal light reflexes. Gross appearance may be misleading, and true ocular position can be assessed by shining a light at the child and observing where the corneal light reflexes lie (figure 13.1). They should be symmetrical. If the reflex appears more lateral or medial in one eye than the other then there is a squint. The type of squint will be elicited by the cover test (see Chapter 13, Cover testing).

Amblyopia

Amblyopia is the development of a lazy eye. Children under five years of age have immature visual systems that are still developing. This is a critical period; any block to clear sight in either eye will result in permanently reduced vision. This poor vision is reversible before about five to eight years of age, but after this age the visual loss will be fixed. During the first five years of life, the visual system is practising and working out how it must be orientated in order to see properly. After this, the ability to adapt and change is lost, and the level of visual development achieved at that stage is fixed.

Any block to the passage of light through the eye and accurate focusing of this light upon the retina, with subsequent transmission to the brain, will result in incomplete formation of the developing visual system. After five years of age, the risk of amblyopia is minimal as the visual potential is already established.

Corneal abnormalities, lens opacities (cataracts) or problems with the media (vitreous jelly) will cause amblyopia if not remedied quickly during the critical period.

Amblyopia may develop as a result of the numerous abnormalities, but only when all potential physical/pathological causes of visual loss have been excluded or treated by, for example, cataract extraction can the diagnosis of amblyopia be confidently made. If the vision remains poor despite a clear cornea, clear lens, clear media, normal retina and normal visual system anatomy, then the patient has amblyopia. In other words, amblyopia is a diagnosis of exclusion.

There are three main forms of amblyopia: visual deprivation, strabismic and anisometropic. Visual deprivation amblyopia is related to cataracts and other problems that stop the light from reaching the retina.

Strabismic amblyopia occurs when the eyes are not aligned correctly. One eye is deviated either continuously or intermittently, and during this time the child's brain cannot put the images from the eyes together because those images are very different (the eyes are effectively looking at different things). In order to cope, the brain concentrates on the image from one eye and ignores the other completely. Because the ignored eye is not involved in the generation of sight, the normal visual pathways related to this eye do not develop. If the problem is not remedied during the critical period, the vision will stay subnormal and the child will have an amblyopic eye.

Anisometropic amblyopia occurs when the two eyes have different refractive errors. For example, if one eye is much more long-sighted than the other, the longer-sighted eye will be at great risk of developing amblyopia. The good eye will develop normal neural attachments because its focusing mechanism, consisting of the cornea and lens, will ensure clear focusing of the light on the macula. Both eyes are linked in terms of their focusing power (accommodation). One eye cannot accommodate more or less than the other eye. Thus both eyes will accommodate symmetrically to compensate for the refractive error of the eye with the least requirements and will stop accommodating once that eye receives a clear image. This is not usually a problem, as most patients have similar refractive errors in both eyes, so if one eye is receiving a clear image, the other will also. If the one eye has a markedly different refractive error from the other, it will not receive a clear image and the normal visual pathways will not develop. The eye will become amblyopic.

Treatment

The success of treatment depends on dealing with the underlying cause of the amblyopia early enough to prevent the onset of permanent visual deficit. If there is a block to the light entering the eye, it must be removed as soon as possible, for example by cataract extraction or corneal transplant. If there is an ocular misalignment, the squint should be corrected surgically or, if it can be controlled with spectacles, these should be worn all the time. If there is significant anisometropia (marked difference in the refractive power of the eyes), this should be corrected with appropriate spectacles.

When the underlying cause for the amblyopia is removed, the visual pathways should develop normally, provided the child is still within the critical age period. Sometimes this process requires a kick-start. By a deliberate blocking of the clear image received by the good eye, the child is forced to rely on the weaker eye, thus accelerating the visual development of this eye and reversing the amblyopia. This process is called penalisation because the good eye is being purposefully compromised to benefit the other. Penalisation can be done by placing a patch over the good eye for several hours a day, forcing the child to rely solely on their amblyopic eye. Alternatively drops such as atropine may be used to dilate the pupil of the good eye, thus blurring its vision (penalising it), and making the bad eye the only one with a clear image and thus the one the brain uses for vision.

It should be emphasised that all organic causes of visual loss should be excluded completely, and these treatment measures should be undertaken aggressively during early life. The later treatment is started, the less likely it is to achieve complete reversal of amblyopia.

29 | Trauma

Corneal foreign bodies

The cornea is protected by the lids' blink reflex, but foreign bodies such as grit or insects still slip past and impact on the ocular surface. Even after impact, the blink reflex will attempt to wipe the foreign body from the cornea and reflex lacrimation will flood the ocular surface with tears to try to wash away any foreign material.

Sharp objects or material travelling at high speed may impact into the corneal epithelium and lodge there, resisting the efforts of the lids to wipe them away and causing significant pain and redness. A small corneal foreign body can feel like a brick to the patient.

Foreign bodies should be removed after anaesthetising the eye with topical anaesthetic drops (e.g. amethocaine or benoxinate drops). This will allow the patient a transient relief from their discomfort and facilitate close examination of the eye without the constant blinking. A moist cotton-tipped applicator should then be used to try to dislodge the foreign object. If this fails, a needle can be used (green 21G, blue 23G or orange 25G) but only by trained hands. Magnification should be used to do this if possible or, even better, it should be done at the slit lamp. Always remember to approach from the side and never point the needle directly at the eye.

Metallic materials (particularly those containing iron) will react with the hydrated cornea to form a rust ring, seen as a brownish 'halo' of staining around the foreign body. The rust ring may be removed with the needle or, if not too big, left to work its own way out. Topical antibiotics should be given to prevent infection and lubricate the eye until the residual epithelial defect heals.

Of particular concern are corneal injuries that occur as a result of grinding, welding or hammering. Any metallic fragment liberated in this way will be travelling at very high speed, and there is a significant risk that it will perforate the eye. A small foreign body can perforate the cornea and lodge in the lens or vitreous with significant sequelae. It is important to X-ray the eyes of patients with a history of grinding, welding or hammering, to exclude a metallic intraocular foreign body. A dilated fundus examination is also essential.

An eye that fails to recover after an apparently 'simple' corneal injury, despite lubrication and antibiotics, should also be assessed for the presence of an intraocular foreign body.

Intraocular foreign bodies

If fast-travelling objects hit the eye, they can pass right through the cornea or sclera and lodge within one of the intraocular structures. There they can cause direct mechanical damage or have an effect that is related to their composition, e.g. an iron foreign body will rust and spread iron throughout the eye, causing marked toxicity. In addition, the foreign body could be carrying micro-organisms that cause infective complications, particularly an infective endophthalmitis.

A large intraocular foreign body (IOFB) will be clinically obvious, as it will have caused significant disruption of the ocular anatomy. Of more concern are smaller foreign bodies that can enter the eye unnoticed. If a fast-moving small foreign body perforates the eye, it can leave a self-sealing wound. If it goes through the cornea, it can leave a small epithelial defect, but no other sign of significant injury. The IOFB may only manifest later when toxicity or infective complications ensue. Injuries sustained while hammering, drilling or grinding carry with them a significant risk of ocular penetration by a metallic foreign body and a high index of suspicion should be maintained.

Patients should be examined carefully, ideally at the slit lamp. If the intraocular pressure is low in the affected eye, this might be a manifestation of an ocular perforation that released some aqueous (thus lowering the pressure) and then sealed. A dilated examination of the anterior and posterior segments should be undertaken. X-rays of the eye may help determine the presence of a metallic foreign body. Significant anterior or posterior inflammation that fails to resolve rapidly with standard treatments should raise the suspicion of an IOFB.

Treatment depends on the nature and position of the foreign body. Antibiotic prophylaxis should be considered, and surgical removal is usually indicated. If the foreign body has punctured the lens capsule, a cataract will almost certainly ensue.

Subtarsal foreign bodies

A foreign body can lodge under the upper lid and subsequently rub up and down the cornea with every blink. This may result in numerous linear abrasions with consequent significant pain and redness.

It is important to suspect the presence of a subtarsal foreign body if no corneal foreign body is visualised, but the history is suggestive. Topical anaesthetic drops will give temporary relief of symptoms and allow adequate examination. The upper lid must be everted and the under surface/upper tarsal plate must be visualised. In order to evert the lid, the patient should be asked to look down to their feet, and the lashes should then be firmly held by the examiner and pulled down. A cotton bud or equivalent is used to press on the upper margin of the tarsal plate and the lid pulled up and rotated over the bud. The foreign body should be removed and topical antibiotics given to lubricate the eye and prevent infection until any corneal epithelial defect has resolved.

Corneal abrasions

Blunt or sharp injury to the cornea can cause the superficial corneal epithelium to be scraped off. This exposes bare underlying stroma and results in significant pain, redness and often photophobia. If the abrasion is over the central cornea, the vision may be reduced. The epithelial defect will stain with fluorescein dye.

Treatment involves antibiotic ointments. The antibiotic prevents super-added infection and the ointment lubricates the ocular surface to allow speedy healing.

Unfortunately, the new epithelial cells never quite stick down as well as their natural counterparts and sometimes they detach after minimal trauma. Indeed, simple drying of the eye overnight can result in the inner surface of the upper lid adhering to these weak epithelial cells. When the patient opens their eyes in the morning, they rip these cells away, and experience sudden pain and a foreign-body sensation. This is called recurrent erosion syndrome, and may be alleviated by applying lubricant ointments before sleeping, thus preventing excessive overnight dryness.

Corneal laceration

Sharp injury can result in a laceration of the cornea. If this laceration is of partial thickness, it will cause significant pain and may allow bacteria to enter, possibly resulting in infective keratitis. If the laceration is of full thickness, the anterior chamber will be breached and the aqueous will rush out. The anterior chamber will collapse and the iris may prolapse and become stuck in the wound. Vision will be markedly reduced, and infection can enter the eye with catastrophic effects. Corneal lacerations require immediate surgical repair to reform the eye.

Injury to the globe

Globe injuries can be caused by blunt or sharp trauma. Blunt trauma sends a concussion wave through the ocular tissues and can lead to significant damage, including rupture (bursting) of the globe. Sharp injuries may result in lacerations of varying severity, depending on the site and degree of the trauma.

Prognosis and management will depend upon the amount of damage. Management usually involves antibiotic prophylaxis and surgical repair. The initial operation is designed to restore ocular integrity, while further surgery may be planned to try to restore any lost vision (secondary repair).

There is always a risk of sympathetic ophthalmia (see below), and thus it may be elected to remove a severely damaged eye that has no visual potential.

Chemical injury

Chemical injury to the eye can result from a domestic or industrial accident. Unfortunately, chemical injuries caused through assault are increasing.

Any chemical applied to the eye can cause injury due to direct mechanical or toxic effects. Whatever the offending material, the most important aspect of management is immediate copious irrigation with water, preferably sterile. By washing out the offending chemical, the damage is limited.

Common chemicals that cause ocular injury are acids and alkalis. Acids tend to be better tolerated than alkalis because they react with the superficial layers of the cornea and ocular surface, resulting in precipitation of proteins and superficial damage, but minimal deeper problems. Alkalis, in contrast, do not immediately react with the superficial corneal layers but pass into the eye, rapidly causing extensive and severe problems.

These chemicals have a direct effect upon the corneal epithelium, resulting in a burn with varying degrees of superficial cell loss and abrasion. If this is the only damage, the cells will rapidly be replenished and the defect will heal, usually with minimal residual scarring. If the damage involves the epithelial progenitor cells situated at the corneal limbus, however, this is of more concern. These limbal stem cells lie in a narrow band circumferentially at the junction of the cornea and the conjunctiva. They are responsible for producing a constant fresh supply of epithelial cells to cover the corneal surface. If they are burnt away, the cornea cannot heal and significant scarring and visual loss results. Recent surgical advances have improved the visual prognosis in these cases, but the situation is still worrying and potentially blinding.

Minor injuries will settle with topical antibiotics, but significant injuries require specialist treatment and follow up. After copious extended irrigation and removal of any residual solid foreign matter, the patient should be referred to an emergency ophthalmology service for further assessment.

NB. Irrigation is the mainstay of treatment for all chemical injuries and should be carried out immediately.

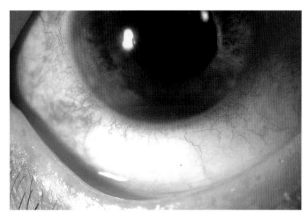

FIGURE 29.1 A traumatic hyphaema. A layer of blood is seen in the bottom of the anterior chamber.

Hyphaema

Bleeding may occur into the front of the eye, either in relation to trauma or, more rarely, spontaneously. The blood will mix with the aqueous and eventually settle to the bottom of the anterior chamber, forming a red layer. This is called a hyphaema, and may be less than 1mm deep or may fill the whole anterior chamber (figure 29.1). If the blood does fill the whole of the front of the eye, it produces a dark red/black appearance, called an 'eight ball' hyphaema.

Spontaneous hyphaemas can occur because of abnormal fragile vascular tufts in the iris or where there are abnormal new vessels (neovascularisation or rubeosis). Patients on anticoagulant therapy or with a bleeding diathesis should have their anticoagulation status assessed.

Hyphaema in relation to trauma may occur as a result of sharp or blunt injury. Sharp injury will result in disruption of the iris vasculature usually associated with significant injury to other ocular structures.

Blunt injury can send considerable force in the form of a concussion wave through the eye. This may cause ruptures within the pupil margin or may directly rupture an iris blood vessel, resulting in a hyphaema. The presence of a hyphaema indicates a significant force to the eye, and so a thorough examination of the anterior and posterior segments should be undertaken to exclude other ocular injury.

The classical history is of injury and then sudden visual blurring that gradually clears almost to normal over the next few hours. The initial visual loss is related to the liberated blood mixing with the aqueous and creating a mist within the anterior chamber. Gradually the blood cells settle to form the hyphaema, and the vision clears.

Treatment consists of strict bed rest and observation. It is important to check the intraocular pressure, as the blood cells may clog the drainage network of the trabecular meshwork and cause a traumatic glaucoma. If the pressure becomes very high, the haem from the red blood cells can be forced into the cornea, resulting in permanent staining and concurrent visual loss.

The initial haemorrhage usually settles and is called the primary haemorrhage. Of more concern is that between three and five days after the injury, the clot formed at the initial site of the bleed lyses and falls away. This can result in another bleed, called a secondary haemorrhage, and is usually more extensive and has a much greater propensity for causing complications (such as glaucoma) and permanent visual loss.

Bed rest should minimise the movement of the eye and prevent excessive exertion, theoretically reducing the risk of further bleeding.

Some ophthalmologists give their patients dilating drops, such as atropine, to stop movement of the iris and thus, again theoretically, minimising the risk of another bleed.

Angle recession

Blunt injury to the globe can cause disruptive forces at the angle of the eye, ripping the normal anatomy of the trabecular meshwork. This damage is visualised with gonioscopy (*see* Chapter 21, Glaucoma) and the angle is seen to be wide (ripped apart), hence the condition is described as angle recession.

Healing occurs, but damage to the anatomy of the drainage systems can cause raised intraocular pressure and glaucoma, particularly if a large part of the angle is affected.

Traumatic cataract

Sharp trauma that disrupts the lens capsule will probably result in rapidly progressive cataract formation.

Even blunt trauma with no evidence of damage to the lens (or even any other ocular structure) increases the risk of a cataract. This is probably related to the subtle effects of the concussion force upon the lens cells. The cataract can develop within weeks or decades later. Such cataracts can be difficult to remove surgically because of subtle damage to other structures, particularly the fine filaments (zonules) holding the lens in place.

Lid lacerations

The lids are the eyes' key line of defence and are thus often forced to sacrifice themselves for the sake of the underlying globe. Blunt injuries may result in traction on the lids, with ripping away or avulsion of part of the upper or lower lids. Sharp injuries may result in full or partial thickness lacerations of the lids.

When significant trauma is sustained to the lids, it is important that the underlying globe is fully assessed to ensure that there are no deeper, sight-threatening injuries.

Once it is clear that the lid injury is isolated, this can be repaired by primary closure in most cases. Standard principles of thorough toilet and suture apply. There are many folds of skin around the eye, and a search must be undertaken to exclude the presence of any residual foreign material prior to closure.

The lid margin must be properly reconstructed as any defect here will persist as a cosmetically poor 'step'.

The canaliculi form the beginning of the nasolacrimal drainage system, extending from the lid puncti to the lacrimal sac by the bridge of the nose. They lie within the lid, one in the superior lid and one in the inferior lid, and thus may be involved in any medial avulsion or laceration. If they are cut and not repaired, they will not heal patent, and the patient will be left with a watering eye. This is particularly likely if the lower canaliculus is disrupted because the most tear drainage occurs through it. Each case should be judged individually, but it is usually elected to repair the canaliculus microsurgically as a primary procedure. The alternative is to allow healing to take place and then undertake a secondary repair at a later date.

Orbital wall fracture

The globe and its surrounding structures are enclosed within the bony orbit of the skull. A significant force applied to the eye, even if the lids are closed, will be transmitted throughout the orbit and thus on to the bony orbital walls. These walls can break, resulting in 'blow-out' fractures. Orbital structures prolapse through the bony deficit and become incarcerated. Usually only orbital fat or, occasionally, small segments of the extraocular muscles become trapped.

The globe will rest slightly backwards (enophthalmos), and the eye movements will be restricted because the muscles and periocular tissues are trapped.

If untreated, permanent scarring will ensue with long-standing ocular motility disturbance, and the patient will be left with double vision.

Patients usually have significant periorbital bruising (a black eye) and obviously reduced ocular movements in the affected eye, particularly in vertical gaze. A good clinical sign of blow-out fracture is the presence of paraesthesia or anaesthesia in the skin under the eye. This is due to pressure on the infraorbital nerve caused by the fracture and orbital prolapse.

These fractures are usually treated in conjunction with the maxillofacial or ear, nose and throat surgeons. Surgery is via an orbital approach, with repair of the fracture with replacement and freeing of orbital tissue.

Sympathetic ophthalmia

Due to the dense blood-retinal barrier, the body's immune system is never normally exposed to some of the ocular tissues and thus ocular antigens. This means the resident white cells have never been exposed to particular ocular antigens and self-immune tolerance never develops.

If the body is then exposed to these antigens, e.g. after trauma, the immune system may react by recognising the ocular antigen as foreign, with a consequent severe inflammatory reaction.

Of more concern is that the injured eye sometimes sensitises the body's immune system to ocular antigens to such a degree that it begins to react to, and attack, the other, perfectly healthy, eye. This is called sympathetic ophthalmia, and may be sight threatening. It is thought that early removal of a severely injured eye – within two weeks of the trauma – will prevent this sensitisation and sympathetic ophthalmia.

It is thankfully very rare.

30 | HIV/AIDS and the eye

The human immune deficiency virus (HIV) is becoming more widespread and prevalent throughout Western society.

There are three main routes of transmission:

- Parenteral intravenous inoculation. This is common among intravenous drug misusers and those who have received blood transfusions with infected blood products (e.g. haemophiliacs).
- Intimate sexual contact: through unprotected sexual practices involving the exchange of HIV-infected bodily secretions.
- Vertical transmission: from infected mother to baby.

HIV infection is usually silent. Gradually, the immune system is depleted and compromised as more and more CD4+ lymphocytes are infected and lost. As the disease progresses, patients are at risk of opportunistic infections and neoplasms. Acquired immune deficiency syndrome (AIDS) is the life-threatening end stage of HIV infection.

A diagnosis of AIDS is made upon the basis of a CD4+ count of less than 200 cells/mm³ or the presence of an AIDS-defining illness in an HIV-positive patient.

These patients are susceptible to opportunistic infections such as those caused by *Pneumocystis carinii*, *Toxoplasma*, *Candida*, *Cryptococcus*, *Mycobacterium*, cytomegalovirus, herpes simplex virus and herpes zoster virus.

Some malignancies are also more common, such as Kaposi's sarcoma (the ocular variety usually occurs in the skin surrounding the eye and manifests as reddish, non-tender nodules) or lymphomas.

Ocular complications

Herpes zoster ophthalmicus (HZO)

Shingles of the ophthalmic division of the trigeminal nerve, particularly in young, previously immunocompetent patients, may be the initial manifestation of HIV infection. The rash can be extensive and severe, and other forms of herpes zoster virus-related intraocular inflammation may be present.

Herpes simplex virus infection (HSV)

Corneal dendritic ulcers can be quite severe. Other HSV-related intraocular inflammation may also be present.

HIV retinopathy

This is the most common ophthalmic manifestation of HIV/AIDS. It may be clinically silent and rarely affects vision in isolation. Patients develop cotton-wool spots, intraretinal haemorrhages and microaneurysms, similar to those seen in diabetic retinopathy.

Cytomegalovirus (CMV) infection

CMV is the commonest ocular opportunistic infection in patients with AIDS. It causes a fulminant progressive retinal infection and inflammation that is vision-threatening if unchecked. This disorder is the leading cause of AIDS-related blindness. Yellow-white patches of retinal necrosis and inflammation are seen throughout the retina, usually sparing the macula until late. The retina becomes atrophic and may peel away, resulting in a retinal detachment.

Treatment

Opportunistic infections are treated aggressively with high-dose chemotherapeutic regimens.

With the advent of highly active anti-retroviral treatment (HAART), the prognosis for patients with HIV is improving and it is to be hoped that the risk of severe ocular complications will reduce as therapy improves.

Appendices

nts

the attention of social services as having needs arising from an impairment of vision.

When the registration documents are received, the social services will arrange:

- An assessment of the patient's needs
- In the case of the CVI only, the person's inclusion on the local authority's register (with their consent) and for them to be issued with a standardised registration card.

So who should be certified as severely visually impaired (blind)?

The National Assistance Act (1948) states that a person can be certified as blind if they are 'so blind as to be unable to perform any work for which eyesight is essential'.

It is important to note that the person should have vision that is too bad for *any* work, not just their own profession.

Three main groups of patients are eligible for registration:

- Vision less than 3/60 (i.e. cannot read the '60' letter on the Snellen chart despite being 3 m away)
- Vision better than 3/60 but worse than 6/60 and with constricted visual fields
- Vision better than 6/60 but with very constricted visual fields, particularly in the lower part of the field.

There is no legal definition of partial sight. Patients may be certified as partially sighted if they are substantially and permanently handicapped by defective vision caused by congenital defect, illness or injury.

People who are certified as partially sighted are entitled to the same help from social services as those who are certified as blind, but they will not be eligible for certain social security benefits and tax concessions that are only available to those registered as blind.

As a general rule, patients with a vision of between 6/24 and 6/60 may be considered for registration as partially sighted.

pital eye services. The patient can be given an LVI at the same time, enabling them to self-refer to social services immediately and/or contact the sources of advice and support mentioned in the letter. This can be quicker than waiting for hospital assessment.

Social needs include the need for information about community services for vision-impaired people, emotional support, practical advice and rehabilitation. Social service departments are keen to be told of any concerns about risk factors or where employment or education is threatened.

The CVI performs the same function as the previous BD-8. That is, it formally certifies an individual as partially sighted or as blind (now using the preferred terms, 'sight impaired/partially sighted' or 'severely sight impaired/blind', respectively) so that the local council can register the person. Patients are entitled to services without registration, but cannot be placed on the formal register on the basis of a referral letter (e.g. LVI) only. The signature of a consultant ophthalmologist is required on a CVI before registration can be offered. Registration is voluntary, but entitles people to various benefits and concessions.

The CVI also acts as a referral for a social care assessment if the person has not previously come to

There are psychological implications for the patient when discussing blind registration. Nearly every patient with significant visual loss fears that they will eventually become blind and locked into a black world. Offering them blind registration can make them feel that they have no chance and that blindness is inevitable. It is important that proper counselling is undertaken before the patient is registered as blind or partially sighted.

APPENDIX TWO

Driving regulations

Fitness to drive is assessed on best corrected vision and on field of vision.

To hold the standard, non-vocational licence, known as group 1, the driver must be able to read in good light, with the aid of glasses or contact lenses if necessary, a standard vehicle registration plate fixed to a vehicle, at a distance of 20.5 m if the letters and figures are in the old font, or at 20 m in the current font. Anyone who cannot do this is not allowed to drive, and a licence will be refused or revoked.

Although this is equivalent to a best corrected visual acuity with both eyes open of between 6/9 and 6/12, the only true way to assess this is to ask the individual to do it.

The regulations for vocational licences, known as group 2, are more stringent. For this group, visual acuity, using corrective lenses if necessary, must be at least 6/9 in the better eye and 6/12 in the other eye, while the uncorrected acuity in both eyes must be at least 3/60.

In addition to visual acuity, the driver must meet the visual field criteria.

For an ordinary licence, the recommended visual field standard is: 'A field of vision of at least 120 on the horizontal, measured using the Goldmann III4e setting or the equivalent. In addition, there should be no significant defect in the binocular field that encroaches within 20° of fixation above or below the meridian. This means that homonymous or bitemporal defects which come close to fixation, whether hemianopic or quadrantanopic, are not accepted as safe for driving. Subject to strict criteria, drivers who have been driving for many years with static fields defects that do not satisfy the standard, and who have non-progressive eye conditions, can be considered on an individual basis.'

Essentially this means that with both eyes open and looking straight ahead, the driver must be able to see 120° from side to side, and 20° above and below the horizontal.

Research is underway into whether these requirements are too stringent. Each case is usually assessed individually, and factors such as how long the patient has been driving, and the groupings of any blind spots and their proximity to the driver's central vision, are taken into account.

Whether the disease causing the visual loss is static or progressive is also considered. All patients who continue to drive or resume driving after a visual disability should be fully adapted to their ocular morbidity.

Patients who lose vision in one eye will still be able to hold a group 1 licence, as long as their other eye is healthy and they can meet the requirements with that eye.

Ocular morbidity

- Cataract. As long as the patient meets the usual visual acuity requirements, they are eligible to drive.
- Monocular patient. Patients with one eye are eligible to hold a group 1 licence if their vision still meets the visual field and visual acuity requirements, as described above. By definition, however, these patients cannot hold a group 2 licence because the vision in their bad eye is worse than 3/60.
- Visual field defects. Patients who are diagnosed with a visual field defect should inform the Driver and Vehicle Licensing Agency (DVLA). They should also stop driving until they are confirmed eligible to drive according to a 'both eyes open' Esterman visual field assessment. In order to hold a group 2 licence, a driver should have normal binocular field of vision.
- Double vision. Group 1 licence-holders may continue to drive once it is confirmed that the diplopia is controlled by glasses or by a patch that the licence-holder undertakes to wear while driving. Those with double vision are not allowed to hold a group 2 licence.
- Night blindness. As long as the visual fields meet the required standards, the patient is eligible to

drive, but cases are assessed on an individual basis.

- Colour blindness. These patients do not need to inform the DVLA about their condition and are allowed to drive.

- Blepharospasm. If the condition is mild, there should be no problem holding a group 1 or 2 licence. Each case is assessed individually, and a report from an ophthalmologist is usually required.

Information from DVLA website □ www.dvla.gov.uk

APPENDIX THREE

Bibliography and recommended reading

Kanski J J. *Clinical Ophthalmology*. Oxford:
Butterworth-Heinemann, 1999.

Vaughan D, Asbury T, Riordan-Eva P.
General Ophthalmology. Stamford, Connecticut:
Appleton & Lange, 1999.

Maclean H. *The Eye in Primary Care*. Oxford:
Butterworth-Heinemann, 2002.

Elkington A R, Frank H J, Greaney M. *Clinical Optics*.
Oxford: Blackwell Science, 1999.

Broadway D, Tufail A, Khaw P T. *Ophthalmology,
Examination Techniques, Questions and Answers*.
Oxford: Butterworth-Heinemann, 1999.

Rhee D J, Pyfer M. *The Wills Eye Manual*.
Philadelphia: Lippincott Williams & Wilkins, 1999.

Useful websites

www.emedicine.com/oph/index.shtml

www.revophth.com

www.mywiseowl.com/articles/ophthalmology

www.eyeatlas.com

www.emedicine.com/oph/contents.htm

APPENDIX FOUR

Common acronyms

AACG ▢ Acute angle-closure glaucoma

AAU ▢ Acute anterior uveitis

AION ▢ Anterior ischaemic optic neuropathy
Ischaemic infarction of a portion of the optic
nerve due either to GCA (AAION – arteritic
anterior ischaemic optic neuropathy) or non-
arteritic (NAAION)

ALT ▢ Argon laser trabeculoplasty
Laser sometimes used to reduce intraocular pressure
in glaucoma

AMD/ARMD ▢ Age-related macular degeneration

BDR ▢ Background diabetic retinopathy

BRAO ▢ Branch retinal artery occlusion

BRVO ▢ Branch retinal vein occlusion

CACG ▢ Chronic angle-closure glaucoma

CCF ▢ Carotid cavernous fistula

CMO ▢ Cystoid macular oedema
A form of oedema seen in relation to inflammation
and after intraocular surgery

CNVM/SRNVM ▢ Choroidal neovascular mem-
brane/subretinal neovascular membrane

COAG ▢ Chronic open-angle glaucoma
Also POAG, primary open-angle glaucoma

CRAO ▢ Central retinal artery occlusion

CRVO ▢ Central retinal vein occlusion

CSMO ▢ Clinically significant macular oedema
A proven threshold of diabetic maculopathy that
requires laser treatment to preserve sight

CSR ▢ Central serous retinopathy

DLK ▢ Deep lamellar keratoplasty (partial thickness
corneal graft)

GCA ▢ Giant cell arteritis

HSK ▢ Herpes simplex keratitis

HZO ▢ Herpes zoster ophthalmicus

KPs ▢ Keratic precipitates
Inflammatory cells collecting on the inner surface
of the cornea. May be related to iritis

NPDR ▢ Non-proliferative diabetic retinopathy

NTG ▢ Normal-tension glaucoma
Also LTG, low-tension glaucoma; LPG, low-pressure
glaucoma
 Special form of glaucoma where the intraocular
pressure is normal but glaucomatous damage still
occurs

NVD ▢ New vessels (neovascularisation) at the
optic disc

NVE ▢ New vessels (neovascularisation) elsewhere/
somewhere within the retina not at the disc

NVI ▢ New vessels on iris
Neovascularisation has developed on the iris usually
due to an ischaemic process in the retina

OHT ▢ Ocular hypertension

PAS ▢ Peripheral anterior synechiae
Adhesions between the iris and the peripheral inner
corneal surface. Can block the trabecular meshwork

PCO ▢ Posterior capsular opacification

PDR ▢ Proliferative diabetic retinopathy

PDT ▢ Photodynamic therapy

PK ▢ Penetrating keratoplasty (full thickness
corneal graft)

PRP ▢ Pan-retinal photocoagulation
Laser applied all over the retina but sparing the
macula, usually to kill off ischaemic retina to prevent
neovascularisation. Commonly used for diabetics

PVD □ Posterior vitreous detachment

RAPD □ Relative afferent pupillary defect

RD □ Retinal detachment

ROP □ Retinopathy of prematurity

RP □ Retinitis pigmentosa

TAB □ Temporal artery biopsy

TED □ Thyroid eye disease

APPENDIX FIVE

Useful contacts

Royal National Institute for the Blind
105 Judd Street
London WC1H 9NE
020 7388 1266
www.rnib.org.uk

British Retinitis Pigmentosa Society
P.O. BOX 350
Buckingham MK18 1GZ
01280 815900
www.brps.org.uk

The Royal College of Ophthalmologists
17 Cornwall Terrace
London NW1 4QW
020 7935 0702
www.rcophth.ac.uk

Driver and Vehicle Licensing Agency (DVLA)
Drivers Medical Group
Longview Road
Swansea SA6 7JL
01792 782341
www.dvla.gov.uk

Diabetes UK
Macleod House
10 Parkway
London NW1 7AA
020 7424 1000
www.diabetes.org.uk

The Partially Sighted Society
Queens Road
Doncaster DN1 2NX
01302 323132

The International Glaucoma Association
108c Warner Road
London SE5 9HQ
www.iga.org.uk

The Macular Disease Society
P.O. BOX 1870
Andover
Hampshire SP10 9AD
01264 350551
www.maculardisease.org

APPENDIX SIX

Algorithm for the early management of diabetic retinopathy in Type 2 diabetes

Adapted from: National Institute for Clinical Excellence. *Management of Type 2 Diabetes Retinopathy – early management and screening* (*Guideline E – html*). London: NICE, 2000.

On diagnosis of Type 2 diabetes, examine eyes:

- Check visual acuity and refer if this is reduced
- Examine for diabetic retinopathy after instillation of tropicamide dilating drops
- Retinopathy present – yes – see below, no – annual review
- Maintain HbA_{1c} below 6·5 to 7·5% and BP<=140/80
- Sudden loss of vision or retinal detachment – refer *immediately*
- New vessels, vitreous haemorrhage, new iris vessels – refer *urgently via letter*
- Unexplained drop in vision, hard exudates within one disc diameter of fovea, macular oedema, severe retinopathy – refer *soon via letter*
- Occurrence or worsening of lesions since previous examination, scattered exudates more than one disc diameter from fovea – arrange recall and review every three to six months.

Index